A

TREATISE ON HEADACHES:

INCLUDING

ACUTE, CHRONIC, NERVOUS, GASTRIC, DYSPEPTIC, OR SICK-HEADACHES; ALSO, CONGESTIVE, RHEUMATIC, AND PERIODICAL HEADACHES.

NOTICE.

To obtain the most rapid yet thorough and practical knowledge of the contents of this volume:

1st. Glance over the *Preface* and *Introduction;*

2d. Read carefully the remarks on the action of the different remedies against headache in the *Synopsis.*

3d. Read the *General Remarks* before, and the *Reviews* and *Notes*, after the cases given in the body of the work.

4th. Look over the *Cases* both in the body of the work, and in the *Synopsis.*

5th. Finally, make use of the *General Review* and *Index.*

A COMPLETE TREATISE ON HEADACHES AND DISEASES OF THE HEAD.

1. THE NATURE AND TREATMENT OF HEADACHES.
2. THE NATURE AND TREATMENT OF APOPLEXY.
3. THE NATURE AND TREATMENT OF MENTAL DERANGEMENT.
4. THE NATURE AND TREATMENT OF IRRITATION, CONGESTION, INFLAMMATION AND DROPSY OF THE BRAIN AND ITS MEMBRANES.

BASED ON T. J. RÜCKERT'S

CLINICAL EXPERIENCE IN HOMŒOPATHY.

WITH INTRODUCTIONS, APPENDICES, SYNOPSES, NOTES, DIRECTIONS FOR DOSES AND MANY ADDITIONAL CASES.

By JOHN C. PETERS, M.D.

NEW-YORK:

WILLIAM RADDE, 300 BROADWAY.

Philadelphia: Rademacher & Sheek.—*Boston:* Otis Clapp.—*St. Louis*, Mo.: D. R. Luyties, M.D.—*London:* Balliere, 219 Regent-st.—*Manchester*, Eng.: Turner, 97 Picadilly.

1859.

H. Ludwig, Printer and Stereotyper,
39 *Centre-street.*

AMERICAN EDITOR'S PREFACE.

I HAVE undertaken the translation and elaboration of "Rückert's Clinical Experience in Homœopathy, or a complete collection of all the cures and practical remarks recorded in the literature of Homœopathy from the year 1822 to 1850;" of which this little treatise on Headaches forms the first part:

(1). Because it possesses much practical value, and will lead to the better homœopathic treatment of the sick;

(2). Because it evinces in every line so much industry and honesty of purpose, that it of itself furnishes strong proof that some homœopathic physicians, at least, are both pains-taking and sincere;

(3). Because Rückert has recorded and compared the experience of all classes of homœopathic physicians with the most wonderful faithfulness and impartiality, utterly regardless of his own preferences and opinions, and without the least trace of a narrow, sectarian or bigoted spirit;

(4). And finally, because I believe that the experience of the numerous physicians he has recorded is as real and true, as the majority, at least, of all that is published in the general annals of medicine.

One is strongly led to wish, that an equally complete collection of allopathic cures, effected by a single remedy in each case, had been compiled faithfully and impartially by some one of the dominant school, who is as honest, well educated, and liberal as Rückert. In default of this, I have occasionally alluded in various notes scattered through the work to the best established old school curative and palliative treatment, by way of contrast with the homœopathic, and for the information of such medical students and young practitioners into whose hands this treatise may fall.

I trust that no excuse will be necessary for enlarging the eighty-five cases of Headache reported by Rückert into the present treatise. Rückert truly says: "There are but few diseases to which the human frame is liable, in which painful sensations about the head do not occur more or less frequently; but few proximate or remote causes which are capable of exciting disease at all, that do not frequently cause headaches; and yet, there are but few monographs on the subject of Headaches; but few works on the Theory and Practice of Medicine in which they are treated of fully and systematically. On the other hand, how frequently is the practical physician called upon to relieve and cure headaches;" and how scanty have been the aids to cure, compared with the frequent demands for cure! It is true that the admirable articles of Dr. Black, in the British Journal, and of Dr. Tietze, reprinted in the Boston Quarterly Journal of Homœopathy, have lately done much towards lightening the labours of physicians in the treatment of headaches; still Rückert correctly judged that it could not prove an unnecessary task to collect and arrange all the cases of cure to be found in the published records of Homœopathy.

As Rückert confined himself to a bald and condensed statement of cases and their treatment, it was regarded as imperatively necessary to add a few general introductory remarks upon the Nature and Causes of the different varieties of Headache. (See page xi.)

As he limited his excerpts almost exclusively to the German Medical Journals, it was felt incumbent to add the cases most easy of access, published in the French, English and American works, and periodicals (see cases, 2, 3, 5, 6, 7, 18, 19, 20, 40, 41, 47, 55, 56, 58, 59, 61, 62, 63, 71, 81, 82, 83, 84, 85, 89, 98, 111, 112 to 114, and 163.)

As his remarks are almost entirely clinical, or drawn from bed-side experience, it was suggested to me to add other indications for the selection and use of remedies against Headaches, to be drawn principally from their well-known pathogenetic and curative effects. (See Synopsis, page 101, and numerous notes scattered through the body of the work.)

Although Rückert has been as minute in his directions about the size and repetition of doses, as a strict adherence to his authorities would allow, still the publisher requested the addition of still more explicit directions. In the notes on doses, I have mainly followed the advice and practice of my lamented friend Dr. Noack, late of the Leipzig Homœopathic Hospital, and of the celebrated Fleischman, of the Vienna Hospital. Personal opportunities of observing their practice have strongly prejudiced me in its favour, corroborated as it then was, and now is, by the successful results of many thousand cases of every variety of disease.

I have also added short articles upon several remedies, viz.: Arum, Carb. veg., Glonoine, Gratiola, Hepar sulph. and Iris versicolor, and regret that time and space would not permit me to allude to a few other well established remedies against chronic and nervous headaches.

Thus Rückert's valuable, but bald compilation and condensation of cured cases, has been gradually enlarged and modified into a more or less complete treatise on Headaches.

I feel constrained, however, to make a few remarks upon the varieties of pain, which have been met in the course of translation. Every English and American physician is necessarily surprised at the infinite variety of pains, which the Germans describe so readily; we admit aches and pains in general, make some distinction between constant and intermitting pains, between dull and sharp pains, fixed and shooting pains, &c., but we know little about the wonderfully numerous, and minute distinctions of pain admitted by the Germans. Still, these trivialities, or profoundly accurate distinctions, whichever they may be, are inherent in the German mind; I shall never forget my first surprise, at hearing these minute distinctions admitted, and fluently spoken of, by peasants and mechanics, not only in the Homœopathic Hospitals of Leipzig and Vienna, but also in the large Allopathic Hospitals of Dresden, Leipzig, Berlin, Vienna, Munich, and others. In Rückert's part of this work I have encountered the following kinds of pain, among others: Klopfend-stechend, or throbbing-piercing; Klemmend, or compressing; Stechend-bohrend, or piercing-boring; Klopfend-reissend, or throbbing-rending, or tearing; Drückend, or pressing, or aching; Betaubender, or stupefying; Glucksender, or clucking pain; Klopfender, or throbbing, or beating; Reissender, or rending, or tearing; Auseinanderpressender, or asunder-pressing pain; Pressender, or pressing; Zerspringender, or bursting pain; Wogender, or dashing-beating; Schwappender, or undulating-dashing; Ziehend, drawing; Spannend, tension-pain; drückend-pressend, i. e. pressing-pressing, or pressing-squeezing, or aching-pressing pain; Schraubender, screwing; Zwängender, pinching; Herauspressend, out-pressing; Zusammen-pressend, together-pressing; Ziehend-wühlend, drawing-rooting pain; and many others, some of which have no real meaning, or are of no practical value to any except a hair-splitting pedant, who doubtless would overlook the state of the most important functions, neglect the most palpable and significant physical signs, and think it of no importance to ferret out the exact seat, or nature of any disease.

Still, to a certain degree, the character of the pain varies according to the nature or seat of the disease, and in many instances is a sufficient guide to a discrimination between some forms of disease, and often enables a homœopathic practitioner to select a curative remedy, which else had been next to impossible. In a forthcoming work, I will take occasion to enter fully into the signification of the principal varieties of pain, and their appropriate treatment.

One great objection may be raised against this and similar works, viz.: that all the cases reported are successful ones. Malaise and Henderson have published several unsuccessful trials, and Dr. Black, in his Article on Headache,* says that he had intended, if space permitted, to report several cases in which treatment proved of no avail; but such statements might merely afford an opportunity for some less honest physician to insinuate that a wrong medicine had been given, or that a better indicated one might easily have been selected. Hence he contents himself with simply stating the fact, that several unsuccessful cases had occurred in his own practice, as well as in that of other physicians, in order that those just commencing homœopathic practice might not suppose, from silence on this point, that all cases admit of at least temporary relief; nor be too much disappointed when they meet with such instances. He says it is advisable from the outset to make the patient fully understand, that chronic headache of many years' standing cannot reasonably be expected to be cured in a few months, and may not even be alleviated in that time, but as a general rule, relief, if not a cure may be looked for in most cases, after the lapse of some months, or one or two years. Of sixty-six cases of chronic and sick headache treated at the New York Homœopathic Dispensary in 1851, eleven were cured, seventeen much relieved, and thirty-eight remained under treatment; in 1848, of eleven cases, seven were cured, one improved, two not improved, and one unknown. In the General Homœopathic Hospital Report,† of fifty-three cases of chronic headache, seventeen were cured, and sixteen much relieved; of fifty-eight cases of nervous and sick headache, fifty-six were cured and two not cured; of one hundred and thirty-eight cases of rheumatic and gouty headache, one hundred and thirty-five were cured, and three not cured. Of two hundred and nineteen cases reported by Kiesselbach of Bremen, one hundred and ninety-nine were cured, and twenty unknown. Thus, of five hundred and forty-five cases of Headache, of all kinds, no less than four hundred and twenty-five were cured under homœopathic treatment, thirty-four were relieved, and sixty-six

* See Brit. Jour. of Hom., vol 5.

† See Annual Report of the New York Homœopathic Dispensary for 1851.

cases were either not relieved, or the result was unknown. Although some of these reports are more favorable than the general practitioner may always meet with in his own practice, still it will be impossible, after consulting some of the cases given in this treatise, to deny that many persons suffering with chronic headaches may obtain permanent relief under homœopathic treatment; see cases 3, 5, 6, 9, 10, 12, 14, 17, 21, 22, 27, 28, 29, 32, 34, 37, 40, 41, 43, 44, 46, 48, 49, 51, 52, 55, 56, 59, 63, 64, 65, 71, 74, 77, 78, 79, 80, 82, 86, 88, 89, 92, 95, 98, 104, 105, and others.

N.B. A volume on Apoplexy, Inflammations and Dropsy of the Brain, similar in design and execution to the above, is in an advanced state of preparation and will soon be published.

J. C. PETERS.

742 Broadway, New York.

ON THE

NATURE AND CAUSES

OF

HEADACHES.

In order to render this treatise rather more complete, it has been regarded as imperatively necessary to make introductory remarks upon the different varieties of Headache, of which cases of cure have been reported in the following pages.

Of the cases reported by Rückert, he has assumed that:

(*a*). Six cases, had a *nervous* character; viz.: cases 9 and 16, cured by Bell.; 72 and 76, cured by Nux; and 96, by Pulsatilla.

(*b*). That twenty-seven, were cases of *Hemicrania*, *Migraine* or *One-sided* headache, viz.: cases 9 and 10, cured by Bell.; 29, by Calc.; 46, by China; 57, by Ignat.; 67, 69 and 70, by Natrum; 74, 76, 77, 78, 79 and 81, by Nux v.; 87, by Opium; 92 and 96, by Puls.; 101 and 102, by Sang.; 103, 104, 107, 108, 109 and 110, by Sepia; 112 and 118, by Spigelia.

(*c*). Eleven cases had a *congestive* character, viz.: cases 14, 15 and 16, cured by Bell.; 30, 34, 35 and 36, cured by Calc. c.; 37, by Camph.; 68, by Natrum; 94, by Puls.; and 104, by Sepia.

(*d*). Nine cases had a *rheumatic* character; viz.: cases 23, 24 and 25, cured by Bryon.; 44, by Causticum; 54, by Dulc.; 61, by Merc.; 101, by Sang.; 108, by Sepia.

(*e*). Five cases, were of a *gastric* nature, or attended with derangement of the stomach, viz.: case 14, cured by Bellad.; 33, cured by Calc.; 43, cured by Causticum; 95, by Puls. ; 119, by Sulph.

(1). With retching to vomit, in case 21, cured by Bryonia.

(2). With nausea and vomiting in general, in eleven cases, viz.: case 4, cured by Arnica; 22, by Bryonia; 42, by Causticum; 57, by Ignat.; 67 and 70, by Natrum; 76, 78 and 80, by Nux; 106, by Sepia; and 121, by Sulph.

(3). With vomiting of bitter substances in two cases, viz.: case 12, cured by Bellad.; and 97, by Puls.

(4). With bilious vomiting in five cases, viz.: case 31, cured by Calc.; 72, 74 and 77, by Nux; and 92, by Puls.

(*f*). Twenty-two cases bore a *periodical* character, occurring in paroxysms, viz.: case 8, cured by Asarum; cases 9, 10, 12 and 16, by Bellad.; case 26, by Bryon.; case 45, by Cham.; case 46, by China; 52, by Coloc.; 53, by Creosot.; cases 65, 66 and 70, cured by Natrum; cases 72, 74, 77 and 79, by Nux; and cases 120, 122, 123 and 124, by Sulph.

(*g*). Fourteen cases were of an *undetermined* character, viz.: case 1, cured by Acon.; 11, 13 and 17, by Bellad.; 27, 28, 32, 35 and 36, by Calc.; 49 and 50, by Coloc.; 73, by Nux; 88, by Phosph.; and 91, by Puls.

1. NERVOUS HEADACHES.

These are generally understood to include periodical and neuralgic headaches, Hemicranias, Migraines, one-sided, or uni-lateral headaches, and some forms of so called sick-headache, viz.: those in which no disturbance of the stomach has been evident before the headache set in, and nausea and vomiting do not occur until after the pain in the head has lasted some time, and become severe. The substances vomited in an attack of *true nervous* headache are generally destitute of acid, bile or any acrid property; while in *sick*-headache, previous derangement of the stomach, bowels or liver is generally evident, and undigested food, bile, or some other offending substance is always vomited up.

Nervous headaches occur most frequently in delicate males, and females of a highly nervous temperament, and are apt to be reproduced by any unusual excitement, by joy, hope, fear, excessive pleasure, anxiety, fasting, fatigue, &c. They are said, generally to depend upon a feeble, disturbed, or irritable state of the nervous system; still, as the Great Sympathetic nerve in some of its ramifications is the most common seat of the disorder, and this nerve also presides over the circulation of the blood, we are apt to have more or less of passive or active congestion, attending the so-called nervous affection. It has long been a stumbling-block in the way of pathologists to explain why a weakened and debilitated state of a nerve should be followed by pain, rather than of loss of sensation; or by congestion, rather than anæmia; but late experiments by Claude Bernard have apparently thrown much light upon this point. He says it has been known for a long time that cutting the medulla spinalis through, or certain other nervous trunks, such as the par vagum, the sciatic nerve and others, will cause a general or partial, but decided diminution of the warmth of the body; but the *reverse* of this is the case when the great sympathetic is cut through. Bernard noticed in cutting through the cervical branch of the sympathetic nerve which unites the cervical ganglions, that there followed immediately, an increase in the heat of the corresponding side of the face, which could very easily be appreciated by the hand, and which was found to be from 4° to 6° centigrade higher by the thermometer. When the superior cervical ganglion of the great sympathetic was entirely extirpated, Bernard found the same effect produced with even greater intensity; and at the same time that the heat was increased, the circulation of the blood became more active. This new phenomenon of increased calorification continued for a long time; Bernard found it to last at times for several successive months, without being attended with, or followed by any appearance of inflammation or œdema, or any other pathological change. If all this be true, it is easy to understand why a feeble state of the sympathetic nerve may be attended by heat and congestion to the head. The occurrence of pain is explained in a similar way:

Bernard asserts, that when a nerve of sensation is cut, every one knows a loss of feeling in the part to which it is distributed is produced; but the *reverse* is the case when the great sympathetic is cut; if the superior cervical ganglion be extirpated, the sensibility of the whole corresponding side of the face is augmented; and it is particularly in the *eye* that this phenomenon can be detected with most ease. Somewhat similar experiments by other physiologists, were cited by the translator as early as 1841, in the second volume of the Homœopathic Examiner, old series, p. 131. If these things be really true, it is very easy to infer, that a debilitated condition of certain parts of the great sympathetic nerve may be followed by heat and congestion to the head, pain about one side of the head, one temple or one eye; in fact, by all the phenomena of nervous headache or hemicrania.

There is one form of *true nervous* headache, which might very properly be termed the *nervous sick-headache*, because it is attended with violent and long continued nausea, retching and vomiting; it is frequently mistaken for the true gastric, dyspeptic, or bilious sick-headache. Although I am very far from denying that some derangement of the stomach or blood often causes headache, still I feel convinced that the nausea, retching and vomiting which attend nervous sick-headache, are always sympathetic and secondary, to a primary disorder of the brain, or nervous system. The true nervous sick-headache probably arises from an affection of the right Corpus Striatum; at least experiments conducted by Budge seem to prove this almost conclusively; after killing a young dog, he removed the skull rapidly, while an assistant laid open the abdomen and exposed the bowels; the hemispheres of the brain were then cut away, the Corpus callosum raised, and the Corpora quadrigemina and Corpus Striatum irritated with a sharp needle, with the effect of producing marked perstaltic action of the stomach and bowels; even when all perstaltic action of the bowels had entirely ceased, it could at once be reproduced by irritating the Corpora quadrigemina, and motions of the stomach could always be excited by irritating the Corpus Striatum, especially on the right side. These experiments throw much light, not only on the vomiting which attends nervous sick-headache, but also explain the early occurrence of vomiting in dropsy of the brain, the presence of obstinate constipation, and we will soon see that they afford an explanation of the slowness of the pulse which attends the same disorder. In fact, every careful observer must have noticed that vomiting does not occur in nervous sick-headache, until the pain has lasted some time and become quite severe, proving that the nausea and vomiting are secondary to the brain-affection. I have regarded it imperative to lay much stress on these points, because all sick and nervous headaches have much too generally been viewed in the light of secondary affections, dependent upon derangement of the stomach and liver, and thus their existence as primary disorders greatly overlooked. Black truly says this error has no doubt rendered the ordinary treatment so uncertain, and will also confuse the homœopathic practitioner, if not sedulously guarded against. Still, I have already willingly admitted that derangement of the digestive organs will often cause headache or neuralgia, which may depend upon the mere presence of acid in the stomach; Dr. Rigby tells us, that having suffered in his own person an intense attack of Tic douloureux which Opium would not assuage, he swallowed, at the suggestion of a friend, some Carbonate of Soda dissolved in water; the effect was almost immediate, carbonic acid was soon eructated, and the pain at once abated. Again, the celebrated Prout, from personal and other experience, concluded that excessive acidity of the cœcum is generally accompanied by a deficient secretion of bile, and sometimes by a complete temporary suppression of the biliary discharge, apparently from spasmodic constriction of the common gall duct; or, may be, of the biliary ducts themselves. In this state of things, all persons, he says, feel more or less of uneasiness; but the point which he wishes to mention is, that certain individuals under these circumstances, experience what is called *nervous* headache. This species of headache is frequently accompanied by nausea, is confined to the forehead, and when severe produces complete intolerance of light and sounds, and a state of mind bordering on delirium. After a greater or less period of time the pain ceases, sometimes quite suddenly, and the remarkable circumstances to be mentioned are, that this sudden termination is preceded by a peculiar sensation, sometimes accompanied by an audible clinking noise in the region of the gall ducts, which immediately after is followed by a gurgling sensation in the upper bowels, as if a fluid were passing through them; in a few seconds after this fluid, which Prout supposes to be bile, has reached the cœcum, the headache at once vanishes like a dream. One of the greatest martyrs to this species of headache Prout has ever seen, invariably experiences the train of symptoms above described; and Prout has witnessed it in a greater or less degree in many instances; and indeed has experienced it in his own person. This variety of headache is generally termed BILIOUS. These facts simply prove, that irritation in the brain and nerves may be propagated down, along the sympathetic nerve to the stomach; and vice versa, that irritation in the stomach may travel up along the same nerve to the brain or face, producing the so-called dyspeptic or gastric headache.

The most superficial knowledge of the anatomy of the great sympathetic nerve, will suffice to explain the readiness with which irritation of the stomach, bowels, liver, urinary or genital organs may be propagated to the brain, viz.: to those parts of it supplied with filaments from the sympathetic nerve. Thus, 1st: the *Pars cephalica nervi sympathetici*, consists principally of two filaments which proceed from the upper part of the superior cervical ganglion; the larger and more anterior being called the *Carotid nerve*, the smaller and posterior, the Jugular nerve. They effect the communications of the sympathetic nerve with almost all the cerebral nerves.

(*a*). The *Carotid nerve* follows the course of the internal carotid artery, passes through the carotid canal into the skull, and divides into an anterior and posterior branch, which, with their twigs form the *Internal Carotid plexus;* from this plexus arise the Inferior and Superior Carotico-tympanic nerves which go to the internal ear, and explain the occurrence of noises in the ears, sensitiveness to noises, &c., which attend many headaches. The Internal carotid plexus of the sympathetic nerve gives off: (1) the deep and superficial Vidian nerves going to the Spheno-palatine plexus; (2) three branches going to the Ganglion of Gasser, situated in the orbit of the eye, and giving off a twig to the Ophthalmic branch of the fifth pair of cerebral nerves; (3) two twigs to the Oculo-motorius and abducens nerves of the eye; (4) a twig which connects with the Ciliary ganglion of the eye; (5) and finally, sends off branches which accompany the Cerebral carotid artery, one of them sinking into the Pituitary gland, and another reaching the interior of the eye and retina, by following the course of the Central artery of the retina. These intimate connections of the sympathetic nerve with the nerves and substance of the eye sufficiently explain the intolerance of light, pain in the eye, dimness of vision, motes, colors, and other phenomena of the eye which so commonly attend nervous and sick-headaches; and the readiness with which excessive use of the eyes will excite headache in some persons.

(*b*) The cervical ganglions of the sympathetic nerve give off branches to the heart, throat, windpipe, to the temporal, maxillary and facial nerves, to the scalp, the vagus and recurrent nerves, &c., sufficiently explaining the occurrence of palpitation of the heart, choking about the throat and windpipe, pains about the temples, jaws and face, tenderness of the scalp, and other sufferings which so often complicate and aggravate nervous headaches.

We are now prepared to understand why such an immense variety of exciting causes, and so many disturbances of distant organs will produce attacks of headache; thus, the effects of mental emotions and passions may be propagated from the brain to the various branches of the sympathetic nerve in, and about the head. The same happens with the eye; at least Piorry has drawn particular attention to the frequency with which one-sided headache, or hemicrania arises from irritation of the retina and iris, excited by excessive use of the eye, bright light, or gorgeous spectacles; in short, he regards hemicrania as originally a neurosis or neuralgia of the retina and iris, confined at first to these parts, but soon extending to the branches of the sympathetic and cerebral nerves connected with them, and then marked by disturbance of vision, pain in the eye, about the orbit and temple, in the head, or on the surface of the skull, and finally followed by nausea and vomiting. Affections of the ears, loud or long continued noises will produce the same kind of headache in those predisposed. I have already referred to other exciting and remote causes of headache; at present we will confine our attention more particularly to some of the peculiarities and symptoms of *Migraine, Megrim, Hemicrania or one-sided headache:*

TISSOT says, when Migraine is hereditary it often commences as early as the seventh or eighth year, or even earlier, but most commonly makes its appearance from the thirteenth to the twentieth year of life, and continues in full force to the fifty-fifth or sixtieth, then almost wholly ceases by the seventieth. If one is not attacked by it before the twenty-fifth year, it is rare to become subject to it afterwards. I have seen boys of three or four years, and girls of five or six years subject to repeated attacks of sick-headache.

Some persons have only eight, or nine attacks a year; and true Migraines, which occur more than three times a month, or less than four times a year, are very rare. The paroxysms have been known to occur with great regularity every fifteen days, or every Monday, or Friday or Sunday, or some other particular day of the week, for years, always at the same hour of the day, and to last at least twenty-eight, and never more than thirty hours; some of these cases are cured by travelling, at least the celebrated FRANK reports the case of a lady in Milan, who was attacked every Wednesday with severe headache; she was cured by going out into the country every Tuesday, and not returning until Thursday. Still, susceptible persons are generally liable to it at any time, and from a great variety of causes; from breathing certain odors, from the influence of stormy weather, from moral emotions, from long continued studies, from an unaccustomed walk in the open air, from the impression of cold on the bare head, from various disturbances of the stomach, difficult digestion, hunger, the use of certain articles of food, reading, studying, or pre-occupation directly after eating, &c. Hence it is evident, from the great variety of the exciting causes which produce headache, that the number of cases which occur at irregular periods must be very much greater than those which re-occur at regular and fixed periods of time. It is rare for a paroxysm of true hemicrania to last less than six hours, and it is not common for it to be prolonged more than two days. Tissot thought, when an attack commenced with a slight sensation of chilliness, the paroxysm was apt to be very severe, and to be confined to the side on which the chill was felt; and that in most attacks the same side of the head was apt to be affected, although they have been known to affect each side alternately, with great regularity. He also thought that those attacks which were preceded with sadness and irritability for several days, were apt finally, to set in severely on the going down of the sun, and to commence with a severe chill. China, Arsenicum and Nux, are said to be almost specific in these cases. Other attacks may be preceded by a degree of deafness for twenty-four hours. See Puls. and China. Piorry thought that nervous and sick-headaches occurred chiefly under one of two opposite conditions of the stomach, viz.: either from a state of too great repletion, or of too great abstinence. The so-called *hungry* headache is sufficiently common in many young persons; it is apt to be preceded by acid eructations, or by excessive hunger, or vomiting of acid or acrid matters, and by an annoying sense of gnawing at the pit of the stomach. Calcarea, Carb. veg., Veratrum, &c., deserve attention.

Some attacks are relieved by spontaneous vomiting; in others, the vomitings are a mere consequence of the severity of the pain, and do not afford relief; C. Pison first drew attention to the difference between the sympathetic and convulsive vomitings, and the curative ones. Ipec., Puls., Cocculus, Zinc., &c., are suitable.

Some attacks are much relieved by sleep; but others, in which the disorder is seated primarily in the brain itself, and extends to the sympathetic nerve secondarily, the more the patient sleeps, the more the brain becomes congested, and the worse he is; improvement only commences when he is fairly aroused, and wide awake. Opium, Hyosc., Coffea, Thea, and other remedies are indicated.

Some paroxysms terminate by profuse sweats upon the fore-arms and hands, and when these perspirations occur regularly every morning the hemicrania will soon cease for ever. Aconite, Arnica, Valerian, Sambucus, Ammon. acet., Nux, and other remedies may be useful in bringing about this desirable result.

Some cease after a slight bleeding of a few drops from the nose. In such cases, Crocus, Carb. veg. and China, deserve attention.

Sometimes an eruption of small pimples terminates the attack, or a sweat on the affected side of the head and face, or a profuse flow of tears, or free discharge of serosity from the nostril. All these varieties of critical terminations doubtless require remedies suitable to aid and produce them, not to check them. See Sulphur, Hepar sulph., Sepia, Gratiola, and Arsenicum.

Although repose is necessary in most cases, some are only relieved by riding in a carriage. Some are relieved in the beginning of an attack by exposure to the fresh air, others are made much worse. See Cocculus, Calcarea, Merc., Natrum, and Hepar s.

In some cases the face of the sufferer is pale and shrunken, in others red, hot and flushed, in others again, pale but bloated. See China, Bellad., Ars., Verat. and Sepia.

When the pain follows the course of the external carotid nerve the scalp becomes excessively sensitive to touch, and the pains resemble those of rheumatism of the scalp; Wepfer has even seen the hair to rise on end during the severity of the paroxysm. See China, Colocynth, Bryonia, Carb. an., and others.

In other cases, the pains extend themselves violently towards the teeth, and sometimes to all the parts supplied by the fifth pair of nerves, so that the patient cannot open his mouth, nor articulate a word; in other cases, the sufferings extend to the neck, shoulder and arm, which remain painful for some time afterwards. I have seen several cases which always pass off when severe pain in the back, one knee, or leg sets in. See Colocynth, Aconite, Aurum, Bryon., Causticum, Rhus, and others.

In other cases the disorder extends down along the sympathetic or pneumo-gastric nerve towards the stomach, liver, and bowels; eructations occur, either inodorous, and without taste, or of an insupportable mawkishness; abundant mucosities and salivary fluid flow into the mouth, intermixed at times with those of a bitter, bilious taste; there is extreme disgust for food; the general malaise is increased by a fatiguing beating of the heart, and by paroxysmal distensions of the stomach with gas, followed by belchings, with transient relief; or vomiting may occur, excited by the swallowing of the fluids which collect in the mouth, and mucus, or a little bile, and much wind may be expelled. From time to time some alleviation may ensue, the distress in the epigastrium be less great, the headache less severe, but occasional aggravations also occur, followed again by intervals of relief, and finally one or two easy loose stools set in, occasionally liquid and bilious, and the whole attack subsides. See Colocynth, Cocculus, Carbo animalis, Caps., Caust., Lachesis, Natrum, Creosote, Pulsatilla, Sepia, and others.

Hence numerous varieties of Hemicrania have been admitted by PELLETAN.

1st. The Migraine stomacale.
2d. " " Irienne, or of the Iris.
3d. " " Uterine.
4th. " " Plethorique, &c.

These divisions are of importance to the homœopathist, as they impress still more forcibly upon him the necessity of selecting a remedy which acts, not only on the part of the head involved by the Hemicrania, but which will also regu late the variously disturbed functions of distant organs.

Hygienic treatment of Nervous Headaches.

A general invigorating mode of life, diet and exercise are considered indispensable. Those who have brought them on by sedentary habits, much mental exertion and loss of sleep, must reform; they must exercise freely and regularly in the open air, sleep sufficiently; and avoid the excessive worry and perplexity of engrossing cares, or they may ultimately be forced to take a journey into the country, or a long voyage, to save their minds from becoming perfectly wrecked. If the patient be in the habit of using strong tea, coffee or tobacco habitually and excessively, he must try the effect of abandoning them, for three or four weeks at least.

It is ordinarily thought sufficient to abstain from the use of coffee and green tea, but WOOD had one striking instance occur to him, in which a patient, after suffering long and severely with nervous headache, obtained an entire exemption from it, by abstaining from the use of *black tea*, which was his only indulgence. The shower-bath, and salt water bathing, either at the sea-side, or in the house, are often useful adjuncts.

BOERHAAVE advised persons who suffered from chronic headaches to use a warm bath frequently, and to rub their feet briskly every morning with a piece of flannel, or cloth dipped in cold water. OSIANDER says, if people would but rise every morning, at 5 o'clock; and continue it during the summer, or take an hour's walk before breakfast, they would get rid of their headaches. He also affirms that simply combing the hair carefully and constantly, just before going to bed, relieved a lady from chronic headache.

Hard rubbing of the feet with rough cloths after a foot bath is one of the best external remedies, according to BUSHAN.

The meals of the patient should be taken regularly, and

when body and mind are refreshed, not wearied by exertion, anxiety or needless worry.

It need scarcely be added that the bowels should be kept regular, costiveness obviated, (and tendency to diarrhœa controlled), as far as possible by attention to diet. The functions of the stomach and liver should be kept in as healthy a state as practicable by the patient, by control of the appetite and tastes in food and drinks; those of the kidneys and skin, by attention to clothing, bathing, drinking of cold water, &c.; and those of the uterus by great care at the monthly periods, favoring the flow, if it be scanty, by avoidance of cold and wet, excessive fatigue or mental emotion, the use of the warm, or mustard foot or hip-bath, &c.; if the flow be excessive and debilitating, absolute rest, cool drinks, cold-water injections, &c., may be used.

Those who will indulge in the dissipations of excessive pleasure, business, grief, or gormandizing, will needs retain their headaches.

2. CONGESTIVE HEADACHES.

These may be active or passive, venous or arterial, arising from too great and too rapid a flow of blood to, or too slow a return of the blood from the head. They may occur singly, or as complications of nervous or irritative headaches, the congestion being secondary; or they may arise from irritation of the brain or neighboring parts; or the brain-trouble may be entirely secondary to an irritated, or sluggish state of the general circulation.

I have already alluded to the frequency with which nervous headaches are attended with congestion, and have cited the experiments of C. BERNARD as affording some explanation of the manner in which congestion follows disorder of the Great Sympathetic nerve. But TURENNE has lately advanced a new theory of nervous headache or hemicrania; he decrees that the pain in the head is caused by compression of the facial nerve, especially of its ophthalmic branch, from accumulation of blood in the sinuses at the base of the brain. He alludes, in proof of this, to the fact, that the ophthalmic nerve and its branches are spread on the external wall of the cavernous sinus, and hence are necessarily compressed whenever this reservoir is crowded with blood. The nausea and vomiting of nervous headache are said to arise from compression of the eighth pair of nerves, at the Foramen lacerum posterius, or somewhere along the neck. The swelling, redness, pain, and watery condition of the eyes, and disturbances of vision in nervous headache, are said to arise from the difficulty with which the ophthalmic vein empties itself into an already over-full cavernous sinus, and from consequent compression of those fibres of the ophthalmic nerve which go to the eye, white of the eye, lachrymal gland and eyelids. Hemicrania is also decided to be most frequent on the *left* side, because the *left* sinuses of the brain are larger and more distensible than the right.

The more common varieties of congestive headaches are so well understood, that it will only be necessary to say a few words about the less common forms.

(*a*). *The Stupid Headache of Dr. Good*

Is said to be marked by obtuse pain, sense of heaviness extending over the whole head, and may arise from various causes, especially from whatever prevents a free evacuation of the right auricle and ventricle of the heart, and contributes to retard the motion of the blood in the veins which discharge their contents on this side of heart. The congestion is supposed to be secondary to nervous debility, or in other words, to arise from the want of a proper and sufficient supply of that nervous power, or may be fluid, on which the feeling of organic comfort, refreshment, and vigor depends. Hence this variety of headache has been decreed to be peculiarly marked by a sense of general disquiet and confusion, rather than severe pain; by a general hebitude of sensorial power which disqualifies the one laboring under it for a continuance of mental labor; the sight is dim, the hearing dull, the memory vacant, and hence it is most common in feeble persons, and in hard students.

The stupid headache from nervous exhaustion is closely allied to that from venous congestion. See Opium, Hyosc., Bellad., Stramon., Coffea, Bryon.

(*b*). *Menstrual Congestive Headache.*

Another very frequent variety of congestive headache is that which occurs near, before, during, or shortly after menstruation, especially when this is scanty, painful or difficult. The state of system previous to the first establishment and periodical recurrence of menstruation tends obviously to a state of general plethora, which ought in due time to be fully relieved by a means which nature adopts for the purpose. But tendency to irritation of the brain, or some other organ, or a loss of balance in the circulatory and nervous system, or other causes, may allow the blood at such periods to rush towards some distant organ; or want of proper and abundant flow from the uterus may leave the system, or some particular organ, oppressed and crowded with blood. Sabina and Stramonium are particularly suited for these menstrual congestions of the head, and many other organs. Almost every variety of headache is aggravated about the menstrual period; but when headache occurs just after the menstrual flow, especially if this has been quite profuse, the headache is probably not congestive, although it may be severe, for nervous headache in excitable persons is apt to be brought on by whatever directly, or indirectly debilitates, viz.: by bleeding, purging, fatigue, loud noises, vivid lights, using the eyes too much, or too closely, and other fatiguing or debilitating causes or losses, such as diarrhœa, excessive perspiration, or profuse menstruation.

(*c*). *Hæmorrhoidal congestion.*

Suppressed, or retarded piles are apt to be followed by irregular hæmorrhoidal congestions to the head, chest, stomach, bowels, liver, spleen, kidneys, uterus, bladder, or any other predisposed organ; hence may arise redness and heat of face, illusions of vision, dizziness, threatening of apoplexy; or constriction and anxiety about the chest, and even spitting of blood, or vicarious bleeding from the lungs; or throbbing and aching about the stomach, with or without vomiting of blood; or aching in the liver and spleen with threatening of dropsy; or venous congestion of bowels with vicarious bleeding from them, or aching in the region of the kidneys with scanty discharge of urine, or tenesmus of the bladder from venous or hæmorrhoidal congestion of it, and bleeding from the kidneys or bladder, or congestion to the womb with more or less profuse and vicarious hæmorrhage from it. In females, the vicarious menstrual and hæmorrhoidal congestions and hæmorrhages are so similar in their symptoms that superficial or careless physicians are very apt to confound, and maltreat them. Sabina is the specific for the former, Aloes for the latter. According to Schœnlein, *menstrual congestion of the head* is frequently marked by stiffness of the neck; dull aching pain in the nape and occiput, from congestion of the cerebellum; by rushing and roaring noises in the ears, hardness of hearing, confusion of the head, momentary loss of consciousness, followed by bleeding from the nose, ears, or Caruncula lachrymalis. Still the symptoms may differ widely from the above description, and very frequently assume the appearance of a most perfect one-sided nervous headache.

According to the same authority true hæmorrhoidal congestion of the head is marked by great heaviness and confusion of the head, the choroid coat is over-filled with blood, and the sclerotica acquires a peculiar blue tinge, owing to a varicose state of this membrane; there are also illusions of the senses, appearances of sparks, figures, motes, flies, spider webs and feet before the eyes, which often cause partial blindness. From time to time violent vertigo sets in, throwing the patient into violent nervous agitation, as he supposes that he is struck with apoplexy.

(*d*). *Throbbing Headache.*

This is generally mistaken for the true congestive variety; the pain is pulsatory, chiefly in the temples, often attended with sleeplessness, and a sense of drumming in the ears; it depends upon an affection of an artery, or part of an artery, without any dependence upon the regular systole of the general circulation; thus, one or both temporal arteries are often disturbed by this spastic irritation, and a pulsation is produced nowise synchonous with the action of the heart, but often half as rapid again. (See Camph., Valerian, &c.)

(*e*). *Anœmic Headache.*

It is well known that excessive loss of blood will produce all the signs of violent congestion to the head. (See China, Ferrum, Manganese, &c.)

3. RHEUMATIC AND GOUTY HEADACHES.

Rheumatic headache is described by some as a chronic headache with vehement pain, but especially characterized by a sense of *tension* of the whole head. If this form be not always rheumatic, it is always dependent upon some local irritation, of which rheumatism is the most frequent. As all rheumatic affections, when they become chronic, have a tendency to intermit and return periodically, we may easily see why the disease before us should do so in many instances. Good says it may be distinguished from other varieties by its being rather limited to some particular part of the head, by its remissions and intermissions; by the acuteness of the pain during the paroxysms, by an intolerance of all motion of the head, far more than of light or sound, both of which, however, are sometimes highly irksome; but especially by a peculiar feeling of tenseness or constriction over the brain, as though its membranes were muscles, and were spasmodically contracted. When the headache is entirely rheumatic, it ceases as soon as another rheumatic pain sets in, in some other part of the body. Frequently the disorder may be detected by attention to its exciting causes; thus, Dr. Parr was for many years a sufferer from irregularly returning paroxysms of headache, for which he could assign no cause, but at last noticed that they frequently returned after having his head shaved; he suffered his hair to grow, and from that time the disease gradually lessened in frequency, duration and violence, and from being a highly serious complaint, and one beginning to affect his memory, its returns became so rare and slight as never to unfit him for any exertion of body or mind. LINNÆUS is said to have cured himself of a severe and obstinate rheumatic hemicrania, which returned every week and continued for twenty-four hours, by merely drinking a draught of cold water early in the morning, and then walking himself into a glowing heat. The majority of those so-called neuralgic headaches which arise from decayed teeth are also rheumatic in their nature, being excited by the frequent alternations of heat and cold which reach the exposed nerve. But the secretions of the skin and kidneys afford the most decided diagnostic signs of the presence of rheumatism; the perspirations and urine are intensely sour, even the secretions from ulcers are unusually acid in rheumatism; the urine in rheumatic affections may seem nearly natural in color, and be perfectly clear, and yet found to redden litmus paper very much more decidedly than in any healthy condition. According to FRICKE the principal cause of rheumatism, as is well known, is the action of cold upon the skin, by which its exhalations are retained, and the lactic acid, instead of passing off as lactate of ammonia, is retained in the blood, finally it becomes oxydized, and is eliminated as carbonic acid and water, but this conversion is produced at the expense of the uric acid, which, thus unoxydized, is deposited about the joints or other parts, causing pain, swelling and fever. Until the pulse loses it hardness, the skin and urine their intense acidity, rheumatic headache will persist, or relapse. (See Aconite, Bryonia, Pulsat., Rhus, and other remedies.)

ON THE

HOMŒOPATHIC TREATMENT

OF

HEADACHES.

The remedies used in the following cases of cure and recovery, were: Aconitum, Agaricus, Arnica, Arum, Belladonna, Bryonia, Calcarea, Camphor, Causticum, China, Cocculus, Colocynth, Creosote, Dulcamara, Gratiola, Ignatia, Lachesis, Magnesia, Mercurius, Nux vomica, Opium, Phosphorus, Pulsatilla, Sanguinaria, Sepia, Spigelia, Silicea, Sulphur, Zincum.

1. ACONITE.

General Remarks.—(*a*). It relieves the most violent headaches when the patient lies as if unconscious, retches to vomit at times, whimpers and complains, fears to die, cannot endure the slightest noise or motion, and in which the pulse is small, or even intermitting; especially when the pain is throbbing and piercing, or compressing, seated over the root of the nose, and the talking and the speaking of others aggravates it very much. Aconite is also useful against headache from taking cold, attended with catarrh of the head, noises in the ears, and pains in the abdomen, or by an annoying sensation as if a ball rose up into the brain, spreading a cool wind around it.

Also in catarrhal headache when relieved in the open air, and increased by talking.

Also in migrane, or one-sided headache, when marked by a violent, piercing, boring pain over the *left* eye, and attended with nausea and vomiting, and aggravated by jarring. In such cases *Acon.* should be followed by *Sulph.*—Dr. Hering, p. 136–140.

(*b*). Aconite is indicated in headaches of a congestive-inflammatory nature, when the patient has a feeling of fulness and tension, as if a band were fastened around his head; in this respect it resembles Bellad., China, Merc., and Sulph.—DR. BLACK.

CASE 1.—A woman, aged 54, of an irritable, complaining, and vicious nature, readily breaking out into complaints and reproaches from slight causes, had suffered for 24 hours, after taking cold, with severe but undefined headache, so violent as almost to drive her distracted. Aconite removed it in 4 hours. Annals, vol. 1, p. 234.—GASPARI.

[NOTE.—*From Fleming's Experiments.*—I infer that Aconite is homœopathic to Headache when attended with numbness and tingling of various parts, and with a sense of tightness and dragging.

Also for headache marked at first by a sense of warmth diffused through the body, with numbness and tingling, and a sense of swelling of the lips and face, and tingling at the roots of the teeth, followed by a feeling of muscular weakness, by slowness of breathing and of pulse, giddiness, confusion of sight, disinclination to be disturbed or to exert oneself, and attended with much chilliness, particularly of the extremities, which become cold to the touch.

Also in headaches attended with numbness of the flesh, lancinating pains in the bones and joints, vertigo, dimness of vision, moisture and coolness of the skin, sickness of stomach and vomiting, and by paleness and a sunken state of the face.

Also in headaches accompanied with a feeling of weight as if a heavy load were resting on the abdomen, bearing one down to the bed; this peculiar symptom was present in five cases, and seemed to resemble closely the feeling of oppression experienced in nightmare, which is said to be owing to congestion of the right side of the heart, from accumulation of blood in venous system, in consequence of a weakened state of the circulation.

In two cases it proved homœopathic to shivering, severe pain in the head and eyeballs, constant lachrymation, intense photophobia, heat of skin, quickness of pulse and general restlessness; to nausea, severe and constant vomiting, with pain and tenderness of pit of stomach, numbness and prickling of the skin, dizziness, dimness of vision, noises in the ears, sensations of weight and enlargement of various parts of the body, but especially of the face and ears, sinking feeling at pit of stomach, &c.

It is also homœopathic to general venous engorgement of the brain and cerebral membranes, and considerable sub-arachnoid effusion.

It has been assumed that the more nearly the headache approaches a neuralgic character, or rheumatic neuralgic, the more readily Aconite will relieve. Still Fleming used it internally in fifteen cases of headache, with complete success in ten; of the successful cases three were nervous headaches, four were congestive or plethoric, and three were rheumatic. Of the unsuccessful cases three were nervous, and two dyspeptic. Relief was usually experienced after the first dose, and a complete cure effected on the first or second day, or at least there was no relapse for several weeks or months. Drs. Burgess and Radly announced to Fleming that they had seen Aconite of incalculable service in relieving the agonizing pain of nervous headache. Professors Henderson and Miller, of Edinburgh, informed Fleming that they had employed it with marked benefit in headache. Storck and Vogel recommend it in rheumatic headache, while Copland found it useful in both nervous and rheumatic cases.

In two cases in which the internal use of Aconite did not afford relief, the external was employed with much benefit; in fact, Fleming, as a general rule, found the external application of the tincture very effectual in the treatment of hemicrania, both when the pain affected a circumscribed portion of the head, and when it extended along the course of a nerve. Dr. Patterson, of the Royal Infirmary at Edinburgh, corroborates this assertion.—PETERS.]

CASE 2.—[E. W., aged 43, had suffered for three weeks with a more or less constant pain extending over the temporal and frontal regions of the left side of the head; firm pressure lessened the pain; exposure to cold, wet feet, or anxiety of mind usually brought on an attack if it was absent, or increased its severity if present. She had taken Opium with but partial relief; was ordered to rub in a teaspoonful of the Tincture of Aconite thrice daily. The first application afforded much relief, and in five days she was quite well; ten weeks after, at last accounts, there had been no return of pain.—*Fleming on Aconite.* English edit., p. 139.—PETERS.]

Dose.—In *acute* cases, and for adults, in the beginning of an attack, put from two to five drops of tincture of Aconite in a tumbler half full of water, and give from a tea to a tablespoonful every one, two, or four hours, according to the severity of the symptoms. If the paroxysm becomes more severe, and is not owing to an aggravation by the remedy, give a dose every quarter, half, or one hour, until some relief ensues, and then lengthen the interval of time between the doses to one, two, or more hours. Or six globules may be solved in a wine-glassful of water, and one teaspoonful given as often as above directed. Frequently, however, in sick headache, the stomach becomes so irritable that it will not bear even a teaspoonful of water, then three or four globules must be given dry upon the tongue, or one or two drops of tincture of Aconite given per dose, upon a bit of sugar, as often as above directed. One half, or one quarter the above quantities will suffice for children. A dose of Aconite may also be given regularly, night and morning, in appropriate *chronic* congestive cases, and in those with a *chronic* inflammatory tendency, for three or four days in succession; then a dose of four globules may be given at night, dry, for three days more; then every other night, until three doses more have been taken; then, every third night, for three doses, and so on, until the case is entirely cured, or it becomes evident that Aconite will not relieve it.—PETERS.

2. AGARICUS MUSCARIUS.

GENERAL REMARKS.—Agaricus is indicated in nervous and congestive headaches, in which fulness, sleepiness, frequent and irresistible inclination to yawn are present, attended by relaxation and soreness of the whole body, pain in the back, and a feeling as if the joints were dislocated.—Genl. Hom. Journal, vol. 26, p. 223.—DR. BLACK.

[NOTE.—It is homœopathic to congestion of the head, with pulsation in all the vessels, redness and heat of the face, and elirium; also to catarrhal headache, with aching in the forehead over the eyes, drawing pain in the forehead extending to the root of the nose, rending pain in the forehead above the root of the nose as if the brain were lacerated, with burning pain in the nose and eyes, great dryness of nose, profuse bleeding of the nose, and abundant discharge of thick, viscid nasal mucus, followed by frequent dropping of water from nose.—PETERS.]

[CASE 3.—D. C., aged twenty-five, had been subject to headache every six weeks for seven years. The attacks commenced with acute pain over the eyes and sense of fulness, gradually extending through the head, but most severe in the forehead, soon becoming oppressive and violent, when the eyelids drooped, pulse rose, face flushed, tongue became dry and brown, the skin dry and hot. The attacks lasted from two to four days, and after the first or second day copious vomiting, principally of a bitter, bilious fluid, took place; urine was scanty and high colored. After a day or two the pain extended from the head down the spine, the neck often became stiff, he felt bruised all over, and his joints painful; the whole being followed by great exhaustion, wakeful nights, and tendency to delirium.

Treatment.—Lach. 6 and Ars. 6 effected some improvement during the whole of six months; then a severe attack was promptly relieved by Agaricus 6, and a continued use of Agar. 3 kept the paroxysms off entirely for five months. Finally Agar., aided by Sulph. and Stramon., cured him effectually at last accounts, three years after.

Dr. Ker says the symptoms which led him to select Agaricus were the violent oppressive pains, principally in the forehead, often attended with delirium, the sense of languor, feeling as if the body were bruised and the joints dislocated, and the sense of uneasiness and weakness all down the spine. These he thought so characteristic of Agaricus, that he selected and gave it with the most happy results.—DR. KER, Brit. Jour. Hom., vol. 5, p. 436.—PETERS.]

Dose.—Same as directed for Aconite.—P.

3. ARNICA MONTANA.

CASE 4.—A man, aged thirty-five, after receiving blows upon the head, was attacked with the following sufferings, which daily increased in severity.

Symptoms.—Pressing pain in the forehead; painful but dull aching upon the edge of the right orbit; heat in the head, with coolness of the rest of the body; pain in the head, increased after eating; heat in the face, noises in the ears, contracted pupils, nausea every morning; disgust for tobacco smoking; tenesmus, with constipation; anxious dreams; evident fever every evening; irritable and complaining disposition.

Treatment.—After taking Arnica 6, all the above disorders disappeared in the course of two days.—Archiv., vol. 5, part 1, p. 68.—Dr. Baudis.

[Note.—According to A. T. Thomson the flowers of Arnica contain Igasaures Strychnion, and some of the full effects of Arnica are similar to those of Nux vomica; thus it not unfrequently causes a sensation of formication, and a prickling, piercing, spasmodic feeling, which may be compared with that produced by slight electric shocks.

It is homœopathic to disorder of the chest marked by anxiety, oppression, palpitation, dry irritating cough, with symptomatic headache and vertigo.

Also in the headaches, flushings and perspirations which attend the change of life in women.

It deserves attention in the headaches which precede or follow attacks of apoplexy. Schneider did wonders with it in such cases.—Peters.]

Dose.—Comparatively larger doses of Arnica may be given than of most other remedies, except Camphor; to adults one or two drops of tincture of Arnica may be given in a teaspoonful of water, or on a bit of sugar, every one, two, four, or more hours, in acute cases; or two or three times a day in *chronic* cases. For children, or very sensitive and delicate adults, from three to six globules may be put in a wineglassful of water and given, a teaspoonful as above directed.—Peters.

4. ARSENICUM ALBUM.

General Remarks.—(*a*.) Tietze says it is indicated in persons who suffer with the signs of abdominal plethora or fulness, in which the whole appearance of the patient reminds one of liver complaint, and in which bilious colics often occur in alternation with Hemicrania.

The pain itself in these cases is of a very indefinite character, so that the patient cannot describe it accurately; but throbbing and rending pains, or pressing or stupifying ones, are the most common, generally most severe in the anterior portion of the head, which is unusually sensitive to the fresh air. The patient cannot find any ease, must move his head to and fro, even toss his feet about, and imagines he receives relief from these restless movements; external warmth also affords relief; he is very weak, thinks that he must die, seems to be bloated, is chilly, and seeks the warmth of the fire, and finds relief from covering and compressing the head with warm cloths.—Genl. Hom. Journal, vol. 34, p. 13.

(*b*.) According to Black it is useful in the headaches of emaciated persons, who suffer with disease of the heart, or of the digestive organs. He saw the most marked curative effects in a lady who had suffered for twenty years with attacks of the most violent Hemicrania, lasting for the most part at least three days, during all of which time the patient generally lay almost unconscious, and tortured by the most violent vomitings.—Genl. Hom. Jour., vol. 36, p. 223, and Brit. Jour. of Hom.

(*c*.) Hering recommends it in throbbing, rending pains in the head, when increased in the warm room and relieved in the open air.

[Note.—In the second number of the N. A. Hom. Jour., Dr. Marcy has given two cases of periodical headache successfully treated with Arsenic; but it seems to have been used much more successfully in old school practice than in the homœopathic. Watson (see Practice of Physic, p. 391) says: "Arsenic is considered by many to have a specific power over the complaint, and believes that four to six drops of Fowler's solution, given three or four times a day, will be almost sure to remove Hemicrania in nine cases of ten in which it occurs." Still it is very certain that the majority of patients will not bear such doses, and that much smaller ones will suffice.

Arsenicum is homœopathic when the eyes are inflamed during the attacks of headache, when the lids are swollen and face bloated, when a pricking sensation is experienced in the tarsi, the eyes are suffused with tears, and the conjunctiva is inflamed.

It is also particularly suited to those patients who have liver spots, and pityriasis, in many of whom those parts of the skin protected from the light also acquire a brownish, dingy, unwashed appearance. Dr. Hunt cured many such cases with one-fourth of a drop of Fowler's solution three times a day.

It is also useful in headaches attended with chronic diarrhœa, or gastric irritation.

In headaches from suppressed eruptions, especially of the scaly kind.

In those dependent upon or attended with scanty urine, or with dropsy; or arising from the incautious healing of ulcers.

It has also been found specific against the headaches which attend an irritable state of the uterus and ovaries, marked by constant pain, with heat, varying in severity, in the lower part of the sacrum, in the left groin and under the pubes, and by bearing down pain, much increased by walking, standing or sitting upright, almost forcing the patient to stay in bed, or recline upon a sofa, the uterus being tumid and tender. Such cases may be cured radically by Arsenic, without any local treatment applied to the uterus.

Schœnlein says, in the worst cases of chronic headache we must have resort to Arsenicum, which often cures the disease, even when of years' standing, better than any other remedy. Bright says that the periodicity of Hemicrania has suggested some similarity between its nature and that of genuine intermittents; however this may be, he says it is certain that Bark, Iron, and Fowler's Solution, remedies which are most successful in ague, are equally efficacious here.

Chapman says so many cases of cure of periodical headache occur to homœopathic physicians, that it may be superfluous for him to cite any, but two may be briefly stated:

CASE 5.—A gentleman had for many years been subject to periodical headaches, always occurring once a week, sometimes twice, and lasting several hours. The headache was stunning, rendering him incapable of all movement, or ot attention to any subject; he could only rest his head on something, and bear the pain as best he could.

Treatment.—Arsen. was given him, and during many months he had only one or two slight paroxysms, and has had none lately.—CHAPMAN, Brit. Jour., vol. 7, p. 398.

CASE 6.—The wife of a physician was subject to distressing periodical headache, with boring, circumscribed pressure on a small spot in one temple.

Treatment.—A few doses of Arsen., of 12th and 30th dilution, cured her as if by magic, and five years have passed without a return of the headache.—CHAPMAN, Ibid, p. 399.

CASE 7.—A weak, thin, poor woman, who had nursed a child for eleven months, had had headaches for six months; the pain commenced over the left eyebrow and temple, and lasted, without intermission, for twelve hours, after which she generally vomited a quantity of yellow, bitter, or tough matter; during the headache, and for some days after, she could not touch food on account of irritability of stomach; as soon as she recovered from one attack, another came on, periodically, every ten days; bowels regular, but loose and bilious after a headache.

Treatment.—Child to be weaned. Arsen. 30 and 18 was given with most decided improvement in three weeks, and entire cure in a month.—MADDEN, Brit. Jour., vol. 5, p. 438. —PETERS.]

Dose.—This powerful remedy must be given with the precautions due to its great power for good or evil. *Noack* advises for adults one or two drops per dose, of the second, third, fourth, sixth, or twelfth dilutions, to be repeated every two, four, six, eight, twelve or more hours in acute cases; or, as much of the powder as will go on the point of a penknife may be taken as often as above directed. Children and delicate adults may take, of a solution of three or six globules in a wine-glassful of water, one teaspoonful every two, four, six, eight or more hours. In *chronic* cases, one dose may be taken every twelve hours, or night and morning until six doses have been taken; then every night only, for six nights in succession; then every second, third, fourth, or sixth day.—PETERS.

5. ASARUM EUROPÆUM.

CASE 8.—A young lady of good constitution, but plethoric, had suffered for several years with the following head-affection.

Symptoms.—Sharp pain over the left eye, with lachrymation; could not read with that eye; bright light increased the pain; the left side of the head was sensitive to touch, and the hair would not bear combing; in violent attacks, both eyes became painful, and nausea was superadded; constipation; menses regular, still the attacks were apt to come on just before or after menstruation.

Treatment.—Asarum europ. $\frac{1}{200}$ given during the interval of relief, removed the whole disease.—New Archiv., vol. 2, part 1, p. 49.—DR. GROSS.

Dose.—*Noack* advises one or two drops per dose of the pure tincture, or first or second dilution, every two or more hours, in acute, or one or two times a day in chronic cases.—P.

6. ARUM.

Bergius asserts that when Arum is taken in doses of half scruple of the compound powder, he has never known it fail of giving relief in nervous headache, even after the most celebrated remedies had proved useless or injurious. Noack advises it in headache from weakness of the stomach.—PETERS.

7. AURUM.

GENERAL REMARKS.—Gold has frequently relieved the sense of rushing and roaring in the head, such as occurs at times in hysterical females from disorder of the uterine system; it not only relieves this permanently, but often improves the whole general disorder connected with it.—DR. HARTMANN, by Rückert, p. 132.

NOTE.—It is suited to that form of headache which, commencing early in the morning, is increased by meditation and reading, but especially by talking and writing, to an extreme degree of violence, and attended with perfect confusion of mind.

It is also useful against congestion to, with rushing and roaring in the head, bloating, glowing and shining of the face, with protrusion of the eyes, especially when followed by a feeling as if all the blood passed suddenly from the head to the legs. When there is great heat of the head and face, with coldness of the hands and feet; heat, pain, fulness of the head, sleeplessness and anxious dreams; congestion of the head increasing to delirium; throbbing of the carotid and temporal arteries. It is also indicated against a twisting, boring, acutely throbbing, one-sided headache, commencing immediately after waking in the morning, increased by coughing and bending the head backwards.

It is particularly useful against hæmorrhoidal and menstrual headaches.—PETERS.

Dose.—One or two grains of the first, second, or third trituration, dry upon the tongue; or, for children and delicate adults, from three to six globules in a wineglassful of water, one teaspoonful every two, four, six, or eight hours, in *acute* attacks, or every two or three days in *chronic* cases.—P.

8. BELLADONNA.

GENERAL REMARKS.—(*a*.) It is indicated against headaches attended with pressure, fulness and heat of the head, transient redness of the face, roaring in the ears, dulness of hearing, dilated pupils, &c. It is suitable for persons predisposed to active congestions; for plethoric persons of sanguine temperament, with great irritability of the uterine system; in the headaches of scrofulous children who learn to walk with difficulty, and are inclined to convulsions.—Genl. Hom. Jour., vol. 36, p. 223.—DR. BLACK.

(*b*). Heichelheim says that several forms of headache may be cured by Bellad.: 1, those occurring after taking cold, attended with visible congestion of blood to the head, red, bloated face, hard beating of the carotids, violent pain, as if the head would burst; 2, in other cases, in which the face is pale and cold, the pain resembling a dull, insupportable pressure in the brain, as if the latter had not sufficient room in the skull, often attended with vomiting.—Hygea, vol. 5, p. 209.

(*c*). According to Tietze, Bellad. is indicated in Hemicrania under the following circumstances: when there is a characteristic one-sided pain over the eye-brow, extending down into the ball of the eye and into the bones of the nose, and attended with increased secretion of tears; the pain is apt to be severely pressing in the forehead and upon the eye; at times it seems as if the affected parts were forced or pressed outwards. Every motion of the head or eyes increases the pain to an insupportable degree, especially when light also falls upon the eyes; every noise or movement of others in the sick-room has a like effect; the affected eye is often reddened, and waters. Sympathetic affections of the stomach, such as pressure in stomach, nausea, eructations, or even vomiting may be present; but when dyspepsia is the primary affection, and the head affection a secondary affair, Bellad. will never afford certain relief, but generally merely palliates.—Genl. Hom. Jour., vol. 34, p. 7.

(*d*). Dr. Schwarze says that he has treated several migranes, some not very severe, and some of not very long standing, occurring in not very robust or plethoric males, and cured them all, without exception, with Bellad.

(*e*). Griesselich has found it useful, when the scalp was very tender, the veins of the head and hands much distended, with sense of rushing in the head, roaring in the ears and darkness before the eyes; also against the most violent pains in one half of the head, extending to the eye and nose, with a sense of pushing, bursting, rushing and beating, increased by every motion, by moving the eyes, by every noise or jarring, and by the moving about of others; and attended by a sense of moving and beating in the head and forehead at every step, especially when going up stairs.

It is also useful against those pains in the head which set in every afternoon, last till midnight, and are aggravated by the warmth of the bed. Also in pains which commence suddenly, change into a sharp stitch, which seems to penetrate so deep into the brain that one almost loses consciousness.—Hygea, vol. 5, p. 136.

CASE 9.—A young, slender man, aged twenty-six, suffered with attacks of Hemicrania on the right side for fifteen years; commencing in the morning, increasing until midday, and subsiding in the evening; the pain being drawing and pressing, beginning about the right orbit and extending to the ball of the eye, to the forehead and temples; increased by stooping, reading and writing.

Treatment.—Bellad. 30, 1 drop, every four or five days for four weeks cured him perfectly.—SCHWARZE, p. 7.

CASE 10.—A gentleman, aged fifty-six, of medium stature and phlegmatic temperament, suffered twenty years with attacks of headache, occurring every Friday. The pain was always on the right side, attended with sense of pressing outwards, bursting and tension, with dizziness and loss of memory; the paroxysms lasted twenty-four hours, the face was hot, red and bloated; there were stitches of pain in the eye, with acrid tears and sensitiveness to light.

Treatment.—Old school remedies had been used in vain; *Nux vom.* was given without effect; then he was cured by *Bellad.* 30, given every Thursday for some time.—Practical Observations, vol. 1, p. 183.—DR. SCHUBERT.

CASE 11.—A lady, aged forty, suffered two weeks with severe headache of indefinite character; she could not keep still an instant, but moved her head and the upper part of her body to and fro constantly.

Bellad. 24 cured her on the first day it was used.—Genl. Hom. Jour., vol. 17, p. 242.—DR. FIELIZ.

CASE 12.—A maiden, aged seventeen, suffered several years with attacks of nervous headache, commencing early in the morning, increasing till midday, and ceasing in the evening; often attended with bitter or bilious vomits, with violent pressure upon the vertex and temples, with dizziness from raising or moving the head, with coldness of the hands and feet, rush of blood to the head, heat and redness of the face. Was cured by two doses of Bellad. 30.—Genl. Hom. Jour., vol. 5, p. 65.—DR. KNORRE.

CASE 13.—A young lady, aged nineteen, suffered with throbbing pains in the forehead, of which she was cured by Bellad. 400 and 800.—Genl. Hom. Jour., vol. 29, p. 275. —DR. HAUPTMANN.

CASE 14.—A plethoric, sanguine, young man, aged nineteen, suffered three years with spasmodic twitchings, and latterly had kept his bed for four weeks, on account of violent throbbing, piercing pains in the forehead and occiput, great heat in the head, and vertigo increased by motion; accompanied by noises in the ears, heaviness of the arms, and swelling of the veins; his eyes were fixed, his pupils very movable, and he had various gastric derangements.

Treatment.—Bellad. 2, one drop every two hours, cured him quickly, after previous aggravation.—Genl. Hom. Jour., vol. 21, p. 66.—DR. NOACK.

CASE 15.—A woman, aged fifty, otherwise healthy, suffered four years with headache, marked by rending pain in forehead to the right temple, with transient pains in the whole head, with heat therein, worst in the morning, with sleepiness during the attacks, rush of blood to, and heat in the face, and chilliness over the whole body. She also had leucorrhœa, especially when walking.

Treatment. Bellad. 300, in solution, one spoonful a day, cured her in sixteen days; the leucorrhœa was relieved by Sepia, 18.—Genl. Hom. Jour., vol. 35, p. 222.—DR. PERRY.

CASE 16.—A young lady, aged twenty-five, suffered eight years with periodical headaches, generally occurring every eight days, commencing with chilliness over the back and shoulders, soon attended with violent nausea, disgust and vomiting, with violent aching, pressing and rending pains in the whole head, especially in the forehead, increased to an insupportable degree by the slightest motion of the head or eyes; the softest bed seemed too hard, and only the greatest rest and quiet brought the slightest relief. Finally the pain extended to the whole front head, a glowing hot spot was to be felt in the forehead, and the bones of the nose became painful; she was obliged to lie in a dark place, as even a ray of light irritated the eyes and increased the headache; her limbs felt as if bruised, and she had palpitation to such a degree that every pulsation jarred the head.

Bellad. 24 followed by Bell. 30 cured her.—Archiv., vol. 6, part 3, p. 84.—Dr. Hartmann.

CASE 17.—A young lady, aged 24, of sanguine temperament and regular menstruation, had suffered for three years, almost uninterruptedly, with the following

Symptoms.—Burning and pricking in the gums, which soon swelled up and became blanched; in a quarter of an hour the upper lip and right side of face commenced to swell, with twitching, pricking and drawing therein; then followed screwing, boring, rending, pinching and piercing pain in the right ear, with noises therein; piercing and drawing pain behind the ear; piercing and rending pain in the occiput, and feeling as if it were screwed or pressed apart; boring and piercing pain in the right temple; extreme painfulness of the scalp. These attacks occurred in the afternoon, lasted until three in the morning, were increased by the warmth of the bed and by laying the head down. She often seemed almost unconscious; the sub-maxillary glands were somewhat swollen; she had great despondency.

Treatment.—Bellad. 30, one drop per dose, moderated the attacks up to the fifth day; from the fifth to tenth day she was quite well; a slight attack on the eleventh was treated with Pulsat. 15, after which she remained well for four months. Subsequent slight returns were treated with Bellad. 30, and she was perfectly cured.—Archiv., vol. 3, part 1, p. 85.—Dr. A. Schubert.

Besides the above cases, Bellad. was often used as an intercurrent remedy in other and in the following additional case.—PETERS.

CASE 18.—A gentleman, aged 50, very subject to attacks of headache and blindness, lasting the greater part of the day, and headache generally for two days, was relieved by Bellad. 18, in a quarter of an hour, and almost entirely cured of one attack in half an hour.—HENDERSON AND FORBES, p. 70.

CASE 19.—A married lady, aged 37, had suffered for six hours with severe pain across the top and middle of her head, extending to both temples; the pain was heavy and crushing; there was a sense of tightness across the eyes and root of nose, with constant pain; the eyes were painful to motion and to light, which produced frequent flashes in them; she also had ringing in the ears.

Treatment.—Bellad. 6, two doses at intervals of twenty minutes, almost entirely removed the attack.—HENDERSON.

CASE 20.—A spinster, aged 40, subject to severe attacks of headache, coming on gradually, lasting all day, keeping her awake a great part of the night, and not usually ceasing till the day after, and often not for several days, had been suffering for six hours with severe headache on right side of forehead and in right eye, with great increase of pain on moving the eye.

Treatment.—Bellad. 6, afforded no relief in twenty-five minutes; twenty minutes after a dose of Lachesis 6, was taken, not a trace of uneasiness remained.—HENDERSON.

Henderson reports several other brilliant cures in which Bellad. and other remedies were used.—PETERS.]

REVIEW.—Of the nine cases reported by Rückert, three were in males and six in females, their ages varying from 18 to 56 years. Schwarze found Bellad. most useful in males. [Of the three additional cases, two were females and one was a male, their ages varying from 37 to 50 years.—PETERS.]

The temperament of the patients was phlegmatic in one case, sanguine in two, and Dr. Black found Bell. most useful in those of a plethoric, sanguine temperament, while Schwarze cured many migranes in males who were not robust or plethoric.

Tietze noticed that the pains which Bellad. relieved most rapidly were those seated in the ophthalmic branch of the fifth pair of nerves.

The pains were one-sided in cases 9, 10, 15 and 17, and in § c, d, e; they involved the whole head in case 17; the back of the head in cases 14 and 17; the forehead in cases 9, 13 and 16; the orbit, brow, and root of the nose in § c and e, and cases 9 and 16; the temples in cases 9, 15 and 17; the vertex in case 12.

As regards the *kind* of pains, they are described as a dull, insupportable aching, pressing out and pressing asunder in § b, c, and e, and cases 10 and 16; as drawing and aching in cases 9 and 12; piercing and boring in cases 14 and 17; as stretching and throbbing in case 13; beating in § e; beginning suddenly and becoming piercing in § e.

Among the accompanying complaints we find vertigo, heat of the head, redness and heat of face, redness of the eyes; noises in the ears, beating of the carotids, and all the signs of congestion to the head. On the other hand, Heichelheim saw the face pale and cold, with dull pressure and vomiting. Many gastric derangements are apt to be present, such as coated tongue, bitter taste, inclination to vomit, vomiting of bitter substances, oppression of the stomach; still Tietze remarks, when the dyspeptic symptoms are primary, and the headache secondary, that Bell. will rarely cure, but at most only alleviate transiently. Further, the pains may be attended with loss of memory, soreness of the scalp, distension of the veins of the head and hands, coldness of the limbs, and chills.

The majority of the cases belonged to the *chronic* forms of headache; the disease had lasted for at least several years in six cases, in the others several weeks.

The cures in some cases were effected very soon, in others, after three or four weeks.

Of the nine cases, Bellad. effected a cure, unaided by any other remedy, in eight; the dose was 24th or 30th dilution in six cases; the 2d dilution was repeated in one case; the high potencies in solution and repeated, were used in two cases.

Dose.—The most efficient doses are sufficiently pointed out in the above paragraphs. When the high dilutions are used, five or six globules may be dissolved in a wineglassful of water, and one teaspoonful taken every half, one or two hours in severe cases, or only every two, four, six or eight hours in milder ones. When the lower dilutions are preferred, one or two drops of liquid Belladonna may be given every two, three, four, six, eight or twelve hours in mild attacks, or every quarter, half, one or two hours in severe cases, and in such as are not relieved by doses given at longer intervals. In *chronic* cases from two to five globules, or one or two drops may be taken every morning, or every second, third or fourth morning, as Belladonna is apt to cause aggravations when given in the afternoon, evening or night. *Children* may take one globule per dose, or one drop of the second, third, sixth or twelfth liquid dilution at the same intervals of time as above directed. PETERS.

[NOTE.—One of the most frequent forms of Belladonna headache is a dull, heavy frontal pain; a heavy regular pain over the whole forehead; a general, dull frontal distress, usually ushered in by a sense of dryness in the mouth and throat, dimness of vision and slight dizziness, attended with enlargement of the pupils.

It is homœopathic to headaches followed by delirium, especially if it be of an extravagant or pleasant character, accompanied with uncontrollable laughter or incessant loquacity, and the face be flushed and the eyes glistening.

It is also particularly suited for hysterical headache with excessive irritation of the bladder, strangury, bloody micturition, followed by an excessive flow of urine.

Piorry has rendered himself celebrated by his bold use of Belladonna in hemicrania: he assumes the disease to be a neurosis or neuralgia of the iris, or, more properly speaking, of the nerves of the iris, and that it is most frequently brought on by exposure to bright light, or dazzling spectacles, and excessive reading. From thence he assumes that the disorder spreads to the great sympathetic nerve, soon involving the stomach, and to various branches of the fifth pair, causing pains about the head and face. On account of the specific action of Belladonna upon the iris, and its well established reputation against neuralgia, he selected it as the principal remedy in hemicrania, and applied it locally about the eye, using from one to four grains of the extract moistened with a little water and rubbed upon the temples and lids. Piorry avers that he hardly ever fails to check the paroxysms if the Bellad. be applied at the moment of their commencement, or soon after. One drop of a solution of Atropine may also be applied, according to Piorry, to the eye itself, or a small quantity rubbed on the lids, brow and temples. I have witnessed several cases in which patients had found this mode of treatment of almost certain efficacy, the attacks subsiding in a few hours.—PETERS.]

9. BRYONIA.

GENERAL REMARKS.—(*a*). The head-symptoms caused by Bryon., when viewed in connection with the physiological phenomena which it excites in other organs and systems of the human body, point to alterations and disturbances in the nerves of sensation, and in the operations of several cerebral nerves, viz.: of the frontal and temporal branches of the trifacial; in fact it causes an actual hemicrania. In this respect its action is nearly allied to that of Colocynth and Nux vom.; Colocynth, however, does not affect the motor nerves of the face, while Bryon. often attacks the temporal and maxillary twigs of the superior facial branch.—Austrian Hom. Jour., vol. 3, p. 118.

(*b*). Bryon., according to Knorre, relieves headaches affecting the forehead, brows and temples, the pain being aching and pressing out as if the head would burst; attended with penetrating stitches so violent as to force one to cry out; arising from congestion of blood to the head, and increased by stooping, moving the head, coughing or sneezing.—Genl. Hom. Jour., vol. 5, p. 68.

(*c*). According to Black it is indicated when the pain is on one side of the forehead and extends to the neck, arms and face, and is more throbbing in its character the more severe it becomes. It may be given with advantage in alternation with Alumina.—Genl. Hom. Jour., vol. 36, p. 224.

(*d*). Griesselich thought it was most useful in burning and pressing pains, with the feeling when stooping, as if everything would fall out of the forehead; especially when they are increased by walking, and relieved by pressing upon the head, or tying something tight around it. He also advises it against superficial rending pains extending to the face and temples; in aching, boring and rending pains in small spots, occurring in persons of an irritable, angry disposition, and subject to rheumatism.—Hygea, vol. 14, p. 228.

CASE 21.—A lady, aged 30, of relaxed constitution, very irritable and timid, formerly irregular, generally too profuse, but now regular in her menstruation, had suffered for years with violent headaches, occurring especially after depressing mental emotions.

Symptoms.—The paroxysms commenced early in the morning, increased during the whole day, and were so intense by evening that she lay almost senseless. The pain was compressing, and involved the whole brain; her eyes were dull, glassy, contracted, and she could scarcely open them from pain; she could not bear the least noise or light; was irritable, inclined to find fault and scold. During the afternoon palpitation of heart, oppression of chest, nausea and retching to vomit generally set in. If she got some sleep during the night she was generally better the next day, but if fever and wakefulness set in, she was often obliged to keep her bed for several days in succession.

Treatment.—Bryon. 3, one drop, was soon followed by sleep; the next day she was quite well, although a fresh attack occurred seven days after from the reception of distressing news; still Bryon. again brought on sleep, and she remained permanently cured.—Archiv., vol. 1, part 2, p. 104. —DR. MORITZ MULLER.

CASE 22.—A young lady, aged 20, irritable and inclined to anger and vexation, had suffered for a year with attacks of headache commencing in the morning, marked by drawing, boring-aching in the forehead, and by piercing, rending and burning in the whole head, gradually decreasing after vomiting set in.

Treatment.—Nux vom. 9 lessened the attacks, and two doses of Bryonia then cured her entirely.—Archiv., vol. 6, part 3, p. 100.—Dr. Schuler.

CASE 23.—Mrs. P., aged 34, suffered frequently and periodically with one-sided headaches. After taking cold she was attacked, June 2d, with violent headache in the left temple, the pain being pressing and outward-pressing.

Treatment.—Nux 6, two doses, was given without benefit; then Merc. 3, two doses; in the afternoon a violent aggravation set in, the pain shifted from the left to the right side, became piercing and drawing, and so severe that the patient cried out from the slightest touch or motion of the head. At 2 o'clock Bryon. 200 was given, and at eight o'clock the patient was almost beside herself with suffering; then Bryon. 6, four drops in solution, was given every two hours; at 12 o'clock she was relieved, and the next day was perfectly well. —Genl. Hom. Jour., vol. 33, p. 101.—Dr. Kallenbach.

CASE 24.—A tailor, aged 44, slenderly built, with the signs of abdominal disease, had suffered from his youth, after a severe fall, with periodical attacks of pain on the right side of his head. The paroxysms were generally excited by changes in the weather, and often were so violent that he fainted away.

Symptoms.—Violent, piercing headache fixed in a small spot on the vertex, with the feeling as if the coronal suture were forced apart and a cool air passed through the brain; vertigo; illusions of visions; lachrymation; sensitiveness to light; loss of appetite; white coated tongue; feeling of heaviness in abdomen; constipation; turbid urine; drawing pains in the joints, without swelling or redness; emaciation; paleness; dejection; loss of hope; his pulse was generally slow and soft, but became frequent and hard during the attacks.

Treatment.—He had taken every conceivable remedy, in the old way, for six weeks, he then received four grains of Rad. Bryon., divided into six powders with sugar, one dose to be taken morning and evening; after the second dose the pain became so violent that he became unconscious, but the next day it was gone and never returned.—Austrian Hom. Jour., vol. 3, part 1, p. 119.

CASE 25.—A powerful man, aged 50, was attacked with violent pains in his head after a severe cold; the pains involved the right side, and were rending and drawing; the temporal veins were unusually distended, and his eyes glistening; he was exceedingly restless, his tongue coated, he had oppression at the epigastrium, constipation, dryness of the skin, and hard, quick pulse.

Treatment.—After a great variety of allopathic remedies, among others leeching and bleeding, had been used without avail, he received one grain of Rad. Bryon., morning and evening, and was cured in a few days after a violent aggravation.—Ibid., p. 120.

CASE 26.—A servant girl, aged 22, of robust frame, suffering at times with epileptic attacks, was seized almost without exception at every menstrual period, with pains in the head, always commencing in the night, and lasting for several days; the pains were violent and piercing, confined to the right side, and deprived her of all sleep; her eyes were bloodshot and protruding; her face was pale and covered with cold sweat; her tongue coated; appetite gone, and constipation had lasted four days; her pulse hard; skin dry; urine scanty and turbid. She had great anxiety, and complained of crawling and pricking pain in the ankle-joints.

Treatment.—After six days' allopathic treatment without relief she received Bryon. one grain, three times a day, with relief the same day and perfect cure in a few days.—Ibid., p. 120.

REVIEW.—Of the six cases, two were in males and four in females, all middle aged.

In two cases taking cold was the exciting cause; in one case changes of weather; in one case the time of menstruation; in another depressing mental emotions; while, according to Hering, Bryonia is useful in the headaches of rheumatic subjects, and those of an irritable, timid disposition and inclined to anger and vexation.

In two cases the pain was on the right side, in the temples, forehead and vertex; in one case it was on the left.

In two cases the pain commenced early in the morning and increased till evening.

Drawing pains occurred in three cases; piercing pains as often; besides, we meet with penetrating, compressing, out-pressing, rending, boring, burning, and throbbing pains, especially when the attacks become severe. In several cases the paroxysms occurred periodically.

Among the attending affections, we find congestion to the head in case 24; vertigo in case 24; distension of temporal veins in case 25; redness, protrusion and glistening of the eyes in cases 25 and 26; dimness, glassiness and inability to open the eyes in cases 24 and 26; illusions of vision in case 24; paleness of the face in cases 24 and 26; face covered with cold sweat in case 26; coated tongue, nausea, retching to vomit, vomiting, constipation and turbid urine in cases 24 and 26; hardish, hard and quick pulse in cases 24 and 26; drawing pains in the joints in case 24; extension of the pains to the nape, arms and face in § c.

The conditions of increase of the pains were: moving the head, or touching it, sneezing or coughing, stooping, walking, noise and light; the pains generally commenced early in the morning and were worst at night.

Bryon. cured four cases, without aid from other remedies, viz.: cases 21, 24, 25, 26. In two cases Nux vom. was given previously without effect.

Black generally found Alumina useful in alternation with Bryon.

The most of the cases were of a chronic nature, and the cures set in quickly.

The doses were of Bryon. 3d and 6th dilution. In case 23, the high potencies merely excited, while the 6th relieved quickly. The doses given by Allopaths were grain doses of the Root; they cured but caused severe aggravations in two cases.

Dose.—The lower or stronger dilutions seem to be most useful. Noack says one or two drops of the pure tincture, or of the 1st, 2d or 3d dilution may be given as directed for Bellad. in *acute*, or once or twice a day in *chronic* cases. When the globules are preferred two or three may be given per dose, every $\frac{1}{2}$, 1, 2 or 4 hours in severe cases; and every 6, 8 or 12 hours in slighter attacks; or five or six globules may be solved in a wineglassful of water, and one or two teaspoonfuls given as often as above directed.—Peters.

10. CALCAREA CARBONICA.

General Remarks.—(*a*). According to Hahnemann it is most suited when there is heaviness and aching in the forehead, forcing one to close his eyes; in headaches from excessive reading and writing; boring in the forehead, as if the head would burst; throbbing pain in the occiput; pushing in the middle of the brain; hammering headache after walking in the open air, forcing one to lie down; headache and buzzing in the head, with heat of the face, icy coldness of the right side of the head, and sweat on the head at night.—*Chronic diseases*, vol. 2, p. 308.

(*b*). Black says Calc. may be used in some cases in which Bellad. seems indicated, viz.: in those with heaviness, fulness, aching and heat in the face. It may also be given when there is a violent aching pain over the eyes with trembling of the lower lids, especially when the patient is dull and confused in the morning, awakes from sleep unrefreshed, and suffers with nervous debility. Genl. Hom. Jour., vol. 36, p. 224.

(*c*). According to Tietze, Calc. is next to Sepia the most important remedy in chronic migrane, especially in persons who have had to contend much with dyscratic diseases, and in whom a scrofulous predisposition is still evident. The pains which it relieves most readily, are dull aching pains in the vertex, extending towards the forehead; or drawing pains and coldness in the forehead attended with nausea, and arising or being increased by exposure to the free air; or rending pains in the right side of the forehead, with great soreness to touch; or throbbing and pushing in the middle of the brain; or headache generally confined to the right side, from which it radiates to other parts. These headaches may be attended with eructations, inclination to vomit and vomiting; or the menses may appear too early and flow too freely.—Genl. Hom. Jour., vol. 34, p. 19.

CASE 27.—A young lady, aged 23, had suffered for two years with headaches; she had been scrofulous when a child; commenced to menstruate scantily when 12 years old, often with an interval of six weeks.

Symptoms.—Dulness of the head, boring in the forehead as if the head would burst; hammering headache when in the free air, forcing her to return and lie down; buzzing in the head with heat of the face, and falling out of the hair; webs before the eyes, dimness of sight especially when reading; inclination to diarrhœa; during menstruation cutting pains in abdomen, and grasping pain in the sacrum; frequent awaking at night, with weeping and unhappiness. Calc. 30 effected a cure.—*Annals*, vol. 1, p. 74.—Dr. Schroter.

CASE 28.—A woman whose menses occurred too frequently and freely, and who felt worst early in the morning, had suffered for 15 years, with:

Feeling of coldness in the whole head; with vesicles or aphthæ in mouth constantly going and coming; acrid eructations from the stomach, without thirst; drawing pains in the legs, extending up to the back, and pricking in the ankle-joints.

Treatment.—Sulph. 30 merely relieved the pains in the limbs, but Calc. 30 removed the whole trouble permanently.—Archiv., vol. 17, part 1, p. 9.—D. B. in D.

CASE 29.—Miss G., aged 19, had suffered almost daily for 7 years with headache, sometimes affecting one side only, at others the whole head. She had frequent nausea and vomiting, and her menses were rather profuse.

Treatment.—Sepia and Carb. veg. were given without avail, except the pain became more limited to the right side; Calc. carb. 500, was also given without relief; then Tinct. sulph., four doses of two drops each, one dose daily; then Calc. carb. 4th dilut., six doses, two every week, with improvement after

2d dose, so that she had no return of headache for four months; then a slight attack was immediately relieved by one dose of Calc. c. 4th, and she remained permanently cured.—Genl. Hom. Jour., vol. 33, p. 106.—KALLENBACH.

CASE 30.—Miss J. had suffered for a long time with violent pressing pain over the left frontal protuberance, which prevented her from attending to any household duties; it was increased by over-heating and by fright; relieved by binding up the head and by lying down; it commenced early in the morning, persisted the whole day, and then returned again in a few days; she had heat and rush of blood to the head, pain in her eyes, dimness of sight, red, dull spots on her cheeks; also sore throat from every cold, constant pain in her back and stitches in the sacrum; she was annoyed with falling asleep of her feet, and constant drowsiness; her menses were very profuse and attended with pains in the hips. Calc. c., repeated every 8 days, cured her entirely. Practical Observations, vol. 2, p. 5.—DR. SCHINDLER.

CASE 31.—A robust woman, aged 51, had an attack of headache, coming on with every rain-storm, and lasting 24 hours; consisting of constant darting and pricking in the head, attended with much drowsiness, and vomiting of bile.

Treatment.—Sulph. 30 did not relieve; but after taking Calc. c. 30 she had no attack subsequent to the first 8 days of treatment.—Archiv., vol. 17, p. 1, page 8.—DR. B. OF D.

CASE 32.—Mr. J., aged 40, of sanguine temperament, had suffered when a child with scald-head, afterwards with worm complaints, and finally for many years with the following constantly increasing malady.

Symptoms.—Tearing pain, extending from the temples towards the vertex, which then became hot; when the pain increased much, throbbing set in, and was aggravated by mental exertion and spirituous drinks. These attacks were worse every four weeks; and if he ate rather freely in the evening he was generally attacked with spasms of the stomach and vomiting of food. He had burning in the eyes, and purulent discharge from the ears; when reading his head became confused, and painful on one side, with sweat on that side; his hair fell out freely; his nose was filled with offensive pus; he hawked up phlegm from the throat; was constipated; had piercing pain in the left side from motion; shortness of breath from stooping and going up stairs; nocturnal pains in the back and arms; loss of strength; talking weakened him very much; he fell asleep early in the evening, awoke frequently during the night; was irritable and easily excited to anger.

Treatment.—As he had been in the habit of being bled every year, for four years, he first received Aconite; then Nux vom. 30, followed by some relief from headache; then Calc. c. 30, for five weeks, when he was fully relieved of all his complaint.—Annals, vol. 1, p. 236.—Dr. Schroter.

CASE 33.—Chronic headache occurring after suppression of itch; affecting the forehead, most violent in the forenoon, increased or excited by mental occupation, attended with paleness of the face, disordered digestion, and weakness, especially in the morning.

Treatment.—Nux vom. only afforded palliative relief, but several doses of Calc. c. 3, given at long intervals, cured the case permanently.—Hygea, vol. 20, p. 355.—Dr. Maly.

CASE 34.—A young lady, aged 21, of slender make, and taciturn, but irritable disposition, whose menstruation occurred profusely every three weeks, and was preceded by swelling and painfulness of the breasts and leucorrhœa, had suffered for several weeks:

With throbbing pain in the forehead, internal heat in the head and sensation as if it would burst, setting in every afternoon and increasing till evening; during the attacks the blood flew to her face, her cheeks became very red and spotted, and her sleep was heavy with loud, almost snoring breathing. Calc. c. 30 effected a permanent cure.—Archiv., vol. 17, p. 1, page 8.—Dr. B. of D.

CASE 35.—A lady, aged 43, of choleric temperament, had suffered since the suppression of a chronic catarrh of the nose with:

Violent one-sided headache in the forehead over the left eye, attended with feeling of coldness, with stitches in the epigastrium, and pain in the back.

Treatment.—Calc. c. 30, followed in eight days by Sulph. 30, and after eight days more by Calc., cured her entirely in three weeks.—Archiv., vol. 17, p. 1, page 10.—Dr. B. of D.

CASE 36.—A single woman, aged 25, of violent temper and bilious constitution, who had suffered formerly with discharge from the left ear, was troubled with an internal sense of coldness and numbness on the left side of head near the back, accompanied by rending pain, shooting through the left arm down to the hand, and often extending to the left leg, with swelling of the knee, most severe in the evening, and while at rest.

Treatment.—Calc. 30 for four weeks, followed by Nux 30, for eight days, and again by Calc. c. 30, effected a perfect cure.—Ibid.

Review.—Of the ten cases, two occurred in males, eight in females, their ages varying from 19 to 51 years. The temperament is given as sanguine in one case; choleric in one case; venous or bilious in one case; delicate in one case.

The most common exciting causes were previous scrofulous affections, scald-head, suppressed discharges from ears or nose, or suppressed itch. In case 31, the attacks always occurred during rain storms.

In four of the female cases, the menses occurred too soon and too profusely; in one case only, in a scrofulous person were the menses too late and scanty.

The *character* of the pains varied very much; most frequently they were of a hammering, throbbing or pushing nature, as in § a, c, and cases 32 and 33; pressing and dull in § a, b, c; boring with sense of bursting in § a, and cases 27 and 34; pricking in case 31; rending in § c; stretching in case 32; piercing in case 31; radiating in § e.

Quite peculiar to Calc. is the sensation of coldness in the head, the icy coldness of the right side of the head, mentioned in § a, c, and cases 28, 35 and 36; and the night-sweats, § a.

As regards the *locality* of the pains, the majority were seated in the forehead over the eyes, see § a, b, c, and cases 30, 33, 34, 35; next in the middle of the brain § a, c; then in vertex, see § c; occasionally in the occiput, see § a; or in the side of the forehead, § c; or on one side, see case 33, viz.: on the right side in § c, and case 29; on the left side in cases 30, 35 and 36.

As regards the *time of day* in which the pains commence or increase, we find early in the morning in cases 30 and 38; in the forenoon in cases 33 and 34.

Among the accompanying disorders, we find congestion to the head and face in § a, and cases 30 and 34; red spots upon the cheeks in cases 30 and 34; dimness of vision in cases 27 and 30; paleness of face in case 33. Dr. Black mentions quivering of the lower eye-lid. Among the gastric derangements we find nausea, eructations, hot risings from the stomach, vomiting of bile or food, inclination to diarrhœa; also aphthæ in the mouth; and sleepiness.

Among the causes of the commencement or increase of the Calc. headaches, we find mental labor, reading and writing in § a, and cases 32 and 33; household occupations in case 30; speaking in case 32; exposure to free air and walking in § a, c, and case 27; touch in § e; fright and over-heating in case 30; use of spirituous liquors in case 32. Among the causes which alleviate the pain, we find, closing the eyes in § a; binding up the head in case 30; lying down in § a, and cases 27 and 30.

Calc. effected four cures unaided by any other remedy; in several cases Sulph. was given with little or no effect; in one case Calc. was given in alternation with Sulph.; and in one case with Nux.

All the cases were old chronic ones, and the cures were effected in a few weeks.

As regards the *dose*, Calc. 30 was given in seven cases; Calc. 3 in one case; Calc. 4 in one case. Generally one dose sufficed to effect a cure. In case 29, Calc. 500 was given without avail, while four doses of Calc. 4 effected a cure.

Dose.—In *chronic* cases, two or three grains of the 1st, 2d or 3d trituration, or as much as will cover a sixpence, or the top of the cork of the vial, may be taken once or twice a day, or every 2d, 4th or 6th day. Or from three to five globules may be taken as often as above. It is not often used in *acute* cases.—Peters.

11. CAMPHORA.

CASE 37.—A woman, aged 36, with unusual development of the cerebellum, had suffered for several months with:

Throbbing and heavy beating in the cerebellum; pulse irritable and synchronous with the beating in the brain; great redness and heat in the face.

Treatment.—Spirits of Camphor. 1 to 10, ℥ij, of which one or two drops were given every five minutes, removed the who le attack in the course of an hour.—Griesselich.

CASE 38.—A young lady, aged 19, suffered with paroxysms of headache of the following character:

Throbbing in the cerebellum synchronous with the pulse beats. Camphor $\frac{1}{10}$th, one drop per dose, every ten minutes, relieved the attack in a few hours.—Griesselich.

CASE 39.—A man, aged 39, was attacked with throbbing headache in the cerebellum, which he himself described as synchronous with the pulse.

Spirits of Camphor, four or five drops per dose, were given every fifteen minutes, and sufficed to remove the difficulty in the course of two hours.—Hygea, vol. 13, p. 456.

Review.—Camphor is the only remedy which produces and promptly cures throbbing pains in the cerebellum synchronous with the pulse.

[Note.—Judging from Christison's records, Camphor is homœopathic to some varieties of nervous and congestive headaches, when the patient is languid, listless, giddy and confused; when all objects quiver, and sparks appear before his eyes, and his body feels so light that he seems to skim along the floor almost without touching it; when the patient is pale and chilly and his head feels numb; followed by a strange feeling of anxiety, so that without thinking himself in danger he sheds tears, but cannot tell why. These symptoms may be followed by some heat of skin, palpitation, hurried pulse, sense of intoxication, moisture of the skin, and profound sleep for some hours, attended with excessive sweating.—Peters.]

Dose.—The proper dose is sufficiently indicated in the treatment of the above cases. It is a matter of regret that other mild remedies, such as Chamomilla, Coffea, Borax, Ferrum, Ipecac., Lycopodium, Nux moschata, and many others are not given as freely as above recommended for Camphor, instead of being administered in doses as infinitesimal as if these remedies were as powerful as Arsenic., Bellad. or Merc. corrosiv.—Peters.

12. CARBO ANIMALIS.

General Remarks.—According to Black, *Carb. an.* is useful in nervous and congestive headaches, in which pressure in the occiput sets in after eating, attended with soreness of the scalp, and by pains arising from irregular action of the digestive organs, connected with flatulence.—Genl. Hom. Jour., vol. 36, page 224.

13. CARBO VEGETABILIS.

CASE 40.—A young gentleman, aged 8, had been subject for two years to attacks of excruciating headache, commencing with giddiness and sense of fulness, ending in most acute pain. Carb. veg. relieved him entirely.—Dunsford, p. 104.

CASE 41.—A gardner, aged 40, became subject to headaches after a fall upon the head; the paroxysms came on two or three times a day, lasted an hour and were followed by great weakness and palpitation.

Treatment.—Bellad. kept off the attacks for three weeks. Carb. veg. was then given and the pain did not return for six months; it was repeated and the malady was overcome, slight pain only being experienced on sudden changes in weather. —Ibid.—Peters.

Dose.—Carb. anim. and vegetab. may be given in the same doses as recommended for Calcarea.—Peters.

14. CAPSICUM.

General Remarks.—(*a*). According to Hering, Capsicum is often useful against throbbing headaches, or those marked by distending, bursting or out-pressing pains, increased by motion or walking; or against piercing-rending pains, occurring while one is at rest, or when moving the head or eyes, or stooping; when exposure to the free air or cold aggravates the pain; and the attacks occur in phlegmatic, dull, or irritable people, or in children who are very contrary, apt to be chilly, especially after drinking, and are afraid of the free air and of active exercise.

(*b*). Tietze uses Caps. when the pains are throbbing, or aching and piercing and attended with nausea to the point of vomiting; when they are aggravated by moving and bending the head, by moving the eyes, and the patient is very sensitive to the cold air.—Genl. Hom. Jour., vol. 34, p. 32.

Dose.—Capsicum may be given at the rate of one or two drops of the 1st, 2d or 3d dilution, every two, four, six or more hours, according to the severity of the symptoms. Children and delicate females may take one or two globules as often.—Peters.

15. CAUSTICUM.

General Remarks.—According to Hahnemann it is indicated against dull, stupifying aching in the brain; piercing in the head; stitches in the temples; burning piercing in the vertex.—Chronic Diseases, vol. 3, p. 86.

CASE 42.—A delicate seamstress, aged 37, had suffered for a long time with an affection of the head.

It began with stitches in the scalp, shot to the temples, where it also became piercing, and was attended with nausea; the pain was most severe in the morning, soon extended through the whole body, which became chilly and covered with goose-skin, whilst the head and face became burning hot. Her menses were very irregular, at times too early, at others too late.

Treatment.—Bellad. not only did not relieve, but the paroxysms became more severe in the evening. Causticum 30, removed the whole difficulty.—Archiv., vol. 17, p. 1, page 10. —Dr. B. of D.

CASE 43.—A merchant, aged 52, of robust constitution, had suffered for several years with the following complaints:

Violent stitches of pain in the right temple, most severe in the evening when he came out of the open air into a warm room, and attended with giddiness. Irregular appetite, at times poor, at others ravenous; fulness in the abdomen, constipation for several days at a time; at night when in bed he had drawing pains in all his limbs, persisting severely until midnight; chills during the evening, with dejection of mind, and gloomy anticipations about the future; frequent sorrow and care.

Treatment.—Pulsat. afforded but little relief, but Caust. 30, removed the whole difficulty.—Ibid.

CASE 44.—An old lady, aged 75, a great coffee drinker, had suffered several years with:

Nocturnal pains of a rending and digging character, attended with constant roaring and rushing in the head; formication in the arms and rending in all the limbs, increased by motion.

Treatment.—Sulph. 30, one dose every fourteen days for five doses, with the continued use of coffee, removed the pains in the limbs, and Caust. 30, five doses at the same intervals of time cured those in the head.—Ibid.

REVIEW.—All three cases were chronic; the pains affected the temples in particular; they were piercing and connected with rending and drawing in the limbs.

Dose.—Causticum is regarded by many physicians as a very mild or almost inert remedy, still it seems to have been exceedingly useful in the above three *chronic* cases, and that in the high dilutions. Two or three globules may be given two or three times a day at first; then every two, four or six days; if this does not suffice, one or two drops of the first, third or sixth dilution may be used in *chronic* cases once or twice a day, or at the longer intervals above directed. It is rarely given in acute cases.—PETERS.

16. CHAMOMILLA.

GENERAL REMARKS.—According to Hering, Chamomilla is useful in pains from taking cold and from excessive use of coffee; especially when there is rending and drawing in one side of the head extending down into the jaws; stitches in the temples; heaviness, or very annoying throbbing over the nose; especially when one cheek is red and the other pale, or the whole face is swollen, and the patient has a bitter putrid taste in the mouth. It is often suitable for children and for persons who become ill-natured from pain.

CASE 45.—Mrs. P., aged 34, suffered periodically with one-sided headache.

Symptoms.—Violent piercing pains in the left side of the head, extending from the occiput to the upper jaw of the same side; at times she had rending pains in the left ear, the left cheek became red and hot, and frequent slight chills were followed by stitches in the region of the liver.

Treatment.—Chamomilla 200, afforded no relief from early in the morning until 10 o'clock at night; then Chamom. 3, three drops in solution, one teaspoonful every hour was given with relief in the course of an hour, and the next day she was well.—Genl. Hom. Jour., vol. 33, p. 101.—KALLENBACH.

Dose.—Cham. is rarely or never suitable in the cure of *chronic* headaches. It is such a very mild remedy that in *acute* attacks several drops of the pure tincture may be given every half, one, two or more hours; or the same quantities of the first, second or third dilutions may be used for children or very sensitive adults. In the very rare cases in which these doses do not suffice, the higher potencies may be tried, viz.: six globules in a wineglass of water, one teaspoonful per dose, as often as above directed.—PETERS.

17. CHINA.

GENERAL REMARKS.—(*a.*) According to Hering, China is often useful in the headaches of sensitive persons when the pain is pressing and prevents sleep at night, or causes such tearing in the temples that it seems as if they would burst; also against boring pain in the vertex, with feeling as if the brain were bruised; or jerking, rending, sense of fluctuation and bursting pain, aggravated by stepping, walking, by every movement, and by opening the eyes, and relieved by lying down and by quiet. It is also indicated when the scalp is very tender to touch; and for the headaches of discontented and irritable persons, and those of disobedient and obstinate children, who are fond of stuffing themselves with all kinds of improper food, have pale faces, who are only occasionally red and warm, and then become very talkative, or are restless the whole night. Often suitable after Coffea.

(*b*). Tietze thinks China most suitable when the pain is a pressing rending, or tearing pressing, especially when most severe in the temples, worst at night, preventing sleep, the pain being aggravated by the slightest touch, by stepping, draughts of air or wind. Also when there is excitement of the mind and imagination, and the patient is wayward, abusive and angry.—Genl. Hom. Jour., vol. 34, p. 22.

(*c*). According to Black, China is indicated in drawing, rending, pressing headaches, which abate from quiet, but increase from the slightest motion, and do not remain fixed in one spot; also against the passive congestions of the head which follow great losses of blood, violent purgings, and loss of semen; when there is a feeling of emptiness in the head, ringing in the ears, weakness of sight, with rending, drawing and squeezing pains.—Genl. Hom. Jour., vol. 36, p. 232.

CASE 46.—A girl, aged 15, not yet menstruated, had suffered for six months, with longer or shorter intervals of relief, from headache.

Symptoms.—Very painful movement and beating of the brain against the skull; she could not keep her head still, but shook it up and down; severe pain on the left side; feeling as if the upper part of skull would burst off, the pain being increased by motion and stepping; the left eye was affected; the left side of neck was painful and stiff; and she was lachrymose and dejected.

Treatment.—Rhus did not help; but China 12, half a drop, removed the pain in four hours; it returned in six hours more, and was then removed entirely by a second dose of China.—Annals, vol. 10, p. 414. Dr. HARTLAUB.

CASE 47.—Mrs. D., suffered with severe pain on the top of her head, with a flushed face, but not a frequent pulse; consequent upon immense losses of blood after miscarriage, and at other times.

Treatment.—Bellad. 3 was given without relief, and the

pain became distracting. Nux 3 was also given without benefit, as she was worse if possible on the third day; then China 6, one dose, cured her promptly and completely.—Dr. SHARP.—Brit. Jour. Hom., vol. 9, p. 585.—PETERS.

REVIEW.—The pains relieved by China consisted of rending or pressing, or of both combined, attended by a feeling of fluctuation and of beating in the brain as if the head would burst; they were worst at night, aggravated by the slightest touch, by moving or stepping and by currents of air, and relieved by rest and lying down. The mind was excited, irritable, or inclined to scolding and anger. It was also found useful against passive congestions from loss of fluids.

[NOTE.—China and Quinine have been used much more freely in old school practice than in the homœopathic. Wood says: "In relation to the permanent cure of headache, sulphate of quinine should always be employed in intermittent and periodical cases and may be tried with the hope of good in others. In hemicrania he has found Quinine in connexion with Oil of Valerian almost uniformly successful; he gives from ten to thirty grains of the Sulphate and about twenty drops of the Oil daily, divided into six or eight doses, and persisted in, if necessary, for a week or more; and thinks that enough quinine should be given to induce its peculiar effects upon the brain, such as buzzing in the ears, &c." Dr. W. tells us that "it very often happens that the pain is increased for the first day or two, after which it gradually subsides;" and perhaps takes the patient along with it. Johnson says Quinine and Arsenic are the most potent of all remedies in this disease; they seldom fail to put a stop to the complaint.—PETERS.]

Dose.—Noack advises one, two or several drops of the pure tincture of China per dose; or like quantities of the first, second or third dilution, repeated every half, one or two hours in severe cases, or every two, four or six hours in milder attacks. Children and delicate adults may take from one or two, to three or five globules as often.—PETERS.

18. COCCULUS.

GENERAL REMARKS.—(*a*). Hartmann relieved several headaches by it, which were increased after eating and drinking, attended by a sense of emptiness and hollowness in the head, and by pains which the patient could not describe accurately.

(*b*). According to Black, Cocculus is most suitable for hypochondriacal and melancholic persons, inclined to anxiety and fright; for nervous gastric headaches attended with nausea or actual vomiting; for headaches during menstruation, especially when that occurs too soon. Black also says he has had frequent occasion to observe in chronic headache with vomiting, that the remedies first check the latter, and then the headaches become less severe and diminish in frequency. When the headache is severe and attended with vomiting, he has found Cocc. the most useful intercurrent remedy in checking the vomiting; also Ignat. and Eugenia.—PETERS.—Genl. Hom. Jour., vol. 36, p. 232.

The only case recorded by Ruckert in which Cocculus was used, is case 60, in which it was given in daily alternation with Phosphor.

As the English physicians have used it more frequently and successfully I subjoin the following additional case.—PETERS.

CASE 48.—Miss H., aged 35, of full habit, had been subject to headaches for 15 years; they came on shortly after menses first set in and have regularly appeared at that time ever since; the pain was violent and dull, affecting the whole head; she was obliged to lie on her side, and could not rest for a moment on the back of her head, nor bear the least light; while the slightest noise excited nausea and vomiting; the attacks lasted from 36 to 48 hours, generally commencing on the third or fourth day of menstruation; menses were abundant but not painful.

Treatment.—Cocculus 6, from every half to every six hours during the paroxysms, almost freed her from her headaches in three months. Then Bellad. 6 and Cocc. 18 were given and she had no return of pain for twenty months.

The principal indication in this case for the selection of Cocculus was the marked tendency to nausea resembling sea sickness, as if the stomach heaved up and down. So great was this peculiarity that travelling in a carriage made the patient feel ill, and nausea had often been brought on by looking at a vessel pitching up and down on the sea.—BLACK.—Brit. Jour. Hom., vol. 5, p. 430.—PETERS.

Dose.—One or two drops of the first, second or third dilution of Cocculus may be given every half, one or two hours in severe cases; or every two, four or eight hours in milder attacks. When the stomach is exceedingly irritable the doses should not be given in water, but on a bit of sugar, or granules should be prepared and given dry upon the tongue, from one to three per dose, as often as above directed.—PETERS.

19. COFFEA.

GENERAL REMARKS.—(*a*). According to Hering, Coffea is useful in violent one-sided, drawing, pressing pains, as if a nail were driven into the side of the head; or as if the brain were crushed, torn or bruised; arising from slight exciting causes, such as thinking, vexation, taking cold, eating too much, &c., attended with disgust for accustomed coffee, with sensitiveness to noise and music; the pains seeming quite insupportable, forcing the patient to weep; or the patient gets quite beside himself, screams, cries, tosses about, is extremely anxious, fearful of the cold air, and chilly.

The remedy may be frequently repeated, and followed by Nux v. or China, or at times by Ignat. or Puls.

(*b*). According to Tietze, Coffea is useful in migrane when the pain is drawing and pressing as if from a nail driven into one side of the brain, or as if the whole brain were bruised or crushed; when the pains drive one to distraction, force one to walk around the room, and are attended with great sensitiveness to noise, and fresh air, with chilliness; and are increased after eating. If such a headache has been produced by mental exertion in a person who seldom or never takes coffee, then Coffea will almost certainly relieve.—Gen. Hom. Jour., vol. 34, page 21.

(*c*). When the above state of mental irritability is present with headache, Coffea often relieves with wonderful celerity.

[NOTE.—Coffee and tea are also used much more largely for the relief of headaches in the old practice than in the new;

Wood says: "on the whole, he has found nothing more effectual for the relief of severe headache than two or three cups of strong tea; but when the disease depends upon the use of tea or coffee (there is some homœopathy here), they act simply like ardent spirit in relieving the horrors of intemperance, and then should not be employed, as they aggravate the evil in the end." Trousseau (*see Traité de Thérapeutique*) says, common usage has sanctioned the efficacy of coffee in headaches, especially in that form which sets in after eating, in nervous persons; slight attacks of migrane almost always are removed by it. Sandras (*see Traité pratique des maladies nerveuses*, vol. 1, p. 354) says that the only remedies that he has used with any success in migrane are: tea, morphine and emetico-cathartics. Tea, he says, if taken in very strong doses during the first few hours of the attack, will sometimes dissipate it, as if by enchantment; but to obtain this result one must drink several cups of strong tea, with but very little sugar, and no milk or alcohol. Valleix (*see Guide du Médecin practicien*, vol. 4, p. 766) says: In some cases a cup of the infusion of coffee will drive away an attack. Formey recommends an infusion of crude coffee as follows: coffee, finely ground but not roasted, and perfectly dry, 15 grammes; boiling water, sufficient for a cup; make an infusion and drink at once. The regular daily use of the Tinct. of Crude Coffee and the Tinct. of Green Tea, deserve a much more extended trial than they have yet received. Good says, as a general palliative strong coffee has often proved serviceable, and where its own sedative virtues are not sufficient, it forms one of the best vehicles for the administration of Opium; it diminishes in some measure the hypnotic power of Opium and counteracts its secondary disturbing effects; still if Opium be given mixed with strong coffee for the cure of many modifications of headache, tranquillity and ease will often be produced though no sleep follows; but when Opium is taken alone, sleep will perhap follow, but it is mostly succeeded by nausea and a return of pain. For similar reasons the Turks and Arabs make coffee their common vehicle for taking Opium.—PETERS.]

Dose.—Noack advises one, two, or four or more drops of the pure tincture of *raw* coffee per dose at short intervals of time; in some rare cases the first, second or third dilution may be used, or several globules per dose, either dry upon the tongue or dissolved in a teaspoonful of water.—PETERS.

20. COLOCYNTH.

(*a*). According to Hering, Colocynth will help the most severe and raging rending pains; or one-sided, drawing, pressing, squeezing pains; or aching in the forehead, increased by stooping and by lying upon the back; and, finally those attacks which set in every afternoon or evening, affecting the left side, attended with great restlessness and anxiety, especially when the sweat of the patient has a urinous smell; when but little urine is made, and that which is passed at first is very offensive, but becomes very abundant and clear during the severity of the pains.

(*b*). Tietze thinks that Coloc. is most indicated when the one-sided pains are aching and pressing, or else drawing, and attended with nausea and vomiting; when they affect the forehead and left side of head, and the attacks generally set in in the evening, the pain being increased by stooping, moving, shaking the head, moving the eyelids; also by mental emotions, such as indignation, bitter feelings, or mortification about unworthy treatment. Great restlessness and anxiety often attend the pain.—Genl. Hom. Jour., vol. 34, p. 22.

(*c*). According to the Austrian provers, the forms of hemicrania curable by Colocynth depend upon an increase of sensibility, aroused by rheumatic, arthritic or gastric irritations. It cannot cure megrims arising from thickening of the arachnoid, adhesion of the membranes, or other organic changes. Generally, the hemicrania which Colocynth cures most readily is seated in the course of the frontal nerve, is attended with violent pain in the eye, and alternates with neuralgia of the cœliac plexus.—Austrian Jour., vol. 1, p. 148.

CASE 49.—Coloc. 30, cured a violent, piercing pain in the forehead and eyes, shooting from without inwards, and which had lasted for 90 hours, both by day and night; the pulse was hard, thirst excessive, there was a bitter taste of all food, general dry heat and constipation. Entire relief followed in six hours.—Gen. Hom. Jour., vol. 4, p. 13.—ATTOMYR.

CASE 50.—A young lady, aged 24, of delicate constitution, formerly scrofulous, was attacked with intensely violent, pressing, rending, headache; she could not lie still, was constantly getting up, bent herself together, wept and screamed. When the headache abated attacks of suffocation set in, with oppression of chest, gasping for breath, clenching of the hands, &c. The paroxysms recurred every half or one hour. Coloc., six doses, relieved the whole suffering.—Practical Observations, vol. 2, p. 9.—DR. SCHINDLER.

CASE 51.—An old lady, aged 50, had suffered for several years with headache on the left side, occurring periodically in the afternoon about five o'clock. She had been treated allopathically without relief.

Treatment.—Asarum afforded some relief, but Colocynth cured her in a few days permanently.—Archiv., vol. 11, part 2, p. 114.

CASE 52.—Mr. W., aged 29, of robust frame and choleric, phlegmatic temperament, suffered with:

Periodical headache, recurring every morning about half an hour after awaking, being rending, piercing and jerking in its character, and affecting the right temple in particular, but extending from thence over the whole right side of the forehead. He also had dulness of the head; turning out of the right eye, which was red and watery, and seemed smaller than the other; flimmering before and dimness of the same eye. The pains extended to the teeth, where they became raging, aching, and jerking, attended with sensitiveness of the right side of the head, especially about the eye, with soreness to touch; he also had loss of smell; flowing catarrh; cough, with greenish expectoration and increase of headache; white coated tongue; inclination to vomit; contraction of the stomach, with soreness to touch; heaviness of the limbs; coldness and thirst.

The attacks lasted from 6 A. M. to 3 P. M., attended with great anxiety and restlessness, so that he walked about the room in agony.

Treatment.—Nux v., Bell., Bryon., China, Cham. and Sulphur were given without much benefit; then Coloc. 2 was given and rendered the next attack lighter, and seven more doses effected a perfect cure.—Genl. Hom. Jour., vol. 27, p. 293.—Dr. Haustein.

Review.—The above cases presented the following striking peculiarities: the pains occurred in paroxysms, generally lasting from morning till afternoon; they were violent, rending, compressing, drawing, pressing, piercing and jerking. In three cases they were on the left side of the head, in one case on the right, in others more in the front-head and forehead, and were attended with nausea, vomiting, great restlessness and anxiety; with perspiration of urinous smell, with scanty and offensive urine; the attacks were excited by vexation and mortification, increased by stooping and lying on the back, by moving, especially of the eyelids, by shaking the head and by touching it.

[Note.—The use of Colocynth as specific to some forms of neuralgia of the head, hip and other parts, has long been known to the homœopathists, but Watson tells us that Sir Charles Bell, drawing a bow at a venture, achieved a cure of a patient upon whom much previous treatment had been expended in vain, by some pills composed of Extract of Colocynth, Croton Oil and Galbanum. He mixes one or two drops of the Oleum Tiglii, with a drachm of the compound extract of Colocynth, and gives five grains of this mass, with ten grains of the compound Galbanum pill at bed-time. Watson says he mentions the exact proportions and dose because other cases have been since reported, both by Sir Charles and others, in which the same prescription was followed by the same success. The small quantity of Colocynth in the above farrago would probably have been equally useful.—Peters.]

The **Doses** were Coloc., 2d dilution, 6th and 30th; the cures took place quickly. [Noack advises one or two drops of the 1st, 2d, or 3d dilution, repeated at longer or shorter intervals, according to the severity of the headache.]—Peters.

21. CREOSOTE.

CASE 53.—A man, aged 40, strong and plethoric, was attacked three weeks after having the influenza, with :

Violent pain in the whole back head, extending to the nape, and most severe on the right side ; the pain commenced at five o'clock, A. M., with great severity, increased for several hours, then lessened, and finally ceased about eleven, A. M. These paroxysms occurred daily, but anticipated and postponed somewhat. Every movement of the head increased the pain ; the sexual desire was much lessened, and the attacks were more severe after gratification of it. Every kind of cure, together with Bark and Quinine, had been tried in vain.

Treatment.—Creosote 3d, one dose per day, for ten days, produced a marked alleviation, then it ceased to cause improvement, and finally the disorder commenced again to increase in severity. Creosote 2d was given, and after being continued, one dose daily, for some time, the patient was entirely cured.—Vehsemeyer's Journal, vol. 2, p. 228.—REISIG.

[**Dose.**—Noack advises one or two drops of the 1st, 2d, or 3d dilution every two, four, six, eight, twelve or twenty-four hours, according to the acuteness or severity of the attack.—PETERS.]

22. CROCUS.

GENERAL REMARKS.—The pains in the head so frequently occurring during the change of life in women, may often be relieved by Crocus, especially when they are of a pushing, throbbing character, with pressure upon the eyes, attacking first one spot, then another, with distension of the blood-vessels, not confined to the head only, but spreading to other parts of the body ; also when the pains are most severe at the times when the menses used to occur, and persist uninterruptedly for two or three days, having but few intermissions even during the night, sufficiently long to allow of sleep ; becoming less severe and continuous after the menstrual period has passed. Dose. Crocus 3d, repeated two or three times a day, and resumed again at each monthly period.—Genl. Hom. Jour., vol. 18, p. 111.

[**Dose.**—Noack advises one drop of the pure tincture, or of the 1st or 2d dilution, every half, one, two or three hours in severe attacks, and two or three times a day only, in mild cases.—PETERS.]

23. DULCAMARA.

CASE 54.—A healthy woman, aged 40, was attacked with headache on coming to, after suddenly falling senseless to the floor.

Symptoms.—Violent boring burning in the forehead and vertex, with digging in the brain from within outwards; sensation as if a board before the forehead pressed back the brain; increase of pain from every motion, even from speaking; heaviness of the head; accumulation of saliva in the mouth; dryness of the tongue and thirst; hard, tense pulse; great weakness and bruised feeling of limbs; attacks of sickness during damp, rainy weather.

Treatment.—Ten minutes after Dulc. 8, increase of pain set in and lasted an hour, followed by sleep for three hours, from which she awoke well.

See Mat. Med. Pur., Symptoms 11, 16, 23, 27, 34, 37, 59, 95, 97.—Annals, vol. 1, p. 234.—DR. GASPARY.

Dose.—Dulcamara is one of the milder remedies, of which Noack advises one or two drops of the pure tincture, or of the first or second dilution every one, two, four or six hours. In appropriate cases the higher dilutions may be used, or three globules solved in a wineglassful of water, one teaspoonful to be taken per dose as often as above directed. —PETERS.

24. GRATIOLA OFFICINALIS.

[Chapman has used it in sick headache with benefit when there is nausea, disgust for food, giddiness relieved by being in the open air, heaviness of head and constriction of forehead. A drop of the second or third dilution will sometimes cut the attack short, but its effects are generally merely palliative; one patient has frequently succeeded in breaking up the attacks during the course of several years, but still remains subject to them.—Brit. Jour. Hom., vol. 8, p. 226.—PETERS.]

[**Dose.**—Gratiola is an acrid remedy, and apt to cause aggravations, hence Noack advises but one drop per dose, of the 2d, 4th or 6th dilution, once or twice a day, or only every two days in chronic cases. In acute and severe attacks, two or three drops of liquid Gratiola may be put in a wineglassful of water, and one teaspoonful given per dose every half, one or two hours, until relief ensues, and then only every two, four, six or eight hours. For children aud delicate adults, as many globules may be put in the same quantity of water, and one teaspoonful given as often as above directed.—PETERS.]

25. HEPAR SULPHURIS.

CASE 55.—Miss J., aged 17, had suffered with headache almost constantly for three months; she had dull, pressive pain over the root of the nose, and a little over the eye, worst in the morning, increased by reading and mental exercise, generally relieved by rest; also weakness of back and occasional derangement of stomach.

Treatment.—Hepar. 6 caused an aggravation for seven days, then Hepar 15 caused a relief for a month, and Hepar 18 effected a complete cure.—BLACK, Brit. Jour., vol. 5, p. 428.

CASE 56.—Lady A., highly nervous, had suffered more than eight years with severe headache, consisting first of a dull pain in forehead, then becoming acute and extending to the whole head.

Treatment.—Hepar for six weeks, when decided improvement commenced, followed by extreme languor and weakness, which lasted fully more than a month—when this curative weakness, denoting a great change taking place in the organism, disappeared, the headaches were also gone.—BLACK, Ibid, p. 429.—PETERS.

[**Dose.**—Hepar sulph. is generally given dry upon the tongue, one dose of the 1st or 2d trituration every hour or two, in severe attacks; or one or two grains or granules of the 3d, 6th or 12th dilution every one or two days in chronic cases.—PETERS.]

26. IGNATIA.

GENERAL REMARKS.—(*a*). According to Tietze, Ignatia is suitable in hemicrania as a purely spinal remedy; also for sensitive, irritable, hysterical persons of a sanguine nervous temperament; for delicate persons, where there is an inclination for visionary dreaming; when grief is borne silently; when slight clonic cramps are apt to occur after fright and vexation; when the pain is pressing, piercing, from within outwards, especially in the forehead and root of nose, or as if a nail was pressed into the temples or sides of the head.—Genl. Hom. Jour., vol. 34, p. 11.

(*b*). Dr. Black says it is a good remedy in the nervous headaches of hysterical women, when they set in and subside suddenly.—Genl. Hom. Jour., vol. 36, p. 233.

(*c*). According to Hering it cures pressing pain over the nose, when relieved by stooping; pressing from within outwards; jerking and throbbing; rending in the forehead as if a nail were driven into the head; piercing and boring deep into the head with nausea, darkness before the eyes, and dislike for light; paleness of the face, much watery urine; the pains ceasing for a while when one changes his position, returning frequently after eating, coming on again in the evening after lying down, and in the morning soon after rising; rendering the patient very timid and changeable, or silent and dejected.—P. 140.

CASE 57.—A young lady, aged 24, blond, pregnant for the fourth time in seven years, had suffered with migrane before her pregnancy, and been troubled for four weeks with the following:

Symptoms.—Pain beginning in the middle of the forehead, extending down to half of the nose, upwards to the middle of the vertex, where it presses like a weight, followed by nausea and inclination to vomit; most severe from early morning to mid-day, then remitting but at times persisting till night; every noise and loud speaking irritated her very much; she was pale, had a suffering appearance, and great lassitude of the limbs.

Ignat. 6, repeated every four or five days, removed the whole difficulty.—Dr. SCHWARZE, p. 9, see case 90.

REVIEW.—The sphere of action of the remedy is sufficiently given in § a and e; it is especially suitable for nervous hysterical persons, other circumstances not forbidding.

Dose.—Ignatia is a powerful remedy, of which one or two drops of the second, third or sixth dilution may be given every one, two or four hours in severe attacks, or every six, eight or twelve hours in milder cases. Or one, two or three globules may be given dry upon the tongue. In chronic cases the dose should be repeated once or twice a day, or only once every two, four or more days.—PETERS.

27. IRIS VERSICOLOR.

Dr. James Kitchen says it is the most prompt and effectual remedy against sick headache that he has ever given in this truly annoying disorder. The first dose will arrest the trouble in some patients, as he has witnessed in several cases. He has made comparative trials with it and other remedies, telling his patient to observe which medicine would relieve them most speedily; they have invariably, on the return of the attack, pointed out the Iris. This he conceives conclusive respecting this complaint, so that he need not comment on it further than to recommend it very highly so far as his experience goes.—North Am. Hom. Jour., vol. 1, p. 464.

Dose.—Dr. Kitchen recommends an alcoholic tincture of the root, diluted as required from the first to the sixth dilution, a few drops in a tumbler half full of water, a teaspoonful per dose. It is particularly useful in allaying the nausea and vomiting.—PETERS.

28. LACHESIS.

GENERAL REMARKS.—According to Black it is indicated in one-sided tense headaches extending from the occiput to the eyes, with vomiting, stiffness of the neck and soreness of the scalp.—Genl. Hom. Jour., vol. 26, p. 233.

NOTE.—In British Jour. of Homœopathy, vol. 5, p. 404, Black reports several severe chronic headaches mainly cured with Lachesis and Sepia.

Henderson, Ker and Russell, also report favorably of Lachesis in chronic headaches.

CASE 58.—C. B. has suffered severely with headaches after a bilious attack; they commence with dimness of vision, which continued for an hour, then go off, leaving a dullish pain over the eye, causing him to feel exhausted and disinclined for any occupation. Bowels rather costive.

Treatment.—Lachesis 15; had one headache only in a week, leaving deafness, twitching of the lids and lips and twitching and throbbing under one eye. Lachesis relieved his head for a week more, but the twitching still remained. Bellad. 12 and Lach. 15 quickly removed the rest.—RUSSELL, Brit. Jour. Hom., vol. 5, p. 433.

In another similar case Russell found the headaches to disappear entirely under the use of Lachesis for one year, but then they returned again and Lachesis was useful for a few months longer in arresting the vomiting, which attended severe attacks, but the headaches remained. Drysdale found Cannabis useful in such cases.—Ibid.

CASE 59.—Miss B., aged 24, had suffered with headaches for four months, with a general feeling of numbness and faintishness, great giddiness and paleness; the pain was generally shooting and throbbing over one eye, frequently attended with nausea, increased by motion and always worst in the morning; is seldom a day free from headache, and when she is, giddiness takes its place; acid taste in mouth, everything turns sour, fulness and weight in stomach after eating; tongue clean and bowels regular. Menses regular, but attended with pain in back and lower part of abdomen, and more severe headache than common. Lach. 15, almost entirely effected a cure in six weeks. The indications for its use were the one-sided headache, often attended with sickness, the vertigo with paleness, the tendency to faint and general sensation of numbness.—Dr. KER, Brit. Jour. Hom., vol. 5, p. 434.—PETERS.

Dose.—The credit of introducing this powerful remedy into practice is entirely due to the veteran Dr. Hering of Philadelphia; he advises one dose of the 6th, 15th and 30th dilution once or twice a day in acute cases, every two, four, eight, ten or more days in chronic cases.

29. MAGNET. SOUTH POLE.

GENERAL REMARKS.—After the use of Nux vom. (see case 80) the following state remained.

CASE 60.—Confusion of the head, dizziness, tottering and staggering while walking, with rush of blood to the head; formication in the brain, about the root of the nose and in left temple; at 12 o'clock violent but transient stitches set in, with smarting and dryness of the eye-lids, and watering of the eyes.

Treatment.—After stroking the painful part for two minutes with the South Pole of the Magnet the whole was relieved in twenty-four hours.—Archiv., vol. 5, part 1, p. 89.

30. MERCURIUS SOLUBILIS.

General Remarks.—(*a*). According to Hering, Merc. is indicated when the head seems so full that it feels as if it would burst, or as if it were pressed together with a band; worse at night, the pains being rending, burning, boring or piercing.

(*b*). Black says it may be used against rending and drawing pains in the head, seated in the pericranium and bones of the face; also in rheumatic headaches, with vertigo, pain in the forehead, and derangement of liver.—Genl. Hom. Jour., vol. 36, page 233.

(*c*). Schelling recommends it in headaches and toothaches of a peculiar kind, especially when accompanied with an affection of the mouth; with jerking, throbbing pain in the forehead, temples and vertex; with digging in the head, rending and piercing in the teeth, which become loose; the pains extending over the cheek, behind the ear into the occiput, and attended with:

Vertigo, chilliness, shuddering with flushes of heat, thirst, congestions, and inclination to perspire; with moist skin and great sensitiveness to every change of temperature; with yellow color of the face, and blue rings about the eyes, rumbling in the bowels, oppression of the stomach, &c.; the symptoms being most severe in the evening or at night. It cures in from two to seven days.—Hygea, vol. 17, p. 359.

(*d*). Rademacher points out the following kinds of head-rheumatism which Mercury will cure. In general, he remarks, the affection is always periodical, at first perhaps almost as regular as a fever and ague, and the aggravations occur more frequently in the forenoon, than afternoon. When the disorder becomes chronic the paroxysms become irregular, or even continued.

The different forms are:

(1). When the pain has its seat under the skull, and shoots from the region of the eye-brows into the back of the head. When the pain lessens, the scalp becomes tender.

(2). When the pain involves the region of the supraciliary arch of one side and the temporal bone, extending to the eye of the same side, which becomes fiery red and lachrymates during the paroxysms.

(3). Against dull rheumatic pain over the orbits of the eyes. In one case the patient had a dull pressing pain over the eye-brows, lost his sight entirely, and the pupils became sluggish and immovable; he was also weak minded, and repeated one thing very frequently.

Merc. solub. given to the point of salivation restored him entirely.

CASE 61.—Mrs. N. had suffered for nine days with:

Violent rending in the left side of the head, extending to the teeth and muscles of the neck of that side, with piercing pain in the left ear; either cold or warm things taken into the mouth, or the slightest touch, aroused the pains; she had three severe paroxysms per day, followed by chills without heat or thirst; was relieved by lying down, and she staggered when she attempted to walk. On the eighth and ninth days delirium set in during the attacks, with perspiration in the palms of the hands, and fits of partial unconsciousness; she had no appetite, got no sleep, and her mood was irritable and lachrymose.

Treatment.—After an evening attack Bryon. 30 was given, and only a few slight attacks occurred, always in the morning; after the lapse of fourteen days more severe attacks again set in, in the evening, marked by rending pains in the forehead, shooting with the speed of lightning into the teeth, forcing her to get up and walk about. Profuse salivation set in, but she was able to hold both warm and cold things in her mouth; violent chills occurred after the paroxysms, and she became very weak, irritable, and inclined to anger. Merc. 12 was given with rapid relief to all the pains.—Annals, vol. 1, p. 235.

[CASE 62.—Lady J. D., aged 30, when weakened by nursing, was attacked with pain on left side of the face, from decay and filling of a tooth; she had severe pain in the lobe of her right ear, extending down into the jaws, over the side of her head, and into one eye; it commenced with slight jagging, and then became severe and shooting; it generally came on at night and left a sense of throbbing. Cured by Merc. 6, 15 and 3d in about 6 weeks.—RUSSELL.—Brit. Jour., vol. 5, p. 431.

CASE 63.—T. F. had suffered with rheumatic pains in the head and gums for six weeks, also with slight pains in the legs. He generally awoke at 7 A. M., with pain in the head, followed by soreness of the gums when it ceased; the pains were most severe in the back and top of the head, and in the right side of upper jaw; aggravated in the morning and when in bed, relieved by getting up and by pressure. Merc. 6, three or four doses, removed the pains entirely for five months.—MADDEN.—Brit. Jour., vol. 5, p. 438.

CASE 64.—A spinster, aged 30, had suffered for seven or eight months with severe pain in her head, arising from inflammation of the bone or periosteum; the pain was dull and constant over both occipital prominences, but on the left side it extended along the side of the head as far as the eye; she was unable to turn her head to the left side; the pain was worst in bed, aggravated by motion, and attended with great tenderness to pressure, and occasional throbbing. Merc. 3 and Ruta 3 effected a cure in two months.—MADDEN.—Ibid, p. 438.—PETERS.]

REVIEW.—The headache for which Merc. is most suitable is generally of a rending character, although at times it may be piercing, boring, burning or drawing; with feelings as if the head would burst, or as if it were bound with a band; involving the pericranium, bones of the face, region of the eyebrows and temples, and from thence extending to the back of the head, or into the teeth, or muscles of the neck; occurring periodically at times, attended with flushes of heat intermixed with chills, inclination to perspire, with bilious derangement, yellowness of the face, dark rings around the eyes; being worst at night, and relieved at times by lying down. The bilious and rheumatic character of the whole disorder is not to be mistaken at times.

Dose.—This should always be comparatively small; I have noticed several times, even in headaches which were evidently connected with decided bilious derangement, that a dose of Mercurius sufficiently large to act on the liver and bowels would always be followed by more frequent and severe attacks of headache. One or two grains of the 2d or 3d dilution of Merc. viv., Merc. solub., or Merc. corros., or from two to four globules may be given night and morning in chronic cases. In acute cases the same quantities of Merc. solub. or Merc. corros. may be put in a wineglassful of water and one teaspoonful given every half, one or two hours until relief ensues, and then every two, four, six or eight hours. For children or delicate adults the same quantities of the medicine may be put in a tumbler half or quite full of water, and from a teaspoonful to a tablespoonful given per dose.—PETERS.

31. NATRUM MURIATICUM.

GENERAL REMARKS.—According to Hahnemann, this remedy comes in play against daily headaches, especially when seated in the back of the head and forcing one to close his eyes; also when there is a pressing in the whole head and temples; in headaches with feeling as if the head would burst, commencing early after awaking in the morning; against rending, piercing pains in the head, forcing one to lie down; against stitches and pressing over the eyes, and beating, hammering and throbbing in the head.—Chronic Diseases, vol. 4, p. 349.

CASE 65.—Miss L., aged 30, of delicate frame and inclined to sorrow and melancholy, had suffered for many years with periodical headaches, especially after taking cold about the head.

Symptoms.—Violent stretching, drawing, rending pain, extending from the top of the head towards the temples and cheeks, and persisting without cessation for several days, although not always equally severe; always attended with toothache and violent salivation, the spittle often gushed violently out of her mouth, her gums were reddened, the whole cavity of the mouth sore, and her teeth painful, especially the front ones. She often had stretching pains in the whole of her face, the scalp was sore to the touch, as if ulcerated, especially when she was dejected and sorrowful. Her menses returned somewhat too soon; she complained of continued excessive lassitude and a certain uneasiness in the whole body, as if everything within her were in motion, and trembled so that she could not sit quietly in one place. These attacks had become more frequent during the last eight months, and arose from the slightest cold.

Treatment.—Cham., Bell. and Merc. were given without relief; then Natrum Muriaticum, 22, one dose, night and morning, sufficed to cure the disease in a short time. Three weeks after, a slight return of the old trouble occurred from a violent cold, but disappeared rapidly and permanently under the use of the same remedy.—Austrian Hom. Jour., vol. 4, p. 1, p. 169.

Here belong also the following interesting cases cured by the so-called "Sool," or Saline Baths.

CASE 66.—A lady, aged 28, in whose family head affections with congestions were hereditary, received an accidental blow three years before, upon the left temporal bone; this spot remained sore and sensitive, and the slightest touch of it caused trembling of the whole body; the pains persisted night and day, and were attended with general cramps of the limbs.

After the use of twelve general, and daily foot baths at the "Sool" baths of Ischl, in Austria, she was entirely cured. —Austrian Hom. Jour., vol. 10, p. 1, p. 173.

CASE 67.—A lady, aged 32, without children, of a mild but irritable disposition, and disposed to melancholy, suffered with paroxysms of one-sided headache, attended with sudden distension of the abdomen, rumbling in bowels, inclination to vomit, fainting fits, and cramps of the limbs.

Thirty "Sool" baths relieved her considerably, and a repetition of the baths the next year cured her entirely.—Austrian Hom. Jour., vol. 10, p. 1, p. 174.

CASE 68.—A spinster, aged 34, had suffered with daily attacks of headache, ever since she had got rid of a tape worm, by heroic means, several years before.

Symptoms.—Violent pains with congestion of the head, to which were added cramps, pains in the breast and limbs, and distension of the abdomen. During the intervals of relief she had great nervous weakness, and constipation.

The use of the Ischl "Sool" baths for six weeks restored her entirely.—Austrian Hom. Jour., vol. 10, p. 1, p. 174.

CASE 69.—A young married lady was attacked with varioloid after confinement, followed by necrosis of the leg, after the cure of which she was visited with one-sided headaches, recurring frequently with increased severity.

Symptoms.—She had suffered for thirteen years with these headaches; for ten years with very profuse leucorrhœa of bad appearance, attended with pain in the region of the ovaries, in the loins and thighs; her menses had been suppressed for several months; the os uteri was beset with ulcers with a grayish base. Her appetite was poor, digestion slow, she had desire for acids and farinaceous food; her abdomen was distended, the mesenteric glands were evidently enlarged and indurated, and she had obstinate constipation.

Treatment.—She took two or three glasses of Wildegger water per day, with meat diet, and in a few weeks all the morbid symptoms and appearances ceased, and she recovered perfectly.—Austrian Hom. Jour., vol. 4, p. 1, p. 175.

CASE 70.—A forester, aged 40, was attacked with violent headache after a severe cold, which headache continued to return periodically every eight or fourteen days, for five months, with such severity that the previously robust man was reduced to a skeleton.

The pain extended from the middle of the left temporal bone over the left eye-brow, and from thence to the cheek, so violently and suddenly that he often fainted away; in the course of a few hours with the increasing severity of the headache, violent retching and vomiting usually set in, and a slimy, watery fluid was ejected from the stomach, after which the pains diminished.

The use of twenty-eight baths at Kissingen, in the course of four weeks did not produce much relief; in the sixth week of this treatment improvement commenced, in the seventh week he was almost, and in the eighth week, quite restored. —Ibid, vol. 4, p. 1, p. 172.

[CASE 71.—A young lady had been subject to headache for eight years. The pain generally commenced in the morning on getting up, was incessant, dull, wearing and aching, seated in the forehead over the eyes, and attended with intolerance of light, tenderness of the scalp, and such trembling of the hands that she could not lift a cup without spilling some of the contents. She was seldom free from the pain at any time, although a walk in the open air often relieved it *somewhat.* Her menses were irregular and painful; she always had much thirst.

Treatment.—Pulsat. and Graph. restored the menses to a natural state, but left the headaches unabated in severity. After using Natrum Mur. she was so completely relieved, that with one or two exceptions she had remained free from headache, for six years, at last accounts.—Dunsford's Practical Advantages, p. 103.—PETERS.]

REVIEW.—In the above cases we find old chronic headaches, some of them hemicranias, cured by Natrum Mur. in the form of "Sool" baths; in two cases only, a homœopathic preparation, the 22d dilution, was used.

[NOTE.—The experiments of M. Plouviez throw some light upon the action of Natrum Muriaticum when taken in large quantities. From careful chemical analysis it seems to diminish the quantity of the water or serum of the blood quite decidedly, thus rendering the blood thicker; it also increases the quantity of blood globules in a marked degree, viz.: from 130.08 to 143.00; and these effects were always most decided in feeble and lymphatic subjects. It increases the quantity of fibrin in the blood in a slight degree, and diminishes the quantity of albumen in about an equal proportion; i. e. it tends to cause a fibrinous dyscrasia rather than an albuminous. Finally, it slightly increases the quantity of fat and iron in the blood. It is said to increase the appetite, but its most frequent and certain effect is increase of strength, while the heat of the body is more readily generated, and exposure to cold is better borne. M. Plouviez increased in weight under its use to the amount of 13⅓ lbs. Troy in about two months, and repeatedly became so plethoric, with fulness about the head, that he felt himself obliged to be bled.—PETERS.]

Dose.—One or two grains of the 2d, 3d or 6th dilution may be taken night and morning; in appropriate cases the higher dilutions may be tried. When salt baths are used in conjunction with the internal use of the remedy, more massive doses must be given, viz.: from two or three, to five grains of the 1st, or decimal dilution. Children and very delicate adults may take from two to five globules per dose, every one, two or four hours in acute attacks; or once or twice a day in chronic cases.—PETERS.

32. NUX VOMICA.

GENERAL REMARKS.—(*a*). Schröen says as follows about the use of Nux vomica in general:

Youths and maidens who have weakened themselves by masturbation often suffer with headache of the following kind:

Suddenly that part only of an object on which their sight is directly fixed appears steady, while all the rest of it seems to move and float around the fixed part: thus, of a hand they will see only a finger, of a chair only one leg; they can spell printed letters with some exertion, but cannot see a whole word at a time; they often see luminous appearances like a fire-wheel, reaching from the external angle of the eye towards the pupil. Watering of the eyes often precedes the commencement of a frightful, gradually increasing headache, lasting for 24 hours and attended with vomiting.

Nux v. 12, a few drops per dose, will soon lessen and finally cure this disorder.—Hygea, vol. 5, p. 197.

Nux v. will also often cure the headaches of hysterical women, when taking the form of boring Clavus hystericus, or of a dreadful pressure upon the temporal region, forcing one to lie down, and attended with retching to vomit.—Ibid.

Nux will also help, or cure the headaches of men in the prime of life, arising from sedentary pursuits, or great mental exertion, especially when there is an aching in the forehead and temples, commencing soon after awaking in the morning, attended with noises in the ears when they sit up, and synchonous with the pulse; it is most useful in those who have weak digestion, sluggish bowels and an irritable temper.

Dose.—Nux v., 6th or 12th, a few drops repeated every three or four days.—Ibid.

(*b*). Knorre found it useful in headaches from congestion of blood to the head, attended with pressing and squeezing in the forehead, especially over the eyes; with dulness and heaviness of the head, vertigo when walking or stooping, heat and redness of the face, and vomiting of tasteless substances, night and morning.—Genl. Hom. Jour., vol. 5, p. 274.

(*c*). Knorre also found Nux useful in periodical headaches, beginning every morning soon after rising, increasing till mid-day, and then diminishing; the pain being aching and rending, attended or not with pain in the region of the liver, with nausea, inclination to vomit, bitter eructations and vomiting, constipation and choleric disposition.—Ibid.

(*d*). According to Tietze, Nux is most useful in males, when the headache or hemicrania proceeds from an affection of the ganglionic system, especially if the patient be subject to hæmorrhoids, is of a choleric temperament, apt to indulge in drinking, or is studious and sedentary in his habits.

The pain is most frequently of a drawing, aching character, with the feeling as if a nail were driven into one half of the head, on which side the brain seems bruised or jarred. It is also useful in the headaches of women who are apt to have their menses too frequently and profusely, especially when the attacks set in early in the morning, or immediately after eating, or after mental exertion.—Genl. Hom. Jour., vol. 34, p. 11.

(*e*). Lobethal thinks Nux most useful against headaches from excessive drinking, and from mental exertion when attended with congestion to the head; especially when they occur in sanguine, excitable persons and consist in a dull confusion of the head, and are complicated with aching in the pit of the stomach, or pain in the hypochondria, with nausea, eructations and constipation.

Nux v. also relieves more readily than any other remedy, those congestions to the head, dependent or not upon habitual constipation, which arise from a plethoric state of the abdominal blood-vessels. Such conditions are most apt to occur in men who lead a sedentary life, and who by constantly renewed mental efforts, induce repeated congestions to the head. —Genl. Hom. Jour., vol. 13, p. 274.

(*f*). According to Hering, Nux is useful in headaches from constipation and excessive use of coffee; also against pains as if from a nail driven into the brain, or consisting of a succession of piercing throbs, attended with nausea and sour vomiting; or of stitches and pressing on one side of the head, commencing early in the morning and increasing in severity until the patient becomes unconscious or half delirious; or of pains which increase until the head feels as if it would burst whenever one attempts to think; also when the brain aches as if it were lacerated, the face being pale and distorted, the head heavy with noises therein, attended with dizziness or trembling when walking; the pains being increased by motion, even of the eyes, in the open air, early in the morning, after eating, or from stooping; and finally when the head is sore to the touch, increased by cold.

CASE 72.—An active woman, aged 40, had suffered for nine years with hysteric headaches, occurring paroxysmally every ten or fourteen days, and had been treated allopathically for five years, without benefit.

Symptoms.—The attacks commenced with dull, aching pain in the whole head, but most severe in the vertex and forehead; attended with vertigo, dulness of the head, violent pressure over the eyes, sensitiveness of them to light, and increased secretion of tears; followed by paleness of the face, with distortion; nausea, bitter-sour taste in the mouth, vomiting of bile, asthma, palpitation of heart; finally, when the pain became most intense, a heavy sleep set in, from which she could hardly be aroused.

During the intervals of the paroxysms she had frequent, but endurable headaches, constant feeling of coldness in the head, and gastric derangements; but mental emotions, and the neighborhood of disliked persons, would bring on an attack immediately. Nux effected a cure.—Genl. Hom. Jour., vol. 5, p. 274. DR. KNORRE.

CASE 73.—A lady, aged 27, of sanguine temperament, apt to be violent, and excessively irritable, had the following:

Symptoms.—Sensation of wavering in the brain, dulness of the head, as after a debauch; pressing pain in the occiput, almost as soon as she awoke in the morning; pressing, pushing headache from the slightest exertion of the mind, increased by the use of coffee and wine. After eating she had drawing pains in the teeth and temples; looseness of the teeth; bitter taste in the mouth. Nux v. 24 effected a cure in 6 days.—Annals, vol. 1, p. 73. DR. SCHROTER.

CASE 74.—A blooming maiden, aged 11, had suffered for half a year with headaches, recurring periodically, every four or five days, affecting one side, being pressing and boring, commencing early in the morning, forcing her to lie down, and attended with bilious vomiting. Nux v. 18, two doses, effected a cure. DR. DIEZ, p. 180.

CASE 75.—A powerful man, aged 52, had suffered for ten days with severe headache on the left side. Nux v. 24, one dose cured him in two days.—*Ibid.*

CASE 76.—A delicate man, aged 48, had suffered for twelve years with intermitting nervous headache, occurring every four or six months, lasting from three to four weeks, and persisting every day from 7 to 12 A. M. It affected the left side of the forehead, and left eye, in particular; was attended with much eructation, nausea, and vomiting. Nux

v. 18, two doses, broke up one attack entirely; a later attack was cured by Nux v. 9, and he remained well subsequently. DIEZ, p. 181.

CASE 77.—A man of powerful constitution and choleric temperament, had suffered for years with periodical headaches, affecting the left side, recurring every ten or twelve weeks, lasting from sixteen to twenty days, commencing early in the morning, increasing gradually to an almost insupportable degree, then ceasing about 2 or 3 P. M., but returning on the following morning with renewed violence.

They were preceded by oppression of the chest, anxiety, and palpitations. The pain was boring and rending; it extended over the left side of the head and eye, concentrating itself in the region of the left orbit, in a spot about the size of a sixpence which became slightly reddened, swollen, and sore to the touch. The headache was attended with nausea, bitter eructations, vomiting of bile, and by constipation. Nux v., 24th, given on the fourth day of the attack, removed it in twenty-four hours, and it never returned again.—DIEZ, p. 180.

CASE 78.—A man, aged 30, of healthy but irritable constitution and sedentary life, had suffered for five years with periodical headaches.

Symptoms. The attacks came on daily, very early in the morning, forcing him to lie down; increased in severity till mid-day, and often were so violent that the patient was in the greatest despair. He had a piercing pain over the left orbit, at times also a pressing pain which shot into the eye, and was increased by pressure; contraction of the eyelids from sensitiveness to light, and lachrymation; heat about the whole of the eye, obstruction of the nose; the attacks were relieved by sneezing, which it was hard to provoke; he also had an inclination to vomit; confusion of thoughts from the severity of the pain; great irritability, and dislike for all noise. Nux v. 24, two doses effected a cure.—Archiv., vol. 2, part 1, p. 146. DR. WISLICINUS.

CASE 79.—A woman, aged 35, of choleric, irritable and vexatious disposition, had suffered for three years with vertigo and periodical headache on the left side.

Symptoms. The pain involved the left side of the forehead, as if from an ulcer, or a wedge pressed into the head, or as if the left side would press asunder, or burst; it always set in suddenly, early in the morning, continued until 1 P. M., and then ceased quickly; it was most violent in bad weather, and attended with constipation.

Treatment.—Nux v. 9, effected a speedy cure, after a previous aggravation.—Archiv., vol. 5, part 3, p. 31. DR. H. in Z.

CASE 80.—A lad, aged 14, had suffered with headache from his fourth year, after a fall.

Symptoms.—Almost every day, and sometimes several times a day, he was attacked with an undefined pain, or a heavy, dull pressure, extending from the back of the head to the top, and attended with nausea, obliging him to keep very quiet; the pain set in almost every morning, just after rising, and was also brought on by mental exertion.

Treatment.—Nux vom., 1st, one dose every other day, effected an improvement in fourteen days, and twenty-two doses in all, effected a cure.—Hygea, vol. 6, p. 499. GRIESSELICH.

CASE 81.—A powerful man, aged 40, of fiery, angry disposition, had suffered for eight days with violent headache, on the right side.

Symptoms.—The pain was pressing and piercing; it commenced every morning early, about 7 A. M., above the root of the nose, and extended from thence over the right eyebrow into the right temple; it increased in severity from 9 A.M. to 12 M., to such a degree that the patient tossed about frantically in the bed; his face became pale and covered with cold sweat; when he stooped forward it seemed as if a ball would fall out of the root of the nose; the scalp was painful, and he had a dry catarrh of the head.

Treatment.—Nux v., 15, one dose removed the majority of the sufferings in four days, and the south pole of the magnet removed the rest.—(*See case* 59.) Archiv., vol. 5, pt. 1, p. 89. DR. PLEYEL.

[CASE 82.—A pale little boy, aged 6, had suffered for six months after an attack of hooping cough, with frequent attacks of the most violent pain in the forehead, coming on suddenly, and lasting ten or fifteen minutes. He took Nux in the evening and had an attack at night, which had never occurred before; in less than a week the headache had entirely ceased, and did not return for two years.—DUNSFORD, p. 104.

CASE 83.—Professor Fourdrin was attacked suddenly with severe pressing pain in the eye and brow, attended with nausea, and straining to vomit; his pulse was feeble and quick, his agitation extreme; he was forced to move his head about from side to side; his eyes were weak and fatigued. Prolonged study was the exciting cause.

Treatment.—Nux 30, three globules; the next day he was well. A similar attack, three months after, was relieved by the same remedy in ten hours. After great fatigue he had alternate chills and heat, severe pain in left temple, heaviness of the eyelids, and heavy pain over the brows; nausea and vomiting.—MALAISE, p. 11.

CASE 84.—A young lady had suffered for four years with great heat in the forehead, tearing and lancinating pains in the skull, occurring at short intervals, and attended with beating in the forehead and temples; the pains were always most severe after dinner and after mental exertion; she also had pain in the loins, palpitations and sleeplessness.

Treatment.—Nux vom., 30, effected a cure in a month.—MALAISE, p. 14.

CASE 85.—Baroness L. had suffered for five days with pain, principally in the forehead, increased after dinner, with painful commotion in the nape when walking, and her face and eyes were slightly bloated.

Treatment.—Nux effected a cure in three days.—MALAISE, p. 17.

CASE 86.—Miss C., aged 11, languid, sallow and tall, had suffered almost every day for four years with severe headaches, causing great prostration, with inability for physical or mental exertion; the pain was chiefly over the eyes, causing her to frown, and producing dimness of vision; her eyes were dull; head, heavy and aching; she was relieved by lying down and by pressure; her pains were aggravated by motion and intellectual exertion; her tongue was pale and slightly coated, bowels costive, abdomen swelled, but not painful; sleep heavy, with dreams and starts, her pulse slow, feet very cold, and appetite capricious.

Treatment.—Nux 30; on the second day after commencing treatment the headache left her, and did not return for three months, at last report.—Ker, Brit. Jour. Hom., vol. 5, p. 434. —Peters.]

Review.—Of the ten cases, by Rückert, six were in males and four in females, all of different ages; with one exception all the patients were of robust constitution; or sanguine, see § e, or choleric temperament, § c & d; they were active, irritable, and inclined to anger.

According to Schroen, see § a, Nux cures the faulty vision, with pains in the head and vomiting, which are apt to occur in both sexes, when weakened by masturbation. Schroen says it cures clavus hystericus, see § a, also Hering, see § f; and the headaches of women with too frequent and copious menses, see § d; also of men who sit much, study hard, see § a, d & e; after the abuse of coffee and spirituous liquors, see § d, e & f; headaches of hæmorrhoidal subjects, see § d & e; from constipation, disorders of the ganglionic system, and consequent congestions of the head, see § d, e & f.

As regards the *locality* of the pain, we find it affecting the back of the head and extending to the top; but most frequently it attacks the forehead, temples, the parts over the eyes, and the root of the nose. Of the ten cases cured, no less than seven were one-sided headaches, and of the seven, no less than five were on the *left* side, see § a and f.

The paroxysms occurred periodically in six cases; were intermitting in one case, and returned in longer or shorter paroxyms.

The *pains* were generally pressing, violent or dull; aching and pushing; aching and boring; aching and piercing; but the piercing pains were the least frequent; besides, in a few cases they were boring and rending, involving a small spot which became red; or felt as if a wedge was pressed into the head, or like an ulcer, or as if the brain was torn, or pressed outwards.

In the majority of the cases the attacks commenced early in the morning, increased during the day, and lessened towards evening.

The pains were excited by mental emotions, from the approach of disliked persons, from mental exertion, by bad weather, and were increased by bright light and noise, by exposure to the free air, and after eating.

The accompanying disorders, were: confusion of thought, intolerance of light, dimness of vision, flow of hot tears, dry catarrh of head, toothache, paleness of face, bitter-sour taste in the mouth, eructations, nausea, vomiting, especially of bile, constipation, asthma with palpitation, chilliness and coldness of the body, and finally perspiration at the end of the attacks.

In two cases the disease had lasted only eight or ten days; in eight cases it had persisted for a half, five, or twelve years. The cures took place rapidly in most cases, and decidedly.

As regards the dose:

1 dose sufficed to effect a cure in 5 cases.
2 doses " " " 4 "
22 " " " " 1 "

The 1st, 9th and 15th potencies were used each in 1 case.
18th potency was " " 2 "
24th " " " 4 "
30th " " " 2 "

Dose.—The proper dose is sufficiently indicated in the above cases and review. It seems that cures have been effected with the every dilution from 1st to the 30th. No cures have as yet been reported from the exceedingly high dilutions. One or two drops of the 1st, 2d or 3d dilution may be taken by adults every one, two, four or more hours in acute and severe cases until relief ensues; then every six, eight or twelve hours until a perfect cure follows. Delicate adults and children may take like quantities of the 6th, 12th or 30th dilution, or one or two granules, as often as above directed. In chronic cases, one dose may be taken night and morning, or every second or fourth day.—Peters.

33. OPIUM.

General Remarks.—The headaches which can be relieved by Opium, are both those which have their seat solely in the brain, and those which are essentially connected with other disturbances of the body; the latter is the case in the so-called migranes.

CASE 86.—A lady had suffered with headaches for many years, occurring at uncertain periods of time. Many remedies had been used in vain, but the severity of the attacks and the length of time which they continued (generally several days) always obliged her to seek fresh relief from medicine.

Symptoms.—The pain occupied the left supra-orbital region, and was pressing, stitching or piercing; motion, noise or fresh air increased it, hence she always sought rest, solitude and darkness; her pulse was feverish, she had chills, yawnings, loss of appetite, and an irritable state of mind, both previous to and during the paroxysms of headache; also nausea and vomiting. Her urine was at first clear and spasmodic, afterwards it became darker, with a sediment. The temperature of her skin alternated at first, then became moderately and permanently increased, and finally a gentle, general perspiration set in with evident relief to all the symptoms. The attacks occurred at irregular periods of time, and the menses had less influence upon them, than the state of the weather. The intervals were characterized by an uninterrupted state of good health.

After trying almost all other means, the patient finally took nothing but Opium during the attacks, which then ceased in a few hours, and became much less frequent in their occurrence.—Hygea, vol. 14, p. 147.—Dr. Schmid.

CASE 87.—Dr. Schmid himself had suffered for several years with attacks of headache, which were violent, and if left to themselves lasted from four to eight days; they incapacitated him for any unusual exertion, and at one time verged closely upon a decided affection of the brain, when he finally concluded to use Opium. Among all the remedies which he had used, Opium was the only one which relieved him, not only certainly, but quickly.

It is to be regretted that Dr. S. did not describe the character of his headache, but he seems to have thought more about the dose than the peculiarities of his case. Whenever the attacks reached a considerable degree of severity, he took from five to ten drops of the concentrated tincture; one or two doses sufficing to relieve the attack rapidly. But after the cessation of the headache, constantly recurring disturbances of the abdominal organs always set in.—SCHMID.

[NOTE.—Opium is of course used far more frequently and freely in the ordinary practice, than in the homœopathic. SANDRAS (*see Maladies nerveuses*, vol. 1, p. 355) advises the use of from $\frac{1}{30}$th to $\frac{1}{15}$th of a grain of the Muriate of Morphine, to be taken every quarter of an hour, at the commencement of an attack of nervous or sick headache; and says, that he has not only frequently noticed a very decided relief from present suffering, but that subsequent attacks would be less frequent and severe. He always expects relief to follow by the time that the third or fourth dose has been taken, and never pushes the remedy beyond the fifth or sixth dose. MAGISTEL asserts that he has succeeded in more than fifty cases by the endemic use of Morphine about the brow and temples. Others, speak highly of the regular use of two or three drops of Morphine, night and morning, between the intervals of the attacks; also of giving a larger dose, say, from five to six, or more drops, immediately at the beginning of a severe paroxysm, and smaller ones occasionally, during the first few hours of suffering. I have heard of several cases in which this treatment was apparently very useful, and others in which the suppression of the disorder plunged the patient into a profoundly melancholic, or some other nervous state.

Still Morphine and its Acetate exert a remarkable and specific action upon the *right* side of the head. According to the experiments of Chevallier and Beraud it is homœopathic, when there is an intolerable pain on the *right* side of the head, with redness and perspiration of the face, heavy and dull expression of the countenance, and excessive itching of the skin. Also, when there is a violent burning in the occiput, redness of the eyes, heaviness and fulness of the head as if it would burst, increased by reading and mental exertion, attended by coldness of the extremities and back, sour eructations and acid vomiting; all followed by hot perspiration and excessive itching of the skin.

Opium and China are both homœopathic to congestive headaches, but Opium is specific against passive congestive, or venous headaches, China to the active or arterial congestive form. Again, China and Quinine exert as decided an action upon the *left* side of the head, forehead and *left* temple, as Opium and Morphine do upon the *right* side and occiput. China and Quinine are homœopathic to violent semi-lateral, periodical and intermitting headaches, particularly when involving the *left* side of the head, and attended with throbbing of the temporal arteries, ringing in the ears, partial deafness, with excessive hunger and thirst, followed by eructations, nausea, great flatulency upwards and downwards, and excessive debility, similar to that which succeeds a long fit of illness.—PETERS.]

34. PHOSPHOR.

GENERAL REMARKS.—(*a*). According to Dr. Lobethal, Phosph. is often very useful against stormy congestions of blood to the head, especially of the vessels of the eye and ear, when they are either too obstinate to give way before the use of Acon., Bellad. and Nux v., or depend upon a general erethism of the system.—Genl. Hom. Jour., vol. 13, p. 291.

(*b*). Hahnemann recommends it in stupefying headaches, congestions of the head, morning headaches, and against piercing pains externally on the side of the head.—See Hahnemann's Chronic Diseases, translated by Dr. Chs. J. Hempel.

CASE 88.—A man, aged 30, several weeks after falling from a scaffolding, was attacked with the following sufferings, shortly after being thoroughly wet through.

Symptoms.—Burning in the nape of the neck, and between the shoulder-blades, but most severely in the back and top of the head. Throbbing, raging and pressing forwards towards the forehead, as if the head would burst and the eyes be forced out; the eyes then becoming fixed and staring; every motion increased the pain, so that he was obliged to hold his head perfectly stiff and creep about gently; when eating he only dared to move his jaws very gently; changes of weather also aggravated the suffering; pressure upon the second cervical vertebra increased the pains and the formication, which was almost constantly present in the arms; he was feverish, with profuse night sweats.

Treatment.—Arnica, Bryon., Silex and Hepar. were given without benefit. Rust's inunction cure was then tried for a time, with relief at first, soon followed by an increase of the whole disorder. Phosphor. 1st was now given, two drops per dose, in alternation with Cocculus 1st, two drops per dose, one remedy only each day, and continued for three months. In fourteen days signs of improvement commenced, which gradually increased, so that at the end of three months a perfect cure was effected, and the patient could return to his work.—Hygea, vol. 20, part 2, p. 160.—Dr. Bosch.

[Note.—Phosphor. is also one of the best remedies against the headaches which attend the so-called *irritative dyspepsia;* especially when there is a periodical twitching, beating pain in the forehead and about the root of the nose, for many days in succession; commencing every morning about 9 o'clock, becoming most violent towards noon, and followed by vomiting. In many morning-headaches, particularly when the patient has a capricious appetite, sense of weight and fulness in the stomach after meals, irregular bowels, severe lancinating pains darting between the shoulder-blades from the pit of the stomach, and much flatulence; white tongue, often with red points on its tip and edges, quick and irritable pulse, dull heavy aching pain over the loins, excessive depression of spirits, and despondency so intense as to excite the most painful ideas. Phosphorus enters so largely into the composition of the brain and nervous system, and exerts so specific an action upon the sexual and urinary organs, that it deserves particular attention in nervous headaches and in those arising from, or connected with derangements of the kidneys, ovaries, &c.—PETERS.]

Dose.—Noack advises one or two drops of the tincture, or ethereal solution of Phosphor., or of the 1st, 2d or 3d dilution in severe cases every half, one, two or four hours; or the same quantities of the 6th or 12th dilution, in milder cases, every six, eight, twelve or twenty-four hours. Very sensitive males, delicate females or children, may take two or three globules as often, or solve from three to five pellets in a wineglassful of water, and take one or two teaspoonfuls per dose as often as above directed.—PETERS.

35. PLATINA.

GENERAL REMARKS.—(*a*). Dr. Seidel recommends it in violent compressing pain in the forehead, especially over the root of the nose, attended with heat and redness of the face, lachrymose disposition, too frequent and profuse menstruation. —Archiv., vol. 12, part 3, page 148.

(*b*). According to Black, Platina is suitable for headaches, connected with excessive leucorrhœa, the pains being nervous, stretching and spasmodic, and involving the forehead and eyebrows.—Genl. Hom. Jour., vol. 36, p. 234.

[CASE 89.—Miss C., aged 18, had been suffering for about seven or eight months, with severe but dull pain, commencing behind the ear, extending to the side of the face, lips, forehead and crown of the head; it was increased by light and touch; was preceded by coldness of the feet; commenced on waking in the morning, gradually increased in severity until about noon, then became sharp, and continued so for two or three hours, when it gradually declined till evening; her tongue was apt to get red and dry, she had oppression of the stomach, her bowels were costive, appetite poor, with dislike for animal food; her menses regular and natural, and the pains always ceased during them.

Treatment.—Platina 6, was followed by increase of pain for seven days; then Plat. 12, produced almost entire relief; still her bowels remained costive and passages clay-colored, or white. Digitalis quickly corrected the state of the bowels, and she had no return of pain for more than one year.—Russell.—Brit. Jour. of Hom., vol. 5, p. 432.—Peters.]

Dose.—Noack recommends one or two grains per dose, of the 1st, 2d or 3d dilution in severe cases, every two, four or six hours; or of the 6th or 12th dilution every eight, twelve or more hours in milder attacks. Delicate adults or children may take two or three pellets as often as above mentioned; or night and morning only in *chronic* cases. —Peters.

36. PULSATILLA.

General Remarks.—(*a*). According to Hering, *Puls.* is useful against rending pains, which become worse in the evening; or throbbing, piercing pains soon after rising in the morning, and in the evening after lying down; against pushing, piercing and rending in the temples, especially when the pains are confined to one side; or are attended with vertigo, inclination to vomit, heaviness of the head, darkness before the eyes, and great sensitiveness to light; by roaring in the ears, or pricking, jerking and tearing pains in them; or by pale and tearful face, no appetite or thirst, but with chilliness, anxiety, bleeding of the nose, and palpitation of the heart. Also, when all the above complaints are worst when quiet or sitting, are relieved in the open air, and the headache is lessened by pressing on the head, or tying something around it. It is most useful in the headaches of slow, good-natured people.

(*b*). According to Tietze, *Pulsat.* is especially indicated when the pains are rending, throbbing, piercing or jerking, affect the temples and back of the head most severely, and are accompanied by the well-known general indications for the remedy.—Genl. Hom. Jour., vol. 34, p. 21.

CASE 90.—A puerperal woman, aged 24, was attacked with headache after taking cold; her gentle nature, inclination to weep and pale appearance indicated *Puls.* After the fruitless use of *Bellad.*, she was relieved by Puls. 30—Revue Hom. Mar. 1846.—Dr. Sollier.

CASE 91.—An obstinate, censorious and irritable woman, aged 30, who menstruated profusely, always suffered with severe headaches, both before and after menstruation; the pain was on the very top of the head, pressing, boring and digging there until she was almost driven to distraction; she could not bear anything upon the head, which seemed as if festered, still she could not avoid carrying her hand involuntarily to the painful part. Bowels not constipated, but difficult to move; her sleep was full of dreams; she was chilly, but not thirsty. Puls. 200, relieved the pain in half an hour. —New Archiv. vol. 1, part 3, p. 59.—GROSS.

CASE 92.—A girl, aged 8, of gentle lachrymose disposition, had suffered for six months with headache on the left side. The pain involved the left side of the forehead, was throbbing and piercing; occurred alternately either early in the morning, or in the evening soon after lying down; was relieved by external pressure and by the open air; increased in the warm room, by lying down, by stooping and by moving the eyes; it lasted several hours, and then increased to an almost insupportable degree, so that the little patient tossed about in agony. When the pain lessened severe stomach-ache set in, followed by sour and bilious vomiting; which was succeeded by griping, pressing and squeezing pain in the bowels. At times these three varieties of pain occurred in alternation, and at other times, on successive days. After the use of Puls. 3, the whole disorder ceased on the fifth day of treatment, for ever.—Archiv., vol. 5, part 1, p. 93.—Dr. PLEYEL.

CASE 93.—A lady, aged 43 years, troubled with irregular menstruation, thin, pale and of a gentle disposition, was attacked with permanent headache after using mercurial ointment for the cure of sore throat.

Symptoms.—Persistent headache, increasing towards evening, relieved at night, but not allowing of sleep; the pain seemed to rise up from the nape of the neck, and extend to both temples, leaving the neck cramped; the attacks were violent, forcing her to lie down, were attended with noises in the ears, dizziness when walking, and appearance of black gauze before the eyes; the pains were boring and piercing, occasionally slightly tearing, and extended at times between the shoulder blades; or were attended with twitching of the left eye-lid, by smarting, aching and weeping of the left eye, with piercing pains in the limbs, with chilliness, and constipation. Bryon. did not afford relief; Puls. 6, one drop per dose, effected a cure in eight days.—Archiv., vol. 3, part 2, p. 115.—Dr. SCHNIEBER.

CASE 94.—A young lady, aged 24, of strong constitution but gentle disposition, and subject to irregular menstruation, was attacked with headache; at first it affected the forehead and then the whole head, which finally seemed as if screwed up into a vice; she also had vertigo, and heaviness of the head when she attempted to sit up in bed; the pain was increased by thinking and reading; lassitude, trembling and shaking of the limbs were present, with alternating paleness and redness of the face, nausea, sense of crawling in the pit of the stomach, dryness of the mouth without thirst, disgust for food, tightness of the chest, transient shivering, weak, scarcely perceptible pulse, excessive sensitiveness, weeping, &c. Pulsat. 12, one drop, cured her in twenty-four hours.—Archiv., vol. 2, part 2, page 135.—Dr. HARTMANN.

CASE 95.—A man, aged 25, had suffered for two months, in consequence of taking cold, with piercing, boring headache, extending from the right temple to the back of the head; increasing to a frightful degree in the evening and at night, and shooting into the ear and towards the side of the neck. His head seemed numb, his mind as if paralyzed and unfit for any occupation. Pulsat. 24 in solution, one dose every morning, cured him entirely in eight days.—Genl. Hom. Jour., vol. 37, p. 96.—Dr. RAMPAL.

CASE 96.—A lady, aged 30, eight days after confinement was attacked with chills, heat and headache from taking cold. She had an insupportable tearing pain in both temples, attended with vomiting of bitter substances; vertigo and constant nausea, compelling her to maintain a half sitting, half recumbent posture, with closed eyes and the greatest quiet. Every movement, even opening the eyes, increased the pain, as if the head would burst; her pulse was frequent and full, skin hot but slightly moist, and the lochia were not suppressed. Bryon. 200, caused improvement up to the fourth day; then the pains returned again, and were so much relieved by Puls. 200, that she was quite well on the fifth day.

CASE 97.—A lady, aged 30, of healthy constitution, but suffering for several years with attacks of cramp in the stomach, and used to being bled, had been nursing a child for three months, when she was attacked with headache persisting for several weeks, and for which she had already been bled without relief.

Symptoms.—Violent one-sided headache consisting of piercing pain in the forehead, temples and right ear, extending into the teeth, and attended with general throbbing in the head, as if from the beating of the pulse. The pain lasted the whole day, and became especially violent in the evening, and at night after lying down. She had thirst, constipation, chills, and evident loss of strength.

Treatment.—Puls. 6, removed the headache and chills entirely; but transient gnawing pain in the stomach and constipation, required Nux v. 12, for their removal. She then continued to nurse her babe in health and comfort.—Annals, vol. 1, p. 85.—Dr. RUCKERT.

[CASE 98.—A woman, aged 54, had suffered with headache for three weeks; she had tearing pains in the forehead, worst in the evening and at night; it seemed to her as if her head must burst if she did not tie something around it; the pains were so violent as to force her to cry out; she had various strange noises in the head, also photophobia, bruised and tired feeling in the limbs, sleeplessness and despondency.

Treatment.—Bellad. was given for one day, without benefit; then Pulsat. effected a cure in twenty-four hours.—Malaise Clinique, p. 9.—PETERS.]

[NOTE.—Pulsatilla acts especially upon the eye, like Bell., but on quite different parts; it acts primarily upon the mucous membranes of the lids and ball, and upon the nerves and bloodvessels which supply them; while Bellad. acts upon the Iris and Retina and the nerves and bloodvessels which supply them; to be more precise, Pulsat. acts upon the ophthalmic branch of the fifth pair of nerves, Bellad. upon the optic, or second pair of nerves. Pulsat. has been found almost specific by Herz and Hufeland against nervous headache when attended with the following very peculiar affection of the eye, viz.: when there is a spasmodic affection of the eyelids, commencing at the external angle of the eye, and attended with a peculiar flimmering, so that all objects whose rays fall upon the eye from that side, seem to be in a very rapid and waving motion; or the patient seems to look through very rapidly moving water, or through rapidly vibrating air, which appears heated to an intense glow; accompanied with a number of light colored, circular, serpentine, or zig-zagged appearances, especially about the external angle of the eyes. The above mentioned authorities say that this peculiar disorder will yield rapidly, to a few grains of Extract of Pulsatilla, although it will obstinately withstand even massive and heroic doses of Bellad., Hyosycam. or Opium. Again, while *Bellad.* is specific against the purely *nervous* and *congestive* headache, *Pulsat.* is a principal remedy against the *sick* headache, strictly so-called. We have already seen that in the Belladonna headache sympathetic affections of the stomach may arise, but when indigestion, or irritation of the stomach, or dyspepsia, is the primary affection and the head disorder a secondary affair, Bellad. will never afford certain relief. Exactly the converse of this holds true with regard to Pulsatilla. The headache which Pulsatilla most readily relieves, is one which has its starting point in the stomach, brought on by the use of indigestible, rich, or fat food, or from excess in eating or drinking, or from indigestion produced by great bodily fatigue, loss of rest, extraordinary mental inquietude, or exertion just before or after meals. The pathological state of the stomach, is irritation of the mucous membrane induced either by an excess of acid, by undigested food or regurgitated bile, or by venous congestion arising from a sluggish state of the liver. Under all these circumstances the affection of the brain is secondary; the predisposition is said to consist for the most part in debility of the stomach, and in a peculiar state of the nervous system which renders the brain especially sensitive to gastric irritation.—PETERS.]

REVIEW.—Of the eight cases reported by Rückert, seven were in females of gentle, delicate and yielding dispositions, and most of them were middle aged.

In two cases, taking cold was the exciting cause of the headaches; in case 92, the pain attended a profuse flow of the menses.

The pains occupied the forehead and temples, as well as the top, a whole side, or the back of the head; in one case it was confined to the right side; and in one, to the left.

The pains were generally pressing, piercing or boring; at times slightly tearing, or throbbing and digging, with the feeling as if the head were festered, or screwed up.

The attacks were especially violent in the evening and at night, but in one case they occurred early in the morning, as well as in the evening; the sufferings were increased by being in a close room, by lying down, by stooping, by moving the eyes; in one case also by thinking and reading; while they were relieved by pressing on the head, and by the free air.

In case 92, the paroxysms appeared on the setting in, and also towards the end of menstruation.

As accompanying complaints, we notice disinclination for food, absence of thirst, presence of nausea, sour, bitter and bilious vomiting; straining at stool, which is not hard; oppression of the chest and chilliness.

In two cases Bell. and Bryon. had been previously used without benefit, and in one case Bryon. had materially relieved the patient before Puls. was given.

The cures took place rapidly in all the cases.

The doses were Pulsat. 3, 6, 12, 24, 30 and 200. In the majority of cases one dose sufficed to cure; still Puls. 24, was given repeatedly in solution, one dose per day.

Dose.—Noack prefers the 2d dilution, which he asserts has proved more serviceable than any other preparation; still he advises one or two drop doses of the pure tincture, or of the 1st, 2d, 3d, 6th or 12th dilution, to be repeated once or twice a day, in *chronic* cases; or every quarter, half, one, two or more hours in severe attacks; or every two, four, six or eight hours, in milder ones. Delicate adults and children may take two or three globules as often; or three, five or more globules may be solved in a wineglassful of watér, and one or two teaspoonfuls given per dose.—PETERS.

37. RHUS TOXICODENDRON.

GENERAL REMARKS.—According to Schelling, in 1849, when the whole epidemic constitution of the period frequently called for Rhus, violent headaches also occurred frequently; they were one-sided, attacked the forehead, temples, ears and teeth in particular, and recurred periodically; the pains were drawing and tearing, as if a sharp knife were run through the affected parts, or as if the eyes, ear or forehead were being cut out; they were severe enough to make the stoutest persons complain loudly, and even to cause cramps in others.

In one such case, *Arsen.* produced relief immediately, but only transiently; in many other cases *Rhus* afforded relief effectually.—Hygea, vol. 17, part 3, p. 274.

CASE 99.—A young man was attacked suddenly, after suffering for some time with pain in the back and loins, with a piercing pain in the forehead soon after rising in the morning; followed by a sense of creeping, dashing and digging in the brain, also by a stupefying dizziness and an indescribable aching and pain in the left temple, forehead and eye, so that he fell back fainting upon his bed again; he also had oppression of the chest, sore-throat and thirst; his tongue and left side seemed partially paralysed; he could scarcely speak intelligibly, and could move the limbs of the left side imperfectly.

Treatment.—Rhus 1st, restored him in 2 days.—Dr. SCHELLING.—*Ibid.*

Dose.—Noack advises one or two drops of the pure tincture, or of the 1st, 2d, 3d or 6th dilution, repeated frequently in acute and severe cases, but to be given only once or twice a day in slighter attacks. Schelling, it will be seen above, also used the low dilutions. Still Rhus is an acrid remedy, and apt to cause aggravations in delicate persons and children, who should use from one to three granules per dose, or for whom from three to five globules may be solved in six tablespoonfuls of water, and one teaspoonful given per dose.—PETERS.

38. SANGUINARIA.

GENERAL REMARKS.—According to HERING, *Sanguinaria* is the best remedy against most cases of Migrane, or sick headache; still it will prove most useful when the attacks occur paroxysmally, viz., every week or at longer intervals; or when the pains begin in the morning, increase during the day and last till evening; when the head seems so full that it must burst, or as if the eyes would be pressed out; or when the pains are digging, attended with sudden piercing, throbbing lancinations through the brain, involving the forehead and top of the head in particular, and being most severe on the *right* side; followed by chills, nausea, vomiting of food or bile, forcing the patient to lie down and preserve the greatest quiet, as every motion aggravates the sufferings, which are only relieved by sleep.—New Archiv., vol 2, part 2, p. 132.

CASE 100.—A man was attacked with frightfully severe headache; the only relief he could obtain, was from pressing the back of his head against the head-board of the bed.

Treatment.—An infusion of Rad. Sanguinar. removed the headaches permanently.

CASE 101.—A lady suffered with frequent and severe attacks of headache, with such sensitiveness during the paroxysms, that no one dared to walk across the room.

Treatment.—The first dose of Sang. 6, produced such an aggravation that the patient became almost beside herself; after the second dose, she fell into a pleasant sleep from which she awoke refreshed. Dr. Helfrig always gave Acon. and Bellad. during the paroxysms of sick-headache, and used Sanguinar. 30, during the interval, unless some other remedy was more indicated.—HERING.—*Ibid.*

Dose.—The proper dose is sufficiently indicated in the above cases. —PETERS.

39. SEPIA.

General Remarks.—(*a*). According to Hahnemann, it is indicated when there is dulness of the head, and inability for mental occupation; in attacks of sick headache, attended with boring pains forcing one to cry out with agony, and with vomiting; against throbbing headaches most severe in the back of the head; congestion to the head while stooping; coldness on the top of the head.—See Hahnemann's Chronic Diseases, translated by Chas. J. Hempel.

(*b*). Hering assumes that Sepia is suitable against piercing, boring, or throbbing headaches, most severe in one temple, or under one frontal protuberance, which is often sensitive to the slightest touch; especially when the paroxysms are so severe as to force one to cry out, and are attended with nausea and vomiting; also when the slightest motion increases the sufferings and the patient is obliged to remain very quietly in a darkened room, with his eyes closed; sleep then being easily induced and the whole attack passing off after a long slumber.—P. 143.

(*c*). Dr. Kreussler found Sepia most useful in the following kinds of headache:

In aching, piercing, drawing, and rending pains, affecting all parts of the head, and attended with heat in the face, noises in the ears, nausea and vomiting, vertigo, and great weakness; all the sufferings being generally greatly aggravated by warmth. The piercing pains, however, were not so severe as those which Acon., Rhus, or Pulsat. relieve so readily, and were not constant, but occurred in paroxysms of longer or shorter duration. The aching or pressing pains were most frequent and severe in the back of the head. —Genl. Hom. Jour., vol. 29, p. 172.

(*d*). According to Dr. Tietze, Sepia acts upon the nervous and vascular system, wherever it finds a passive congestion connected with a dyscrasial suffering; and all diseases to be cured by Sepia must be traced to some such source. In general, we should bear in mind that both Bellad. and Sepia, if they are to cure hemicrania, pre-suppose the existence of congestion of blood to the brain; but for Bellad. the congestion must be decided and active; for Sepia, rather passive; for Bellad. to afford help, there need be no dyscrasia present; for Sepia, a dyscrasia should never be absent. Tietze found Sepia most useful in the headaches of females, especially of hysterical patients; in obstinate and deeply-seated cases, in which derangement of the nervous system had already lasted for a long time; when the pains were piercing and confined to one side; and when leucorrhœa was present during the intervals of the paroxysms. He found it almost specific in cases attended with *Sudor hystericus*, or a peculiarly sweetish smelling perspiration of the arm-pits and soles of the feet. He assumes that it is most indicated against those hemicranias which arise slowly out of an affection of the assimilation, and the whole bearing of the patient expresses the presence of a deep-seated affection; his skin being pale, dingy or sallow, the frame delicate, and the features marked with traces of frequent and severe suffering.

The pains it most readily relieves are piercing or pressing, or aching and piercing, boring, rending, and pricking, and attended with passive congestion to the head.—Genl. Hom. Journal, vol. 34, p. 10.

(*e*). Black contents himself with asserting that it is most suitable against nervous, rheumatic and arthritic headaches, especially when they occur in delicate and sensitive women. —Genl. Hom. Jour., vol. 36, p. 234.

CASE 102.—Mrs. B., aged 21, of venous constitution, suffered in the middle of pregnancy, with frequently recurring rending, piercing pains on the right side of the head.

Treatment.—Sepia 30, removed the pains in 2 hours, permanently.—General Homœopathic Journal, vol. 29, p. 72. —Dr. KREUSSLER.

CASE 103.—Mrs. M., aged 25, of bilious constitution, suffered with drawing, rending pains on the right side of the head, intermingled with sharp stitches; the attacks being most severe every morning and evening, and much relieved during middle of the day. Her menses had commenced to become rather scanty.

Treatment.—Aconit., Pulsat., and Rhus were given without benefit, but Sepia removed the whole disorder rapidly and permanently.—Genl. Hom. Jour., vol. 29, p. 191.—Dr. Kreussler.

CASE 104.—Miss H., of venous temperament, had suffered for some time with headaches, which were becoming more and more severe. She had violent pressing or aching pains in the back of the head, attended with heat and redness of the face, painfulness of the eyes, lassitude and weakness of the limbs, lachrymose disposition, and disinclination to any occupation.

Treatment.—Two doses of Sepia 15, removed her sufferings permanently, although the first dose produced an aggravation.—*Ibid.* p. 172.—Dr. Kreussler.

CASE 105.—A stout girl had suffered for several months with constant headache, frequently attended with nausea; her face was flushed, but her pulse small and weak, and menses regular.

Treatment.—Sepia 30, in solution, cured her perfectly in a week.—Archiv., vol. 20, part 3, p. 58.—Dr. Goullon.

CASE 106.—A lady, aged 32, who had suffered for many years with cramps, and congestions of the head and chest, had had violent headache for 14 days.

Symptoms.—Soreness and pain in the left eye and temple; throbbing, rending, and piercing in the left temple; pricking as if from an ulcer in the left zygoma and in the molar teeth; soreness of the scalp to touch; aggravation of the pains at various times of the day, followed by fainting fits. She also had shivering, coldness of the feet, flushes of heat, thirst, anxiety and despair of recovery.

Treatment.—Seven doses of Sepia 2, were given, one dose every night and morning; she was entirely restored on the 4th day.—Genl. Hom. Jour., vol. 33, p. 23.—Dr. Haustein.

CASE 107.—A young lady, aged 19, a brunette of sanguine temperament, who had been rheumatic for several years, had now suffered for several months, generally after a slight cold, with violent pains in her head.

Symptoms.—Tearing and boring, intermingled with acute stitches, more frequently on the right side, than the left; when the pain was very severe, she was obliged to keep very quiet, close her eyes, and press her hand upon the painful part; chilly weather increased the pains, which were scarcely ever present at night, but occurred at almost any time during the day; she had disinclination for food, her passages were rather loose, her menses occurred too frequently and lasted 5 or 6 days.

Treatment.—Sepia 30, produced a decided improvement about and after the 12th day; she relapsed slightly at the end of 5 weeks, and then was cured entirely by repeated doses of Sepia 30, in solution.—Dr. Hirsch.—Genl. Hom. Jour., vol. 7, page 132.

CASE 109.—A lady, aged 40, and of an hysterical habit, had suffered since her fourteenth year with headaches recurring every 2 or 4 weeks, affecting the left side, commencing early in the morning, with rending and drawing pain under the left temporal bone, passing over into aching and throbbing in the back of the head, and followed by nausea and vomiting; she could not open her eyes or bear light, and had obstinate constipation.

Treatment.—Sepia, several doses, repeated every 8 days, removed the disorder.—Practical Observations, vol. 2, p. 10. —Dr. Schindler.

CASE 110.—A man aged 30, of medium stature, and with blackish brown hair, had been speedily cured of an ulcer upon the leg, by external applications. Since then, he had suffered with headache on the left side, extending to the left ear and eye, commencing with violent stitches in the forehead, recurring every five minutes, day and night, with such violence that his face became distorted, and he screamed out with pain; his scalp became exceedingly sore, he knew not where to lay his head; every noise, even the speaking of others, increased the pain; his tongue was white and he had a bitter taste in the mouth.

6

Treatment.—Sepia 6, relieved the pains in two hours, and he was cured in four days.—Genl. Hom. Jour., vol. 10, page 220.—Dr. S.

[CASE 111.—A nursing mother had suffered with headache for three weeks, characterised by acute pain in the forehead, attended with throbbings which occasioned pain in the teeth, and eyes; with noises in the ears; constipation, nausea, and sometimes vomiting.

Treatment.—Sepia (two doses) was followed by a severe aggravation; the pains changed to one side, and the disorder assumed the form of megrim; but in two days almost all traces of the disorder were removed. A few doses of Nux subsequently removed the constipation.—MALAISE, p. 12.

CASE 112.—Miss V., aged 17, had had headache more or less for eighteen months; the right side of the head was principally affected with violent pulsations, especially severe in the right side of the back of the head, attended with dimness of vision, itching of the nose, dilatation of the pupils, and frequent nausea; her tongue was coated, she had a bad taste in the mouth, and irregular appetite; her sufferings were more severe in the morning than in the evening; scarcely a day passed by without some pain, ordinarily commencing in the occiput. Her menses were regular.

Treatment.—Nux, Bellad., Aconit., Spigelia, China, and Cina, were used for twenty days without benefit; then Sepia 30, (several doses) was given, and effected a perfect cure in fifteen days, which lasted for at least two years and a half. —Ibid.]—PETERS.

REVIEW.—Among eight patients, reported by Rückert, seven were females; of these, three were said to be of a venous constitution, and one of sanguine temperament; two had dark hair, and all were middle-aged.

Among the causes of the headache, we find: taking cold in one case; and suppressed ulcer in one case.

Of the eight cases, six had the pains confined to one side of the head; three times on the right side, and three times on the left.

Among the localities involved by the pain, we find: the forehead, extending to the eye, mentioned most frequently, then the sides of the head, next the temples, top and back of the head.

As to the character of the pain, we find it most frequently rending or tearing, frequently attended with stitches; less frequently we find drawing, aching or throbbing; boring pain occurred only once.

As regards the time when the pains appear, we do not find them confined to any particular period.

The pains were *increased* by rough weather, by moving or opening the eyes, by noise, or the speaking of others, by the slightest touch, by every movement, and by warmth. They were *relieved* in one case by external pressure, by rest in a dark place, by closing the eyes, and by a long sleep.

As accompaniments of the pain, we find: soreness of the scalp, in case 105; heat and redness of the face, in cases 103 and 104; disgust for food, in case 106; white tongue and bitter taste, in case 108; nausea and vomiting, in cases 104 and 107; constipation, in case 107; too frequent menstruation, in case 106; scanty menstruation, in case 102; fainting fits, in case 105; shivering and coldness of the feet, in case 105; anxiety, in case 105; disinclination to work, in case 103; and inclination to weep, in case 103.

Among the indications for the use of Sepia, we find: hysteria, with long-continued derangement of the nervous system, in § d and e; leucorrhœa between the paroxysms, in § d; sudor hystericus in § d; chronic expression of suffering in the features, in § d; pale, sallow, dingy complexion in § d; congestions in § b and d; passive congestions in § d; delicacy of frame in § d and e; and return of pains at intervals, in § c.

Almost all the cases were chronic, and the cures followed very quickly.

Sepia effected a cure in all eight cases without the aid of any other remedy; in three cases, but one dose was used; in two cases, two doses; in one case, nine doses; in one case Sepia in solution was given, in repeated doses.

The 2d, 6th and 15th potency were used each in one case; the 30th, in four cases.

Dose.—Noack prefers one-grain doses of the 2d or 3d trituration, to be given once or twice a day in sub-acute and chronic cases; more frequently in acute attacks. In the above cases the use of the 2d and 6th dilutions was not followed by aggravations, but by speedy recoveries; while the higher potencies, such as the 15th or 30th, sometimes either caused aggravations, or more probably allowed the disorder to progress unchecked to an extreme degree of suffering. Delicate and nervous adults, and children may use the granules or high dilutions, either in solution, or by drops or globules.—PETERS.

40. SILICEA.

GENERAL REMARKS.—(*a*). According to Hering, Silex is useful against pushing, throbbing pains, with heat and rush of blood to the head, especially when they are excited by exertion, speaking, or stooping; in nocturnal pains, extending from the nape, up to the top of the head; against rending pains setting in every forenoon; when it seems as if the forehead would be pushed out; when lumps arise upon the head, the hair falls out, and the scalp is very sensitive to touch; also against tearing pains in the head, p. 142.

(*b*). Hahnemann advises it against headache ascending from the nape to the top of the head, and preventing sleep at night; for daily headache in the forenoon, with tearing pains and heat in the forehead; for heaviness in the forehead from noon till evening; for pain as if the head would burst; sweating of the head at night.—Chronic Diseases, vol. 5.

(*c*). Black advises it against headaches from organic disease, excessive study, or nervous relaxation arising from any other cause, when vertigo and weakness of memory are present, &c. —Genl. Hom. Jour., vol. 36, p. 235.

CASE 113.—A young lady, aged 28, a brunette, of middling stature, had suffered for a long time with violent headaches.

Symptoms.—The pain involved either the vertex, back of the head, or forehead; at other times when it extended over one-half of the head, the one-sided pain consisted in a bruised feeling, so that even external pressure caused pain; in the forehead the pain was of a pushing character, attended with great weakness of the eyes; when the pain became very violent, nausea and vomiting set in; touching the head, walking about, and exposure to the free air caused aggravation; the paroxysms came on every two or three days or weeks, sometimes lasting only a few hours, at others several weeks. At times, all food tasted like clay; bits of tape-worm were discharged; she had trembling of the limbs, and general feeling of weakness.

Treatment.—Silicea 30, in two drachms of diluted alcohol, ten drops to be taken daily, from July 24 to the middle of September. *Result.*—The first four doses always caused aggravations; afterwards a perfect cure was effected.—Genl. Hom. Jour., vol. 22, p. 11.—Dr. Tietze.

Dose.—Trinks says in obstinate and chronic cases he has always used the 2d or 3d dilution, one or two grains per dose, night and morning, for weeks and months together, not only without producing any unpleasant or stormy aggravations, but always with the most gratifying curative results. Those who prefer them may use the higher dilutions and globules, at long intervals.—Peters.

41. SPIGELIA.

General Remarks.—(*a*). Spigelia, according to Tietze, is indicated in hemicrania of the *left* side, the pain often involving the whole of that side of the head, and extending to the face and teeth. Also:

When the pains consist in a digging-tearing, or in an aching-pressing; are increased by stooping, the slightest movement in the free air, and by every loud noise. It is especially useful when gouty affections in various parts of the body are also present.—Genl. Hom. Jour., vol. 34, p. 21.

(*b*). According to Black, Spigelia is suitable against nervous rheumatic headaches, when the pains are aching and piercing, extend to the nape and face, and are increased by touch, motion, and noise.

(*c*). Dr. Nehrer says, in the winter of 1845, he cured six cases of one-sided headache, involving one or the other eyebrow, the pain being violent and throbbing, or else throbbing and piercing, or tearing, and attended with redness and lachrymation of the affected eye; the paroxysms followed a perfectly regular twenty-four hour type; the weather at the time was icy-cold and rainy.—Spigelia 20, afforded relief quickly and certainly.—New Archiv., vol. 3, part 1, p. 63.

(*d*). According to Hering, the typical character of the pains relieved by Spigelia, is remarkable; the head, eyes, face, or teeth may be affected; the paroxysms occur generally in the morning or forenoon, before twelve o'clock; and motion, especially *stooping*, causes an aggravation. Among the other indications for the remedy, are noted: aggravation from stooping; aching and pressing in the head; sensation as if the brain would be forced out through the forehead, &c. The latter symptom occurs in fifteen or twenty other remedies; the first symptoms in many remedies also, especially Ign., Pulsat., Coloc., Bryon., Bell., &c; but in no other remedy do we find so many pains increased by the same causes, and hence this possesses a peculiar significance for Spigelia. In Spigelia-headaches, the face is often pale.—Correspondenz-Blatt, vol. 6, p. 80.

CASE 114.—A man, aged 25, of choleric sanguine temperament, and powerful constitution, had had violent headaches, off and on, for three years.

Symptoms.—Constant, violent and partly jerking or rending pain; partly sawing pain, as if the nerves were lacerated with fine instruments, involving the right side of head and temples, and extending over the eye into the cheek-bones. The right eye was much affected, and wept freely; it pressed and pushed itself forward, and was very sensitive to light; there was a burning heat in the affected part, and in the face; the veins of the temples were distended and pulsating; there was coryza and disturbed sleep.

Treatment.—Bellad. and other remedies were given without benefit, as the pain increased to an extreme degree, and extended to the teeth. Then Spigelia 30, was given, followed by profuse sweat in half an hour, lasting all night, and the patient awoke well after a sound sleep.—Correspondenz-Blatt, 6.—ROMIG.

CASE 115.—A woman, whose menses recurred too frequently, preceded by weakness of the chest with fainting, and with great weakness from the slightest exertion; also complained of violent stitches in the left temple, worse when moving about. A few doses of Spigelia 30, cured her entirely. —Ibid.

CASE 116.—A boy, aged 7, had suffered for several weeks with headache; first here, then there, but especially in the forehead and back part of the head; increased by motion, by running, jumping, even by walking, but especially by stooping, or shaking the head, by coughing, and every concussion of the body, even by noise, and the warmth of a stove. He frequently became pallid in the face, with blue about the eyes, and sometimes became so sick as to vomit.—Spigelia 30, effected a cure.—Ibid.

CASE 117.—It also cured a case in which pains in the eyes occurred every morning, followed by piercing in the head, face, teeth, and throat. In a week after were added, chilliness and heat every night, without thirst; the headache became throbbing on one side, so that he could not stoop, and it seemed as if his head would fall off. There was throbbing over the left eye, burning and piercing therein, commencing early in the morning behind the eye, and finally extending forwards; the eye seemed smaller, but was swollen (Dulcam. and Scilla cause the same); the patient had fever the whole day, with dryness of lips, and whiteness of the tongue. The whole disorder, after lasting three weeks, was cured in a few hours by Spigelia 30.—Ibid.

CASE 118.—Beating and throbbing in the vertex and under the eyes, especially the left, increased by the slightest motion. There was a discharge of thin green mucus from the posterior nares; the gums were swollen, and there was pain in the teeth. Spigelia 30 effected a cure.—Ibid.

CASE 119.—Chronic catarrh of head, violent headache, with feeling as if the head would burst when stooping, worse on the right side, and increased every morning till twelve o'clock, after which it diminished; there was such tearing pain when stooping, that he was obliged to support his head. Cured by Spigelia 30.—HERING.

CASE 120.—A widow, aged 56 (born in the East Indies), of choleric and irritable temperament, with dark hair and complexion, and of large stature, received a blow upon the head many years before, and frequently suffered with headaches since then. After a severe cold, taken at the end of June, 1850, the headache set in, and persisted with greater or less violence, until the last of October. The disorder remained about the same, for, if single symptoms ceased awhile, they were sure to return again.

Symptoms.—Pain, especially in the forehead, where she had received the injury; feeling as if from an internal ulcer on the left side above the eyebrow, extending to the temples, and occasionally to the back of the head; the pain often shot into the eye, rendering it so painful that it could not be moved; it consisted of a sore feeling, or of a boring or heaviness, more rarely of throbbing, especially on laying the head down; it was increased every night and forenoon, also from every movement, especially from stooping, which she could not do without pain, even when free from headache. The pains were also increased by every concussion, by noise, by the loud speaking of others, with nausea from the same causes. The only relief she obtained was from absolute quiet, and from resting the head against something. Otherwise, she was generally well, with the exception of being costive.

Treatment.—She used many remedies, among them Sulph. 30, twice with benefit; still, the increase of pain from stooping remained. Merc. and China produced transient relief. July 13th she received Spigelia 22, with relief for several days; on the 16th, she took Coffea without benefit; the relief afforded by Spigelia was thus neutralised, and the old disorder returned in full force. In August, several doses of China 27, and Bellad. 15, produced some relief, and in September, Merc. 15; but October 21st, the old disorder again returned severely, and she received Spigelia 200, in solution, one dose, soon followed by slight aggravation with toothache, and bleeding of the gums; a repetition of the same dose was followed by a frightful aggravation, more severe than ever before experienced, and attended with chills, shivering of the whole body, and walking round the room in agony. After using Camphor the aggravation subsided, and on the following day the pain was all gone, so that she could even stoop without re-producing it. She then remained free from all pain until March, 1851, when she took Staphysagria 15, in solution, for gum boils; after using Staphysag. for two days, a violent aggravation again set in, followed by severe headache, feeling of ulceration, and as if the eyes would fall out, from every motion or touch; with chills and spasmodic shivering from the severity of the pain; she was again obliged to use Camphor as an antidote; in a few days she was restored, and remains well to the present time, December, 1851.—R CKERT.

REVIEW.—This peculiar and important remedy was used in thirteen cases; two, are described as occurring in those of powerful constitution, and choleric or choleric-sanguine temperament.

The character of the pains relieved by it differed very widely; in some cases it was boring, ulcerating, or throbbing, see § c, e, and g, and case 112; in others it was aching or pressing, tearing or digging, or jerking and rending, see § c and a, and case 112; or finally sawing and piercing. Hering calls particular attention to the fact that no other remedy relieves such a variety of pains arising under the same circumstances. Finally, it also relieves a feeling as if the eyes were pressed, or turned out.

The situation of the pains relieved, was generally in the fore part of the head. In eight cases the pains were confined to one side, viz., in two cases to the right, and in *five* cases to the *left*. In several instances the region of the eyes, and the eyes themselves, were attacked with pain; they even became inflamed and watery.

The regular, typical recurrence of the pains was peculiarly marked, generally in the night or in the forenoon; the pains spread not only to the eyes, but also to the whole side of the face and to the teeth, in § a and case 112 ; to the nape of the neck in § b ; and are apt to be associated, according to Tietze, with arthritic pains in various parts of the body. Dr. Nehrer effected cures with Spigelia when the weather was damp, cold and rainy, and Black thinks it cures nervo-rheumatic pains most readily.

Among the causes of aggravation, *stooping* is the most prominent; then every motion, concussion, loud noise, the speaking of others, straining at stool, &c., see case 112, and § g.

Among the accompanying symptoms, Hering draws attention to a peculiar paleness of the face, see § d and case 114.

The doses were Spigelia 30 and 200 in repeated doses.

The cures occurred speedily and decidedly, in cases more or less chronic or recent.

Dose.—Noack and Trinks as usual prefer comparatively large doses, such as two or three drops of the 2d or 3d dilution, repeated at short intervals, in acute attacks; at longer intervals in chronic and milder cases. Still the high dilutions seem to have been decidedly useful in the above cases, and we can only regret that Romig, Hering and Rückert did not note more carefully the intervals of time allowed to elapse between each dose. The same doses as those recommended for Rhus., may be used.—Peters.

42. SULPHUR.

General Remarks.—(*a*). Hahnemann recommends it against night-headaches, which arise from the slightest movement in bed ; against heaviness of the head, especially in the occiput; daily drawing headaches, with sense of bursting; piercing headaches with buzzing; throbbing pains in the vertex; coldness, and cold spots on the head.—See Chronic Diseases, translated by Dr. Chas. J. Hempel.

(*b*). Hering advises Sulph. against throbbing and rending pains, with fever heat, occurring early in the morning, or in the evening, attended with nausea, aggravated in the open air, and relieved by being in a warm room; also against rending, stupefying pains and aching, occurring every week, followed by falling out of the hair, and occurring after the suppression of eruptions, or ulcers.—Page 142.

(*c*). According to Black, Sulphur is indicated against headaches affecting the forehead and vertex, in which the patient complains of heat of the head and coldness of the feet, and has a sense of compression of the head, with noises in the ears and hammering; also, against the congestive headaches of persons who lead a sedentary life, suffer with constipation or piles, or in whom old ulcers or eruptions, or hemorrhoidal fluxes have been suppressed.—Genl. Hom. Jour., vol. 36, page 235.

CASE 121.—A robust woman, aged 62, was attacked with the following:

Symptoms.—Vertigo, crawling and pricking in the vertex, rushing and noises in the ears, aching in the forehead, tightness around the head as if from a band, piercing pain in the temples and cheeks, mucous state of the mouth, oppression of the stomach, heaviness and anxiety in the præcordia; with irritable disposition, great weakness and emaciation.

Treatment.—Pulsat. occasioned very little relief, which, however, followed quickly when Sulphur was used, and she was cured in 10 days.—Hygea, vol. 15, page 512.—Dr. SCHELLING.

CASE 122.—A lady, shortly after confinement, was attacked with violent tearing pain in the forehead and upper half of brain, especially about the eyes and nose, with the greatest sensitiveness of the affected parts to touch, and feeling as if they were blistered; her head and body felt cold, although the external air was warm, and her pulse was quick; these attacks came on several times a day, and also at night; they were preceded by tickling in the nose, like that which precedes sneezing, by coughing and yawning; and were followed by perspiration.

Treatment.—She was cured by four doses of Sulphur, at intervals of from nine to twelve days.—Annals, vol. 4, page 258.—Dr. HARTLAUB.

CASE 123.—A young man who had formerly suffered with *herpes rodens* on the legs before he was attacked with headaches, had complained for thirteen years with:

Throbbing, tearing headache in the occiput, extending forwards, and attended with nausea, vomiting, and aching of the eyes; the attacks were preceded by flatulence, and the headaches lessened somewhat at the end of two or three days, when fever set in, and canker-sore mouth, followed by sore throat; they recurred every three or four weeks.

Treatment.—Bellad., Merc., Nux, and Pulsat., were given without benefit; but after taking several doses of Sulphur, itching of the legs and perspiration of the feet set in, followed by a diminution of the headaches, and in the course of a few months he was perfectly restored.—Genl. Hom. Jour., vol. 10, p. 136.—Dr. Bernstein.

CASE 124.—A robust youth, aged 18, was attacked, one year after the suppression of itch, every morning about nine o'clock, with violent aching pain in the forehead, fever, rushing and roaring in the head, gradually increasing until noon, and then entirely subsiding by four o'clock in the afternoon. He had already suffered for several months in this way.

Treatment.—Sulph. 30, cured him entirely in ten days.—Genl. Hom. Jour., vol. 4, p. 305.—Dr. Hirsch.

CASE 125.—A girl, aged 11 years, had already suffered for two years with headaches, which had been of daily occurrence for the last three months.

Symptoms.—Aching pain in the forehead and whole front head, commencing immediately upon waking in the morning, and persisting the whole day. She was unfit for thought or study, and much debilitated.

Treatment.—Tinct. Sulph. effected a perfect cure in three weeks.—Annals, p. 271.—Dr. Hartlaub.

CASE 126.—Captain R. had suffered for a long time with headaches; shortly before they set in he had suppressed an attack of itch, with ointments.

Symptoms.—Violent throbbing, pressing pains in the head, especially after partaking of warm food, when in a warm room, or exposed to the heat of the sun; congestion of blood to the head, with vertigo, relieved by the application of cold water. He was troubled with itching about the rectum, with flatulence and derangement of the bowels.

Treatment.—After the use of Sulphur, at first in alternation with Nux, and then of Sulphur alone, one dose every fifth day, he was seized with more troublesome itching and pricking about the arms, and finally with itching of the legs, when his other troubles ceased entirely.—Genl. Hom. Jour., vol. 10, p. 138.—Dr. Bernstein.

Review.—Of the six cases one-half were males; in three cases the exciting cause of the headaches was suppression of itch or herpes, see § b and c; inclination to constipation, and hemorrhoids were also present, see § c.

The pains were most frequently seated in the forehead; their character was generally aching and tearing, or as if there were a band around the head; in one case there was throbbing, pressing, rushing, and roaring. They occurred either daily, at a *particular hour*, or in paroxysms several times a day, also at night; were increased by warm things; they were also attended by various disorders of the stomach, flatulence, nausea, or vomiting.

Of the six cases, Sulphur cured four, without aid from any other remedy.

The size of the doses is unfortunately not mentioned in most of the cases, although we learn that they were frequently repeated.

Dose.—Noack advises one or two grains of the 1st or 3d trituration, or from one to three drops of carefully prepared tinct. of Sulphur, once or twice a day in subacute or chronic cases; more frequently in severe attacks.—Peters.

43. THUYA.

General Remarks.—Tietze uses Thuya against hemicrania when he finds that it has been preceded by sycosis. It is most serviceable when the pains involve the *left* side, extend from thence in rays, and become tearing in their character in the forehead and face, as far as the zygoma. It is especially indicated when a peculiar sensation is present, as if a convex button were pressed upon the head, particularly in the neighborhood of the sutures of the skull, or as if a nail were thrust into the head.

If such pains are present, and we have reason to suspect sycosis; if the disorder has become chronic and inveterate; if the pains are increased by rest and warmth, especially that of the bed, and are relieved by looking upwards and bending the head backwards; and if they have been preceded by rheumatic or arthritic affections, with nocturnal exacerbations, then Thuya will assuredly prove the only curative remedy.—Genl. Hom. Jour., vol. 34, p. 19.

Dose.—Noack recommends one or two drop doses of the 1st, 2d or 3d dilution, every one, two or four hours in severe attacks; every six, eight, twelve or more hours in milder paroxysms; and once or twice a day in chronic cases. It is thought to be most useful by some physicians, in cases attended with the most obstinate constipation, with leucorrhœa or other uterine, or urinary trouble.—PETERS.

44. VERATRUM.

GENERAL REMARKS.—(*a*). Lobethal says that Veratrum is very useful against the nervous headaches of young maidens and hysterical women, when they are attended with nausea and vomiting, and the face is pale and cadaverous.—Genl. Hom. Jour., vol. 13, p. 371.

(*b*). Black recommends it against aching, throbbing, nervous headaches, affecting one side of the head, attended with stiffness of the neck, feeling as if the head would burst, and with vomiting.—Ibid., vol. 36, p. 235.

(*c*). Hering asserts that Veratrum is useful when the scalp is very sensitive to touch, when diarrhœa is present, and the pains become so severe that the patient is rendered quite delirious, or at least very weak and inclined to faint; when the pains are increased by rising up, or lying down, and are accompanied with cold sweat, coldness and thirst. Also, when long continued constipation has produced congestion of blood to the head, with unilateral pains, and aching-throbbing feeling as if the brain were bruised or compressed; with choking in the throat, or pain in the stomach, stiffness of the neck, profuse flow of urine, nausea and vomiting.—Pp. 137 and 140.

Dose.—Noack advises one or two drop doses of the 2d, 3d, 6th or 12th dilution every few hours in severe cases; once or twice a day in chronic attacks.—PETERS.

45. ZINCUM.

CASE 127.—A young lady, aged 24, of robust frame and regular menstruation, had suffered for four years with:

Aching, tearing pain in the back of the head, piercing in the right eye, rending and piercing in the ears, and occasionally in the teeth. These attacks had increased yearly in severity, until they had begun to affect her mental powers.

Treatment.—Bellad. 30, relieved the pain in the eye, but merely lessened the other sufferings; then Zinc. 30, cured her entirely in thirteen days.—Practical Observations, vol. 2, p. 187.—Dr. SCHULZ.

Dose.—Noack advises one or two grain doses of the 1st, 2d or 3d trituration every two or three hours in acute attacks, once or twice a day in chronic cases.—PETERS.

GENERAL REVIEW.

It must be expressly understood that this general review applies mainly to the forty articles and eighty-five cases, supplied by Rückert; a general review of the forty additional cases, numerous additional articles and notes, will be given at some other place.—PETERS.

Spigelia was used successfully in thirteen cases; Bellad., in twelve cases; Calc., Nux, Puls. and Sepia, each in ten cases; Bryonia and Sulph., each in six cases; Arsenic., in five cases; Colocynth, in four cases; Camphor and Causticum, each in three cases; Aconite, Opium, Sanguinaria, China, Cocculus, Carb. v. and Hepar sulph., each in two cases; Agaricus, Arnica, Asarum, Creosot., Dulc., Ignat., Magnet., Merc., Phosph.,

Silex, and Zinc., each in one or more cases. Although no cases have been reported in detail, still Aurum, Arum, Coffea. Carb. an., Caps., Chamomilla, Crocus, Lach., Plat., and Iris versicolor, have been found useful by various observers.

According to Rückert, these forty remedies were used against the following groups of symptoms, and under the following circumstances.

(1). Against NERVOUS headaches in general: Agaricus, Aurum, Carb. an., Cocc., Ign., Plat., Sep., Silex, and Verat. Against ONE-SIDED headaches, or *Migranes* in particular: Acon., Ars., Bell., Calc., Caps., China, Coffea, Coloc., Ign., Nux, Opium, Puls., Sepia, Spigel., and Thuya.

(2). Against CONGESTIVE headaches: Acon., *Belladonna*, Bryon., Calc., Carb. an., Nux, Phosph., Sepia, Sulph., and Veratrum; against *passive* congestions, Opium, China, Sepia.

(3). Against CATARRHAL headaches, Aconit., Cham., Coffea. [Pulsat., Agaricus, and Arsen.—PETERS.]

(4). Against RHEUMATIC headaches: Bryon., Acon., Merc., Cham., Nux, Sepia, and Spigelia.

(5). Against ARTHRITIC headaches: Sepia and Spigelia.

(6). Against headaches attended with GASTRIC disturbances: Bellad., Nux, and Pulsat.; with *nausea* and vomiting in particular: Acon., Arn., Asar., Bellad., Bryon., *Calc.*, Caps., Caust., Coloc., Ign., Lachesis, *Pulsat.*, Nux, Sanguinaria, *Sepia*, Sulph. and Veratrum; with *violent* vomiting: Ars., Ipec., Tart. emet., Sulph., Zinc., Cuprum and Veratrum; with *retching*, Acon. and Nux; with vomiting of *bitter* substances: Bell., and Puls.; with vomiting of *bile*: Calc., Nux, Puls., Sanguinaria; with *sour* vomiting: Nux vom. [Dr. Black prefers Cocculus when the nausea is very great; others advise Creosote; Dr. Chapman prefers Gratiola; Dr. Kitchen, Iris versicolor; while I have given Cuprum acet., with the most marked benefit.—PETERS.]

(7). Against PERIODICAL headaches: Bellad., Bryon., Cham., Coloc., Nux, Sanguinaria, Sepia, *China* and Arsen.

(8). Principally against ACUTE attacks: Aconite, Agaricus, Arnica, Bellad., Bryon., Camphor, China, Cocculus, Coloc.,

Creosot., Dulc., Ignat., Magnet., Merc., Nux, Op., Phosph., Puls., Sanguinaria, Arum, Gratiola, and Iris versicolor.

(9). Principally against CHRONIC and inveterate cases: Arsenicum, Calcarea, Causticum, Carb. animalis, Hepar sulph., Phosphor., Sepia, Silex, Sulphur, Thuya, and Zinc.

---

(10). Principally according to the LOCALITY of the pains.

(*a*). When the pains involved the *whole* of the head: Bryon., Caust., Natr., Nux, Pulsat. and Sepia. (*b*). When they seem to be seated in the *brain:* Arn., Bry., *Calc.*, China, Dulc. and Ignat. (*c*). When they affected the *forehead* in particular: Arn., *Bell.*, Bry., *Calc.*, Coloc., *Ign.*, Merc., *Nux*, Puls., *Plat.*, Silex, *Sulph.* and Thuya. (*d*). When the pains were principally over the *eye-brows:* Bellad. Over the *root* of the nose: Acon., Ignat. and Plat. (*e*). On the *vertex*, or top of the head: Bell., Bry., Calc., Dulc., Nux, Natrum m. and *Sulph.* (*f*). In the temples: Bell., *Caust.*, Cham., *China*, Ign., Nux and Puls. (*g*). In the *occiput*, or the back of the head: Calc., *Camph.*, Carb. an., Creos., Natr., Nux, *Puls.*, Sepia and *Sulph.* (*h*). When the pains were confined to *one side* in general: *Bell.*, *Calc.*, Cham., Coffea, Coloc., Lach., Natrum m., Nux, Puls., Rhus, Sepia, Silex, Spigelia. When limited to the *right side: Bell.*, Bryon., *Calc.*, Coloc., Nux, Puls., Rhus, Sanguinaria, Sepia, and especially *Opium.* To the *left* side: Acon., Asarum, Bryon., Calc., Cham., Coloc., Merc., Natrum, Nux, Puls., *Sepia*, *Spigelia*, Thuya, and especially *China.*

---

(11). According to the CHARACTER of the pains.

Against *sore* or festering pains, Puls. and Sep.; *boring* pains, Calc., Puls., Sep. and Spigelia; boring pains, as if in the brain itself, Ignat.; burning pains, Bryon.; boring-burning, Dulc. Against *aching* pains; Ars., Bell., Bryon., Calc., China, Coffea, Coloc., Natrum, *Nux*, Sepia, Sulph. and Veratrum.

Against aching from within *outwards:* Ign., Caps.
" stupefying aching: Arsen.
" dull aching: Calc.
" digging aching: Bryon.

Drawing-asunder pains: Bryon., Caps. Throbbing, pushing and hammering pains: Bell., Calc., Camph., Caps., Cham., Croc., Natrum m., Pulsat., Sanguin., Sepia, Silex, Spigelia, Sulph., Verat.

Squeezing pains: over the nose, Aconit.; compressing pain, Plat.; aching and compressing, Coloc. Feeling of emptiness, Cocc. Pain, as if from a *nail* driven into the brain, or the true hysterical pain: Coffea, Ignatia, Nux, Evon., Hell. and Thuya.

Pressing pain: Bell., Bryon. and Natrum; pressing-asunder, Arsen., Bell. and Bryon.; aching-pressing, Spigelia; out-pressing, Bryon. and Ignat.; throbbing-pressing, Sulphur; pressing together, Bryon.

Rending, tearing or drawing pains: Bell., Cham., China, Coloc., Ignat., Merc., Nux, Pulsat., Sepia, Spigelia, Sulphur, Thuya; boring-rending pains, Nux; aching-rending, China; throbbing-rending, Arsen. and Spigelia; piercing-rending, Natrum; rooting or digging and rending, Spigelia; rending in small spots, Bryon.; drawing and rending, Rhus.

Stretching or tensive pains: Puls. Piercing, or pricking or sticking pains: Bryon., Caust., Cham., Coloc., Nux, Puls., Sanguin., Sep. and Sulphur; *outwards*, Ignat.; *inwards*, Coloc.; as if in the brain, Ignat; like needle-stitches or lancinating or pricking, Sepia; boring, Acon., Bellad. and Puls.; aching or pressing and piercing, Pulsat.; throbbing, Acon., Bellad. and Spigelia; rending and piercing, Caps.

Sensation of rocking to and fro in the brain, Nux; of wavering, Bellad.; of digging, Dulc. and Sanguin.; drawing, Calc., Cham., China, Coffea, Coloc., Merc. and Sepia; aching-drawing, Nux; twitching or jerking, Coloc.; throbbing-jerking, Ignat.; as if compressed together by a band, Merc. and Sulph.; screwed together, Pulsat. and Verat.; as if torn or comminuted, Coffea, Nux and Verat.; as if the head would burst, Calc., Merc. and Natrum; forcing one to cry out, Acon., Coff., Cham. and Veratrum.

When the scalp was tender, Bellad., Carb. an., China and Natrum m., were found the best remedies; when the hair was sensitive, Verat.; when there were hot spots upon the head, Bellad.; coldness of the head, Calc. and Sulph.; sweat upon the head in the evening, Calc.; rushing and roaring in the head, Aurum, Bellad. and Calc.

---

(12). The following remedies were found most serviceable when the headaches were EXCITED OR AGGRAVATED BY:

Touching the head, Bry., Calc., China, Coloc., Sep., Sulph.

Movement in general, Acon., Bellad., Bry., Caps., China, Creos., Nux, Sanguin., Sep. and Spigel.; at night, when in bed, Sulph.; of the head and eyes, Bellad., Bryon., Coloc., Puls., Sepia; from opening the eyes, Sepia; when rising, Veratrum; from stooping, Bellad., Bryon., Caps., Coloc., Nux, Puls., Sepia, Silex., *Spigel.;* when walking, Bryon. and Caps.; when walking in the free air, Spigel.; after walking in the open air, Calc.; while talking, Calc., Dulc., Ign.

From concussion, or jarring: Acon., Bell., China; from the talking of others, Acon., Bellad., Sepia, Spigel.; from the walking about of others, Bell.; from every pulsation, Bell.; from every step, or going up steps, Bellad.

From noise: Acon., Bellad., Coff., Sepia and Spigel.; from music, Coffea.

From mental emotions in general: Coloc. and Nux; depressing emotions, Bryon.; from vexation, Coff.; from fright, Calc.; from mental exertion, Calc., Coffea, Nux.

After partaking of food: Arn., Coffea, Cocc., Nux; of coffee or wine, Nux; of warm food, Sulph.

From bright *light:* Asarum, Bryon. and Nux; from rays of light upon the eyes, Bellad.

From the influence of *air:* In the open air, Calc., Nux, Spigel. and Sulph.; particular sensitiveness to the free air, Caps., China, Coffea; sensitiveness of the head to air, Ars.; draught of air or wind, China; air of a room, Ars., Puls. and Sulph.; warm air in particular, Caust.

At the *time of menstruation:* Bryon., Coccul., Spigel.

From *rest*, or quiet or sitting: Pulsatilla.

From lying on the back: Coloc. and Verat.

From taking cold: Acon., Bryon., Coffea, Nux v.

(13). The following remedies were useful when the headaches were RELIEVED by:

Closing the eyes, Calc.; binding up the head, and external pressure, Calc., Puls. and Sepia; by vomiting, Bryon.; the free air, Acon., Ars. and Puls.; moving the limbs to and fro, Ars. and Bellad.; the arms, Bellad.; by lying still, Calc., China and Merc.; the pains forcing one to lie still, Calc., Coloc., Nux and Sanguin.; by rest, China, Sepia and Spigel.; by bending forwards, Ignat.; by external warmth, Arsen.

---

(14). When the pains and aches occurred *early* in the morning, Bellad., Bryon., Calc., Ignat., Natrum m., Nux and Sanguin., were found most useful; in the forenoon, Spigelia; in the afternoon, Bell., Coloc.; in the evening, Bryon., Caust., Coloc., Pulsat. and Ignat.; at night, China, Merc., Silex and Sulphur.

Rückert reports eighty-five cases of cure of headache, effected by fifty-one different physicians; in eighty-four cases the exact dose used is mentioned.

Strong doses were used, viz.: from the pure tincture to the 3d dilution, in twenty-one cases; one dose sufficed to cure in five instances; one dose in solution was repeated in one instance; repeated doses were required in fifteen cases.

The *higher* dilutions, viz.: from the 4th to 30th potency were used in fifty cases; one dose sufficed to effect a cure in thirty instances; one dose in solution and repeated in three instances; repeated doses were required in seventeen instances.

The *very high* potencies were used in thirteen cases; single doses in ten instances; in solution, repeatedly in three instances.

Olfaction of the remedies was used in a few cases only. Two-thirds of the cases were cured by the higher dilutions; one-third, by the lower potencies.

SYNOPSIS

AND

ADDITIONAL CASES.

THE original intention of this chapter was simply to furnish a condensed statement of the principal indications, both clinical and theoretical, for the selection of remedies against the different varieties of headache. This had been accomplished, when it was discovered that among the sixty-three cases of headache collected by BEAUVAIS in his *Clinique Homœopathique*, no less than thirty-seven were not to be found in Rückert's; hence, it was regarded as imperative to sacrifice somewhat of the symmetry and methodical arrangement of the present treatise, rather than have it go forth incomplete, or less than it pretends to be, viz.: "A complete collection of all the cures and practical remarks upon the Homœopathic treatment of Headaches, which have been published since the year 1822." A few of the cases collected by Beauvais have been rejected as unfit for republication here, as they required the use of from four to five, or even six or seven different remedies to effect a cure; but ten cases, translated from ATTOMYR's *Primordien einer Natur-geschichte der Krankheiten*, have also been added, and eight cases, cured by Glonoine, reported by Dr. COXE, of Philadelphia.

Of these additional cases, eight were cured by Sepia; eight, by Glonoine; four, by Bell.; three cases, each by Ars., Nux, Puls., Rhus, and Sulph.; one, by Staphysag.; and one, by Sulph. and Sepia.

ACONITUM NAPELLUS.

It has been recommended in headaches from suppressed perspiration, and to induce those critical perspirations which sometimes cure chronic headache;

In severe rheumatic headaches, when attended with pains in the fibrous sheaths of the nerves; in other fibrous tissues, such as the dura mater, falx cerebri and cerebelli, in the fibrous tissue of the scalp, in the periosteum of the skull and bones of the face; especially when severe pains in the back, bones and joints are also present, the urine and perspiration having the well known rheumatic characters. (See Merc., Mezereum, Iod. pot. and Bryon.)

In headaches attended with great and peculiar numbness and tingling in various parts, and tending to falling asleep of the limbs, and night-mare.

In severe one-sided headaches, especially on the *left* side.

In violent congestive and sub-inflammatory headaches, with fever, heat and redness of the face, some contraction of the pupil, and *without* active delirium.

In the most violent *nervous* or neuralgic headaches, when the patient is utterly prostrate and exhausted from the severity of the pain, is cold and almost pulseless, with a sinking feeling and great irritability of the stomach, and coldness of the limbs, with tendency to livor, or blueness of various parts.

AGARICUS MUSCARIUS.

In the headaches of persons subject to nervous twitchings and St. Vitus' dance, with spinal irritation, feeling of great uneasiness and weakness down the spine, especially in those unusually subject to frost-bites, and suffering with derangement, or enlargement of the liver.

In the headaches of those who become delirious whenever they are feverish or in pain, attended with twitchings, startings, grimaces, and a state resembling pleasant intoxication. (See Bellad., Stramon., &c.)

In the headaches of persons suffering with softening of the brain, or spinal marrow. (See Nux, and Iodide of Baryta.)

ARNICA MONTANA.

Against headaches arising from mechanical injuries; those of persons subject or liable to apoplexy; and of women during the change of life.

Against headaches similar to those relieved by Nux, Ignat., Strychnine, the Magnet, and the alternate use of electrical remedies, such as Zinc and Cuprum, Zinc and Argentum, Zinc and Platina, especially when there is heat and burning in the head, with coolness of the rest of the body, pain over the eyes and temples, with feeling as if the integuments of the forehead were spasmodically contracted.

Against aching with lancinating and tearing in the *left* half of the head, *left* temple, or *left* frontal protuberance.

In headaches attended with a feeling of formication or creeping in the limbs, with prickling, piercing sensations somewhat similar to slight electric shocks, and a peculiar feeling of coolness over the body, followed by perspiration which sometimes assumes a reddish hue upon the chest, with scanty urine, and great increase of pain from walking about.

ARSENICUM ALBUM.

Against the headaches of persons inclined to dropsy, or bloating of the face or feet, with scanty and albuminous urine, especially if the eyelids be red, swollen and itchy, the tongue white as if rubbed over with chalk or covered with cream, although the appetite may be ravenous, and tendency to diarrhœa be present. (See Merc. Corrosiv., Camph., and Apis Mell.)

Also when the face is pale and sunken, with blue circles about the eyes and blueness of the lips, dingy appearance of the skin, tendency to boils and eruptions. (See Carb. an. and Hepar s.)

In the headaches of those subject to catarrh of the head, short dry cough, and tightness of the chest. (See Acon. and Antim.)

In the headaches of persons with irritable bowels and subject to frequent diarrhœa; or with sub-inflammatory irritation of the uterus or ovaries, and having a pale or bloated, cachectic, suffering or dyscratic appearance.

In regularly intermitting or periodical headaches, affecting the forehead and *right* side of the head. (See China.)

CASE 128.—A lady had suffered for two years with neuralgic headache, and under allopathic treatment had been bled, leeched, blistered, used opium and had the actual cautery applied three times before she was relieved. The attacks commenced at 7 A.M. and lasted until 2 P.M., and were so severe that the patient was obliged to give up and lie down; she wept and screamed from the severity of the pain.

Treatment.—China was given without relief; four globules of Arsen. produced relief in one hour, the next day she was much better, and on the third day she was well.—Bibliothèque Hom., vol. 3, p. 133.—DR. CONVERS.—Beauvais Clinique, vol. 2, p. 23.

CASE 129.—A gentleman had suffered for two months with violent migraine, commencing every morning at 8 o'clock and lasting till 1 P.M.

Symptoms.—Severe pains, cutting and lancinating in the left temple and forehead; they soon became so violent that he wept and despaired like a child; the left eye became sensitive to light, red and tearful; a corrosive fluid ran from the left nostril during the paroxysms; during the interval of relief he had loss of appetite, debility and great sensitiveness to the fresh air.

Treatment.—He had been leeched and blistered without relief, also had taken anti-spasmodics and anti-arthritic remedies. China 3, and Bellad. 12, were given without much benefit; Arsenic. 30, was followed by suppuration in the nostril, discharge ot a hard polypus, and entire cure in five weeks.—Ibid., vol. 1, p. 569.—DR. HERMANN.

CASE 130.—A maiden, aged 15, suffered with pain in the left forehead and temple, so severe that she wept and whimpered, and could not bear to be touched. Near the left temple there was a small, round, brownish red spot, with a black point in the centre, painful to the touch.

Treatment.—Arsen. 30, three doses per day, cured the headache; but chills and spasms of the arms and legs, which set in afterwards, were removed by Ignat. 12.—ATTOMYR., vol. 1, page 474.

ASARUM EUROPÆUM.

Against headaches which come on just before or after menstruation, with painful weight, tightness and dulness of the head, and throbbing in the occiput. (See Pulsat., Sabina, Crocus.)

ARUM MACULATUM.

In dyspeptic headaches, or those connected with debility of the stomach.

AURUM MURIATICUM.

In the most violent congestive headaches, which will not yield to Acon., Bell., Stramon., or *Phosphor.*, attended with great redness of the face, hard throbbing of the carotid and temporal arteries, great rushing and roaring in the ears, especially when owing to sudden suppression of piles, or of the menses, and when the attacks are apt to pass off with the feeling as if all the blood in the head rushed down into the legs.

It is the great rival of Mercurius in the treatment of headaches connected with disease of the periosteum, or bones of the nose, ears and skull, arising from secondary syphilis, although Hydriodate of Potash and Mezereum will often be required in alternation with it.

In headaches arising from such derangements of the stomach as are always followed by nettle-rash, especially when there is a chronic tendency to congestion of the head, with great despondency.

In headaches which commence in the *morning*, last all day, and are increased to an extreme degree of violence by reflecting, reading, talking, or writing. Headaches of literary persons, especially when their urine is rather profuse, thick, and has a peculiarly offensive smell, while the perspiration is copious and peculiar in its odor. (See Nux and Agar.)

BELLADONNA.

In headaches which always commence in the *afternoon* or *evening;* being dull and heavy, affecting the forehead in particular, attended with active delirium, dilatation of the pupils, partial blindness, and ceasing suddenly on the occurence of a profuse flow of limpid urine. In headache from diabetes.

In the headaches of persons affected with active febrile, or florid scrofula, and having unusually large pupils; especially if there be great irritability of the uterine system. (See Baryta and Stramon.)

Against headaches which always commence about, or in one or the other eye, attended with great disturbance of vision, and excessive dilatation of the pupils, being seated in the retina, optic nerve, or ophthalmic branch of the fifth pair. (See Stramon., Pulsat.)

Some remedies are peculiarly suited to headaches which attack one small spot, as if a nail were driven into the brain, or as if a small part were festered or ulcerated; Bell., on the contrary is most suited for headaches extending over *large* surfaces of the brain. Nux vom. is most indicated when the pupils are contracted, and the various sphincters in a state of spasm, the headaches commencing *early* in the morning and subsiding towards evening; *Bellad.* is most suitable against the exact reverse of all this, although in cases 9, 12, and 15 cured by Bellad. the pains commenced and were most severe in the morning. It is perhaps most useful against headaches affecting the *right* side, especially when the face of the patient has a mottled appearance, from the presence of large red spots.

CASE 131.—A lady, aged 36, had suffered for several years with periodical headache, especially at the time of menstruation; she had been treated without success by a number of physicians.

Symptoms.—Severe pain in the head, with great heat and redness of face, burning heat and throbbing in the head, followed by delirium.

Treatment.—Bellad. 30, caused relief in six hours, and although she continued to have periodical attacks, they were much less severe.—Beauvais' Clinique, vol. 1, p. 514.—Dr. Hermann.

CASE 132.—A pregnant lady, aged 35, had suffered for four days with headache, concentrated especially in the bones and skin of the left side of the forehead; the pains occurred in paroxysms, which were at times exceedingly severe; they were drawing, jerking and rending in their character, and the skin and hair of the affected part became very sensitive; there were noises in the left ear, almost entire loss of hearing; mist before the left eye; the upper lid was sunken, as if paralyzed; the white of the eye was reddened; there was loss of smell and taste; also cough, with some expectoration of blood, tickling in the larynx, and pain in the chest; the throat was red, painful and swollen; the left arm was numb; there was no fever.

Treatment.—Four doses of Bellad. 2, effected a cure.—Attomyr's Primordien, vol. 1, p. 451.

CASE 133.—A student, aged 23, had suffered from his eighth year with headache, which had ceased for awhile, when he was suffering with fever and ague, but had returned again.

Symptoms.—He generally had pain in a small spot, on the left side of the forehead, on the evening before an attack of headache; early the next morning the headache set in, and the above mentioned spot became raised and red; occasionally the attacks affected the right side. During the early part of the night he had unusual wakefulness, and only fell asleep towards 5 o'clock in the morning.

Treatment.—He was cured by Bell. 3, one dose night and morning.—Attomyr, ibid.—Dr. Gross.

CASE 134.—A lady, aged 36, had suffered for two years, with pain commencing over the forehead, extending down the right side towards the nose and jaw, and into the neck; the pain was drawing, throbbing and rending; it generally commenced at 4 A.M., and lasted for half or one hour, and was attended with itching in the eyelids, some swelling of the affected side of the face, with aching and pinching pain in the ear, and with perspiration. At times spots came out on the face.

Treatment.—Bellad. 30, effected a perfect cure.—Attomyr, ibid.—DR. KIRSCH.

BRYONIA ALBA.

Bellad. and other remedies are indicated when the head is *heavy* from great fulness of blood; Bryonia is the best remedy against heaviness of the head from simple debility, or loss of energy in the brain, similar to that heaviness which is felt in an arm or leg that is wearied; just as a debilitated stomach will feel the least weight put in it, or the bowels feel heavy from their own weight, will a weakened brain rest heavily against the skull. It is most indicated in severe headache, the brain feeling very heavy, as if it would incline to all sides of the skull, with pressure in the brain from within outwards, and great desire to lie down. Headache when stooping as if all the contents of the skull would fall out of the forehead; giddiness, and weight in the head.

Also against *morning-headaches* from debility of the brain and nervous system. In this form, the patient wakes unrefreshed from sleep, is languid and weary, but not very drowsy, scarcely able to dress himself, or to exert himself sufficiently to get his breakfast; shortly after this meal, however, he becomes revived and active. Bryonia is indicated when the patient's head aches, and he feels gloomy in the morning, as if he had over-exerted himself; with gloomy compression in the forehead, over the eyes; compressive pain *early* in the morning, with heaviness, intermingled with stitches so violent that the patient can scarcely open his eyes. Headache early in the morning, on waking, in the occiput, extending as far as the shoulders, resembling a weight pressing on a sore spot.

Tearing and drawing pain in the cheek and jaw-bones, early in the morning, just after rising. Beating and heat in the head, early in the morning. Headaches which set in principally *in the morning, on waking;* and those which are aggravated by walking in the open air. (See Nux.)

Also against rheumatic headaches, when the disorder is seated, not so much in the fibrous as in the true muscular tissue, involving the nerves and bloodvessels which preside over the nutrition of the muscles, rather than their motions; while Nux and Ignatia are more indicated when the motor nerves are principally involved. Bryonia is also useful in nervo-neuralgic and rheumatic headaches, in which the pains spread to the frontal and temporal branches of the trifacial nerve, and to the temporal and maxillary twigs of the superior facial nerve; also when the pains extend to the muscles of the face, neck or arms; and are much increased by every motion of these parts. When the paroxysms arise in rheumatic weather, in cold, raw, and wet seasons, and are attended with pains or swelling of the joints.

CASE 135.—Bryon. 9, relieved: vertigo in the morning, throbbing in the head, especially after walking, or being overheated; pain in the teeth and dryness of the throat after swallowing cold food, or drink; constipation; occasional pain and tension in the right side.—Beauvais' Clinique, vol. 1, p. 563.—DR. RÜCKERT.

CALCAREA CARBONICA.

It is principally used in *chronic* and obstinate headaches, attended with great sluggishness and some drowsiness, occurring in torpid, scrofulous persons, with a pale and rather fair complexion, and a marked predisposition towards corpulency.

Against headaches which instead of being relieved by a walk or drive in the open air, are very much aggravated by it. In chronic *morning* headaches, somewhat resembling the *stupid* headache of Dr. Good. In those attended with coldness of the head in spots, and large dull red blotches upon the cheeks; and in females with profuse and frequent flow of the menses, tendency to sour stomach and canker sore mouth.

CAMPHOR.

In sudden and acute headaches from excessive fatigue or debility, especially when attended with throbbing in the back of the head; it is supposed to exert a specific action upon the cerebellum and medulla oblongata.

In headaches from suppressed perspiration, or those attended with warmth of the skin, hot perspiration, congestion to the head, redness of the face, sparkling of the eyes, feeling of intoxication, noises in the ears, great anxiety about the heart, chest, and pit of the stomach, and with nausea and vomiting.

In *apoplectic* headaches, with wandering of the mind, sleepiness, even soporose sleep, with coldness of the skin, paleness of the face, stertorous respiration, twitching, &c.

CARBO ANIMALIS.

This remedy, or *animal* carbon, is closely allied in its action to Carbo vegetabilis, or *vegetable* carbon; to Graphites, or *mineral* carbon; and to Sepia, or *fish* carbon. A careful study of these four remedies in connection with each other will lead to a better application of each of them to the diseases in which they are severally indicated.

It should be remembered in the headaches of some dyscratic subjects, as Wurm regards it as the best remedy to improve the blood, especially in cancerous and bilious subjects, and those with indurations and swellings of glandular organs, especially if they are also subject to boils, or copper-colored exanthems. (See Conium.)

In headaches arising from enlarged parotid, or cervical glands pressing upon the bloodvessels of the neck; and in women who suffer with enlargement of the ovaries. (See Graphit. and Staphysag.

But more especially in *dyspeptic* headaches, when the patient is incommoded by everything he eats, when the occiput and *left* side of the head are most affected, the left side of the scalp is sore to the touch, and the pains are decidedly *lancinating*, and cutting. It is well known that shooting or lancinating pains, and sharp, darting and pricking pains, are chiefly met with in neuralgia and rheumatism, when owing to some acrid humor in the blood, and in cancer; these pains either follow the course of the nerves, or the fibres of the muscular or fibrous parts affected.

CARBO VEGETABILIS.

Especially in headaches connected with indigestion and great flatulence; some persons find prompt relief from the most violent headaches by taking an ordinary dose of charcoal. SANDRAS knew of a case of headache, attended with profuse accumulation of wind in the stomach, always relieved by exposing the epigastrium to the cool fresh air, aided by gentle frictions to expel the gas. Against headache connected with obstinate and chronic fever and ague, of years' standing.

CASE 136.—J. K., aged 32, corpulent, sanguine and swarthy, had been in poor health for some time, and consulted several physicians without relief.

Symptoms.—Painful throbbing from the nape up into the head, commencing before noon with stiffness in the nape, and cold sweat; becoming worse after mid-day, especially after eating, but the pain gradually ceased if he would lie down. He had noises in the ears, dimness before the eyes, slight constipation, smarting pain in the urethra before urinating; rheumatic pains in the muscles of the abdomen, coldness of the knees, fetid sweat of the feet, and frequent crops of boils.

Treatment.—Carb. veg. 18; in two months he was almost well.—Beauvais, vol. 2, p. 22.—DR. TIETZE.

CAPSICUM ANNUUM.

Against headaches connected with neuralgia, or with derangement of the stomach, such as a chronic mucous state, with heartburn, flatulence, flatulent colic, cramps of the stomach, diarrhœa and hæmarrhoids, especially when occurring in persons long afflicted with chronic gonorrhœa.

CAUSTICUM.

In the *chronic* headaches of scrofulous and weakly persons, who have become still more debilitated by long continued grief; when attended with nausea, irregular appetite, chronic constipation, menstrual irregularity, and pain in the back, provided the headaches are most frequent and severe at *night*, and attended with pains in the limbs. We have already seen that the chronic dyscratic headaches most readily relieved by Calcarea, are such as are most frequent and severe in the *morning*.

CASE 137.—A boy, aged 12, after the suppression of itch, was attacked with St. Vitus' dance, from which he was relieved in a month under allopathic treatment, but left with: shooting pains in the forehead, drawing pain in the right arm and elbow, painful tension in the knee, and vertigo.

Treatment.—Three doses of Sulphur and two of Causticum cured him entirely in six weeks.—Beauvais, vol. 1, p. 572.—DR. HARTLAUB.

MATRICARIA CHAMOMILLA.

It is best suited as a palliative remedy against the sudden and acute headaches of hysterical subjects, especially when attended with bilious derangement, bitter taste in the mouth, stitches in the region of the liver, a peculiar feeling of anxiety, nausea, vomiting and bilious diarrhœa, with more or less flatulence, and menstrual derangement, viz., menstrual colic with frequent discharge of coagulæ.

CHINA (CINCHONA).

It causes active congestion of the head; as it increases the whole quantity of the blood and favors an unusual flow of it to the head more than any other remedy, except Iron; it is easy to understand how it may relieve passive stagnations of blood in the head, and those headaches dependent upon a deficiency of blood in the whole system, owing to excessive bloodletting, hæmorrhages, or great loss of any of the fluids of the body.

It is most homœopathic to headaches attended with great restlessness, much chilliness, trembling of the limbs, noises in the ears, some deafness, decided hunger, constipation, frequent pulse, heat of skin, and redness of the face.

CASE 138.—A robust and very active pastor, had suffered for several years with an affection of the head, so violent that he had lost all his former activity; there seemed to him to be a place in his occiput as large as a closed fist, over which the skin was as sore to touch, as if an abscess were beneath; and what was most remarkable, the roots of the hair there were sensitive to the slightest touch, while they would bear hard pressure without pain. He also had pain and stiffness in his loins, so that he was obliged to walk bent over, and could only straighten himself with difficulty.

Treatment.—Tinct. China, in drop doses, removed the head-difficulty in thirty hours; Bryon. 3, cured the pain in the loins in two days more.—Beauvais, vol. 1, p. 550.—Dr. Bethman.

CASE 139.—Madam D., subject at all times to headache, was seized in her forty-eighth year, after an extraordinarily copious flow of the menses, with pain in the head, sickness, inclination to vomit, chills, coldness of the feet, and great debility.

Treatment.—China being indicated, $\frac{1}{6}$th of a grain doses of quinine were given every two hours; in half an hour after the first dose, relief commenced, and progressed so rapidly that by the time she had taken six doses, she was restored to health and strength.—Beauvais, vol. 1, p. 511.—Dr. Gross.

COCCULUS INDICUS.

It is serviceable against the headaches which follow a sudden suppression of the menses; those with excessive dizziness; with an unusual degree of nausea, vomiting and irritability of the stomach.

In headaches peculiarly marked by a feeling of emptiness and hollowness of the head; just the opposite of China, Bellad., and other remedies, which cause a feeling of great fulness, or distension.

It is a main remedy against some forms of dyspeptic headache, viz., when there is a bitter, salt, coppery, slimy or bad taste in the mouth; want of appetite, disgust for food, even for the smell of it; excessive nausea, with great dizziness, and tendency to fainting.

CASE 140.—A lady, aged 28, suffered with frequent pains in the forehead, accompanied with vomiting of bile and pressure in the stomach, as if from a stone; pain in the region of the liver, which became acute when she stooped; constipation, with scanty, painful and hard stools; painful menstruation, lasting from eight to ten days, with flow of grumous blood; followed by piles, great debility, sweats, and disturbed sleep.

Treatment.—Two doses of Cocculus 18, at intervals of eight days, cured her entirely.—Beauvais, vol. 2, page 14.—DR. SCHROEN.

COLOCYNTH.

In headaches which are very apt to pass off with diarrhœa, Heckenberger noticed, when one drop of Tinct. Coloc. was given every morning, fasting, for several weeks, that thin, mush-like, and brownish stools would always follow.

Headaches connected with bilious derangement, profuse menstruation, and frequent and violent colics; especially when the pains are most *severe* in the *left* side of the head, forehead, left eye and upper teeth, occasionally extending to the left shoulder, followed by soreness of the left side of the scalp. In some respects this form of headache resembles that for which Carbo-animalis is most suitable; in obstinate cases, Carbo-an. may be given as a chronic remedy during the intervals of relief, to break up the tendency to the attacks; while Colocynth can be used to produce relief in severe and acute paroxysms. In such cases, China may also be required.

CREOSOTE.

It has been advised in headaches attended with excessive irritability of the stomach, severe nausea and vomiting, although Acid. Hydrocyan. may be required, or the Magnet.

In headaches attended with profuse menstruation, chronic inflammation of the labia and vagina, ulceration of the os uteri, with whitish, yellow, serous or bloody leucorrhœa.

CROCUS.

Headaches of women during the change of life; those which follow obstinate and fatiguing bleeding of the nose; or profuse, and too frequent menstruation.

In violent headaches which last three or four days at a time, the pains being most frequent and severe on the *left* side, attended with great drowsiness, confusion of the head, feeling of intoxication, and dimness of vision.

GLONOINE.

This powerful remedy was introduced into practice by the veteran Dr. Hering, to whose zeal and industry the Materia Medica owes so many contributions, both elaborate and fragmentary. Dr. Vinal has reported two cases of cure, of headache; and Dr. J. Redman Coxe, four cases, with it.

SOBRERO says, a minute quantity of Glonoine held upon the tongue produces a very violent headache for several hours. It evidently exerts a peculiar and decided action upon the head, and will prove homœopathic in certain forms of headache, especially in the highly congestive variety, when there is a feeling of great heaviness and weight in the brain, rush of blood, beating and throbbing, sense of soreness and swelling of the head; particularly when the symptoms are most severe at night.

CASE 141.—Mrs. E. T. C. had complained for several weeks with: throbbing headache, dizziness, with flushes of heat to the head and face, and feeling of soreness internally when moving it.

Treatment.—She had taken various homœopathic remedies without relief; then took Glonoine 9, two powders, with relief in half an hour after the first dose, and no return of the disease for six weeks, at last account.—Brit. Jour. of Hom., vol. 7, p. 421.—DR. VINAL.

CASE 142.—Miss Ann R. had suffered for several weeks

with pulsating headache, and soreness on moving the head, with dizziness and vertigo after stooping.

Treatment.—She had been treated homœopathically for some weeks, without permanent benefit, when she finally took Glonoine 6, four powders, one night and morning; she was relieved rapidly, and had no return of the disorder for a month, at last account.—Ibid.

CASE 143.—Mrs. M. J. C., aged 35, of bilious, sanguine temperament, had suffered since her fifteenth year, with repeated attacks of congestion to the head; had been treated allopathically for five years without benefit; then was almost cured by eight months homœopathic treatment, so that she had no attacks for several years; and for seven years more, had only slight paroxysms, which readily yielded to Acon. 9, and Bellad. 12. In 1848, she had two violent attacks; in 1849, prior to June, she had endured three violent paroxysms, all of which yielded, but not very readily, to Acon., and Bell. On June 26th, 1849, she was attacked with the most violent seizure she had ever experienced.

Symptoms.—Her face was nearly purple; the heat of her forehead, and vertex exceedingly great; her eyes blood-shot and protruding, and the pain in her head most excruciating; her brain felt twice as heavy, and much larger than usual; she became perfectly delirious, knew no one, and repulsed her husband and children; screamed violently, wished to escape from the house, &c.

Treatment.—Glonoine 3, two pellets; followed by a violent aggravation in five minutes, and an equally rapid improvement in five minutes more, so that in ten minutes after the first dose, she was almost well; her head and face were cool, pain gone, and she had no return of the disorder for five months, when a slight attack yielded readily to Glonoine 3. —Am. Jour. of Hom., vol. 6, p. 76.—Dr. J. R. Coxe, Jr.

CASE 144.—Deborah Gray, aged 40, a colored cook, had been subject to violent headaches and congestions to the head, every twelve or fifteen days for many years, and from which she was never relieved in less than twenty-four hours.

Symptoms.—Headache and vertigo so severe that she was obliged to hold her head with her hands; eyes very painful and bloodshot; face and head very hot; she moaned much, complained that her brain was being forced out of her forehead, and that it seemed too large.

Treatment.—Glonoine 3, one pellet; followed by evident aggravation in six minutes, and entire relief in ten minutes; she had no attack for fourteen weeks after, when a slight attack was relieved in fifteen minutes, by one teaspoonful of Glonoine 6, two pellets, solved in four ounces of water.—Ibid.

CASE 145.—Miss S. A. C., aged 8 years, of bilious, nervous and choleric temperament, had been subject to bleeding of the nose, pain and fulness in the head with vertigo, and slight palpitation, three or four times a year for several years, when she was suddenly attacked with violent headache, great heat and flushing of the face, bloodshot state of the eyes, and full, quick pulse.

Treatment.—Glonoine 9, one pellet, without any effect; she then recovered in six hours under the use of Acon. and Bellad. Three weeks after, for a similar attack, she took Glonoine 12, two pellets; followed by an aggravation in seven minutes, and a cure in twelve.—Ibid.

CASE 146.—Master L. S., aged 12 years, of bilious, nervous and slightly lymphatic temperament, after being over-heated, was seized with violent headache; his face was flushed, head hot, pulse 106, full and strong; he had violent beating of the arteries of the head, congestion and protrusion of the eyes, feeling as if his head was larger than usual, and as if his eyes were being pushed out, so that he could not sit upright, and was obliged to keep his hand pressed upon his forehead.

Treatment.—Glonoine 12, one pellet; followed by a very slight aggravation for eight minutes, and entire recovery in seventeen.—Ibid.

CASE 147.—Mr. B. M. S., aged 32, of large stature, and bilious sanguine temperament, after taking a violent cold, was seized with severe headache.

Symptoms.—Severe pain in head; face much flushed, and

very hot; whole head extremely hot; eyes very much bloodshot, and with a rather wild expression; trembling of the legs and knees; slight quivering of the hands and wrists.

Treatment.—Glonoine 9, two pellets; followed by a slight aggravation in nine minutes, and perfect recovery in twenty-six.—Ibid.—Dr. J. R. Coxe.

GRATIOLA OFFICINALIS.

In headaches attended with a peculiar biting-burning in the face and other parts, great languor in the arms and legs, often followed by an equally peculiar *coldness* in, and on the head, and in the stomach and bowels.

In the headaches which attend jaundice, bilious diarrhœa or dysentery, with yellow, yellowish green and bilious stools, discharge of brown, fetid and acrid mucus, with great smarting and burning in the rectum.

HEPAR SULPHURIS.

Especially in those headaches which commence *early* in the morning, as soon as one wakes, and are *relieved* by exposure to the open air. The Calcarea-headaches are also morning-headaches, but they are very much *aggravated* by the fresh air. Hepar is used even more frequently than Carbo-an. in headaches arising from an unhealthy state of the system marked by the frequent occurrence of pimples, boils, felons, glandular indurations and suppurations.

IGNATIA AMARA.

In the headaches of those who are a prey to long continued and deep-seated grief; although Arsenicum, Aurum, or Causticum may be required in alternation.

In beating pains in the *left* side of the *occiput*, and especially against those which are most severe over the root of the nose.

LACHESIS.

From Hering's experiments it seems most suited to oppressive headaches, attended with nausea and giddiness; those brought on by slight exposure to the sun, soon becoming violent and throbbing, with nausea, vomiting of green bile, bad taste in the mouth, loss of appetite, flatulence, excessive restlessness, &c. In headaches which last three days, become severe and congestive, with great drowsiness. In violent beating and throbbing headaches just before the menses set in, with nausea, bad taste in the mouth, heartburn, and *scanty* menstruation.

LYCOPODIUM.

CASE 148.—A lady, aged 50, had suffered for a long time with painful and violent pressure on the left side of the top of the head, attended with redness of the face, heat, agitation, loss of sleep, aching and cramps in the stomach, periodical vomiting, and constipation.

Treatment.—She had been treated allopathically in vain; Lycopod. 30, followed in twenty-one days by Nux 30, cured her entirely in three months.—Beauvais, vol. 1, p. 574.—Dr. Kramer.

MERCURIUS.

Especially in simple, recurring, and bilious headaches, arising frequently from the slightest cold, and being decidedly most severe at night.

In pains about the head connected with irritation of the fibrous tissues, although Iod. pot., and Aurum, or Natrum m. may often be required in alternation.

Against rending and tearing pains, and especially against burning on the top of the head.

MAGNESIA CARBONICA.

CASE 149.—A lady, aged 23, had suffered for several years with an affection of the head, marked by shooting pains in the temples and forehead, coming on every morning, but ceasing after mid-day. These pains were particularly violent during the period of menstruation; then they forced her to lie down, and were attended with vomiting. Her menses were always scanty; she was constipated; and had a feeling of anxiety, and palpitation of the heart almost every evening, after lying down.

Treatment.—She took Magnes. carb. 30; her menses set in sooner than usual, were more copious, and not attended with headache or vomiting; followed by frequent bleedings of the nose, with relief from oppression of the chest; her stools became regular. Very slight returns of headache, &c., were removed by Lycopod. 30.—Beauvais, vol. 1, p. 553.—Dr. Hartlaub.

NATRUM MURIATICUM.

In headaches connected with obstinate and protracted chlorosis; defective nutrition; dingy, flaccid, torpid skin; with much nausea and tendency to fainting. Ferr., Calc. or Plumbum may also be required.

In *daily* headaches persisting for 20 days, *relieved* in the open air, but increased by exercise. (See Hepar and Calc.)

Throbbing headaches every morning, especially during menstruation, commencing in the nape and back of the head, extending to the forehead, followed by eructations, nausea, vertigo, and dimness of vision.

NUX VOMICA.

For the fullest information, and a most admirable *résumé* of the action of this, and many other remedies, see Noack and Trink's remarks, reported in Jahr's New Manual, or Symptomen-Codex, translated by Chas. J. Hempel, M.D.

CASE 150.—M. R., a teacher, had suffered for a long time with severe pain in the head, frequent eructations, with inclination to vomit, and actual vomiting, sometimes of mucus, at others of food, followed by more or less relief; his pains were most violent in the morning, aggravated by smoking, and his appetite was often poor.

Treatment.—Nux 24, relieved him entirely.—Beauvais, vol. 1, p. 552.—Dr. Junghansel.

CASE 151.—J. D., aged 52, a thick-set, healthy working man was attacked suddenly, without known cause, with pain on the left side of the head, attended with drawing and shootings; it returned every day at a certain hour, became more and more violent, especially after dinner, and then lasted for about three hours; during the paroxysms he had an entire loss of appetite, became feverish, with a quick and hard pulse, redness of the skin, and was obliged to lie down; towards the end of the attack he perspired a little; he had a bitter taste in his mouth, but little appetite, no thirst; his stools were regular and urine normal. He had already been sick for ten days, and was becoming irritable.

Treatment.—Nux 24, one drop; the next paroxysm was lighter; the second very slight; and he had no subsequent attack for at least six months.—Beauvais, vol. 1, p. 568.

CASE 152.—A lady, past the critical age, had suffered for twenty years with severe headache, which changed its locality frequently; it consisted in drawing and cutting pains, more or less intense, with throbbing and aching in the temples; it often commenced in the back of the head, then suddenly spread to the whole head, attended with pain in the eyes; her head was hot; urine pale and spasmodic, rarely of a natural color, but often slightly red during the attacks. The paroxysms were most severe when the weather was cold and wet, and most frequent in winter; her hair was becoming gray, and fell out in abundance after each attack.

Treatment.—One dose of Nux every six hours, followed by some relief; then other remedies were used without benefit, until Nux was again administered; when Nux was omitted again, the attacks became more frequent and severe; when it was resumed every two hours, relief again followed, and lasted for two months.—Beauvais, vol. 2, p. 30.—DR. SCHMID.

OPIUM.

Has been fully treated of at page 66.

PHOSPHORUS.

Against obstinate tendency to congestion of the head, which resists Acon., Bell. and Opium.

Chronic irritation of the brain—and headache from the slightest vexation.

Headache in the forehead over the eyes, for two days in succession, lasting from morning until evening.

Headache every morning on awaking.

Periodical jerking-throbbing headache over the root of the nose, for eight days in succession, always commencing about nine o'clock in the morning, and most violent about noon, when vomiting sets in.

Headache as if the head would burst, so severe as to force one to cry out—lasting from 6 A. M., until evening.

Headache in the forehead and over the left eye, every morning for twenty-one days in succession, waking one from sleep, and gradually ceasing after getting up and walking about.

CASE 153.—Miss K., aged 24 years, had suffered from early youth with an affection of the head, marked by constant slight pain; and by violent paroxysms several times a week, lasting for a day and night, especially if she had been exposed to a current of air; in the severe attacks the pain became lancinating, commencing in the forehead, extending to the right temple and occiput; her head became heavy, she was obliged to lie down; the pain was increased by eating; she was not able to stoop, as her sight became confused, and the blood rushed to her head; she had but little appetite in general, and often none at all; her bowels were regular; menses scanty, although they lasted eight days, during all of which time the sufferings in her head were much increased.

Treatment.—Sepia 30, was given without effect; Calc. c. 30, with partial relief; but after taking Phosphor. 30, she was entirely cured.—Beauvais, vol 1, p. 566.—Dr. HARTLAUB.

PLATINA.

In headaches of females with an excitable vascular system, too frequent and copious menstruation; especially when the pains increase in severity up to 10 o'clock at night, and are attended with great anguish, burning heat, bright redness of the face, and violent thirst, followed by perspiration.

PULSATILLA. (See page 74.)

CASE 154.—A young lady, aged 23, had suffered with headache for twelve days, after her second confinement.

Symptoms.—Extremely severe pain at intervals, every day, lasting from six to ten hours, attended with cutting pains in the top of the head, and burning in the eyes; nausea soon set in, her mouth became dry and her face flushed; she was obliged to keep the recumbent posture, and dared not make the slightest movement; it seemed as if her head would burst; her pains had increased in severity every day; at first they had been relieved by tying a handkerchief around her head, but now, only the most violent pressure by a stout person, with both hands on her head, afforded her any comfort.

Treatment.—She had been treated allopathically without benefit, for twelve days; then one dose of Pulsat. was given; the next day she only felt a little confusion and heaviness of the head, and on the second day she was well.—Beauvais' Clinique, vol. 1, p. 556.—Dr. Bethman.

CASE 155.—A robust woman, aged 32, had suffered for several months with a disagreeable drawing and twitching pain in the *left* temple; it ceased during the day, but returned regularly every evening and deprived her of rest at night; she had constant noises in the ears and head, both by day and night, both when at rest and when in motion, but more severe in the evening, and then attended with a sensation as if the left side of the vertex were lifted up, and off. This affection of the head, and especially the accompanying sleeplessness, had weakened her very much, and her memory in particular had suffered. She also had twitchings in the left ear, dimness of vision, and for six weeks had been annoyed by a discharge of acrid blood from the vagina; her pulse was small; her temper quiet and patient, but if she closed her eyes she fell into a state of mournful reverie.

Treatment.—She had been bled without relief; then *Pulsat.* 3, was given, and in the course of six days she was almost entirely well. A relapse, three weeks after, from taking cold, was cured in nine days by Rhus.—Beauvais, vol. 1, p. 551.—Dr. Bethman.

RHUS TOXICODENDRON.

In headaches which set in *after every meal*, from the least chagrin, or from exercise in the open air, lasting from 5 P. M.

till bed-time, commencing in the occiput and nape, and extending to the ears, nose, cheek-bones and teeth. Against a peculiarly severe degree of heaviness in the head.

CASE 156.—Mrs. F., aged 37, always subject to headache, had suffered almost constantly for two months, with throbbing, aching, and tearing pains on the top of the head, and in the temples, often accompanied with general trembling of the body; the pains were more severe in the morning, than in the evening; menses regular; general health good.

Treatment.—Bryon. caused some relief, but Rhus cured her entirely in five weeks, after an aggravation lasting several days.—Beauvais, vol. 1, p. 573.

CASE 157.—Mrs. E. suffered with incessant pains in the whole of the head, in the nape and shoulders, with excessive debility, and entire loss of sleep.

Treatment.—She had been treated in vain by an able allopath with anti-spasmodics, narcotics, vesicatories, &c.; one dose of Rhus removed the pains in the head and nape, and restored her sleep; several doses restored her to health. —Beauvais, vol. 2, p. 24.—Dr. Peschier.

SANGUINARIA CANADENSIS.

In sick-headaches with excessive vomiting, water-brash, vomiting of bitter substances; in throbbing headaches with congestion to the head, noises in the ears and fever; in headaches attended with chills, nausea, rheumatic pains and stiffness in the nape and limbs, pain in the whole *left* side of the head, and in the left foot.

SEPIA.

(See page 78.) In the headaches which attend scanty or suppressed menstruation, watery, mucous, sanguineo-mucous, whitish and milk-like, yellowish or purulent, and greenish-red leucorrhœa, with induration of the neck of the uterus. (See Arsen., Creosote, Platina, and other remedies.)

CASE 158.—Miss N., aged 25, blond and thin, had suffered for five years with an affection of the head, which had become especially severe during the last two. It commenced with aching in the left supraorbital region, so that she was obliged to press forcibly upon the eye with her hand; she also had a feeling of dryness and roughness in the eye, and an indescribable pain in all the head. She had such an attack every week, but the approach of her menses, or any unusual emotion, rendered them very severe. She generally waked in the morning with pain, then had no appetite, and was obliged to keep her bed if the sufferings were severe; the paroxysms lasted five or six days, were attended with inclination to vomit, and at times with sudden but transient vertigo, which almost caused her to fall to the ground.

Treatment.—She took ten doses of Sepia 30, at intervals of ten or fourteen days, and although she had two severe attacks during the three months' treatment, she was then entirely relieved of her headaches.—Beauvais, vol. 2, p. 8.—GRIESSELICH.

CASE 159.—Mrs. L., a delicate but healthy brunette, had suffered for several years with attacks of migraine, generally once a week or month, and lasting from twenty-four to thirty-six hours. The pain commenced in a small spot above the right or left eye, extended to the back of the head, where the scalp became very sore to the touch; she was obliged to lie down and avoid the light, had inclination to vomit, and a bad taste in the mouth, as if from indigestion. She had had Tinea capitis in her youth, and had been subject to pimples on the face; her menses were frequent and copious; her sleep was light and disturbed; she had a tendency to congestion to the head; and the soles of her feet were inclined to burn.

Treatment.—She took twelve doses of Sepia 30, at intervals of seven or ten days, and was entirely cured of her headaches in three months, although Sepia rather increased a leucorrhœa with which she had been annoyed for a long time.—Beauvais, vol. 2, p. 9.—DR. GRIESSELICH.

CASE 160.—Miss J. C., aged 10, had suffered for a long time with attacks of headache, especially after active exercise, such as running or jumping; the paroxysms came on at night, as often as every two or three weeks; they consisted of pain above one eye, attended with copious vomiting of mucus.

Treatment.—Bellad. and Nux were given without much benefit, but three doses of Sepia 30, cured her entirely. The attacks at first became milder, and were not attended with vomiting, then ceased entirely.—Ibid., p. 10.

CASE 161.—Mrs. P. R., aged 33, had suffered with headache since her youth, but more severely for the last six months; the attacks came on every five or six weeks, always commencing in the morning as soon as she rose; then the pain became more and more severe, unless she lay down, when it terminated in sleep; she had a pressure and heaviness in the forehead, eyes and root of the nose, attended at times with beating in the head, extending occasionally as far as the occiput. For two days after an attack she was so feeble that she could scarcely rise. For the last six months the headaches had been attended with retching to vomit, always occurring about seven or eight o'clock in the evening. During the intervals of relief, she had confusion of the head with pressure upon the eyes, often attended with heat in and congestion to the head; she had but little appetite, and drank but seldom; had been constipated from her youth; her sleep was heavy, often with troubled dreams, and a paroxysm was generally preceded by a very deep sleep, and by very frightful dreams. Her menses were regular, but rather scanty, and she was often troubled with leucorrhœa. She was becoming inclined to melancholy; and was rather subject to coughs.

Treatment.—She took four doses of Sepia 30, one every eight days; then two doses, one every fifteen days; at the end of which time she seemed cured, as she had had no headache for two months, her general health was improved, and her spirits good.—Ibid., p. 11.

CASE 162.—Mrs. K. R. N., aged 46, stout and strong, had been subject to attacks of headache every three months, ever since she became regular for the first time, but they were becoming more violent, and her physician had announced that he could not cure her. The attacks for the last year had come on every month, at the menstrual period, two days before which she always felt a vague but very severe pain above the right eye; her head became hot; speaking, light, and noise augmented her pains, so that she was obliged to lie down in a room with closed doors and shutters; she suffered night and day without cessation; had sleeplessness and vertigo during the whole period of menstruation, after which the headache changed to a pain in the left temple attended with such acidity of the stomach, that it seemed as if she were under the influence of some corrosive poison, from which, however, she was soon relieved by vomiting. If the headache did not come on before, it was sure to set in during menstruation; the attacks lasted about eight days, but occasionally left behind them a pain on the top of the head, as if it would be forced open, often extending to the occiput, and plunging her into despair. Her menses anticipated two days, and were very abundant, attended with urgency to urinate, and with diarrhœa; at other times she was rather constipated; she had had an attack of gout eighteen years before, of which traces were still present about her hands.

Treatment.—Six doses of Nux 30, at intervals of five or six days, exerted no effect upon her head, although her menses became less copious, and her gouty hand improved; then three doses of Sepia 30, at intervals of eight days, relieved her so much that she only felt some heaviness of the head at the next menstrual period; two doses more of Sepia 30, at intervals of fifteen days, cured her entirely.—Ibid., p. 12.

CASE 163.—A lady, vigorous and brunette, aged 30, had suffered with migraines ever since her youth, and before she became regular for the first time. For the last six or eight years they had become more frequent and severe, so that a day scarcely passed without some suffering, which, however, was most severe during menstruation. If she rode in a carriage, or looked at any object attentively for some time, she was sure to have an attack; the paroxysms generally commenced in the morning; she was soon obliged to lie down, and if she could get asleep, she would wake up well; inclination to vomit and actual vomiting often set in; the pain generally attacked one side of the head, although at times it settled in both temples; menses, and general health normal.

Treatment.—She had but one or two slight attacks after commencing the use of Sepia 30, one dose every five days.—Ibid., p. 13.

CASE 164.—A servant girl, aged 19 years, had suffered for five years with headache, which had increased in violence during the last two; formerly she had attacks only every week, now almost every day, especially in the afternoon or evening.

Symptoms.—She had throbbing in the head, especially on stooping; tearing and lancinating pains in the forehead and face, as if her head had been bruised, often so violent as to oblige her to lie down, when vomiting of bile relieved her for some time. Her menses were always scanty and infrequent, coming on only every five or six weeks; her stools were also scanty, and took place only every second day.

Treatment.—Pulsat. 12, relieved her head somewhat, and her menses became more free; Nux 24, rendered her less costive; and Sepia 30, restored her entirely to health, the cure lasting for at least two years, at last accounts.—Beauvais, vol. 2, p. 28.—DR. SCHULL.

SILICEA.

In headaches attended, or followed by severe pain in the small of the back, with heaviness and uncomfortable feeling in all the limbs.

Obstinate morning headaches, with chilliness and nausea.

CASE 165.—Miss N., aged 26, had suffered for several years with a periodical affection of the head, the paroxysms of which lasted several entire weeks. Her former physician had declared her incurable.

Symptoms.—She had lancinating and drawing pains, sometimes commencing near one temple, at times in both, from whence they extended down into the bones of the face and lower jaw, where they generally attained their greatest intensity. The pain became lancinating in the chin and extended to the teeth, which were in an imperfect state. The pains were present during the day, were often felt in the evening, and commonly awakened her after mid-night. Changes of air did not influence the pains in the head, but exposure to a current of air would. At times the localities of the pains were exceedingly sensitive to touch, at others pressure lessened them. She had long suffered with decayed teeth; was otherwise healthy, and not subject to eruptions.

Treatment.—Bellad. 30, produced no relief in two weeks; then Silex 30, was followed by relief, more or less great for a fortnight; in two weeks more, the pain ceased entirely and did not trouble her again for at least nine months, at last account. —Beauvais, vol. 1, p. 567.—DR. HARTLAUB.

SPIGELIA MARILANDICA

Is a main remedy in the headaches of very hysterical subjects with excitable circulation, subject to violent pain in the back of the head, vertigo, dimness of vision, dilated pupils, to the peculiar hysterical spasms of the eye-lids and face, and even to general convulsions.

Headaches attended with fatiguing palpitations of the heart.

STAPHYSAGRIA.

CASE 166.—An elderly lady had suffered for a long time with violent headache; she awoke in the morning without pain, but while engaged in dressing, washing, or brushing her teeth, throbbing and boring pains set in, in the forehead and part of the left temple; they were increased by lying down again, but gradually became more supportable after sitting down quietly for some time; the pains also diminished gradually in severity during the morning, and disappeared entirely during dinner, but recurred immediately afterwards, although in a moderated degree, and soon ceased entirely for the day, if the patient did not indulge in an afternoon nap.

Treatment.—One dose of Staphysag. removed the disorder immediately and it did not occur again; she soon could dress with comfort, and indulge in her after dinner nap with impunity.—ÆGIDI.—Attomyr, p. 477.

SULPHUR.

In the most obstinate and chronic rheumatic headaches, with *tearing* pains.

In chronic periodical headaches, occurring every other morning, at 8 or 9 o'clock and continuing till bed-time; or every eight days, attended with tearing pains and stupefaction; or violent headache on the top of the head, lasting for twelve hours, and recurring every morning like a periodical fever.

Headaches followed by fetid perspirations.

CASE 167.—A man who worked daily in brass and tin, and who also used paint and varnish occasionally, had suffered for several years with a kind of periodical headache. Every Sunday he experienced a pressure, aching and heaviness of the head, which lasted the whole day and was attended with lassitude, and loss of appetite. On the other six days, he felt nothing of the kind.

Treatment.—Bryon. and Nux were given without benefit; then one dose of Sulph. 3, every six weeks, cured him completely.—Beauvais, vol. 1, p. 551.—DR. SCHULER.

CASE 168.—SCHELLING cured two cases of regularly intermitting Hemicrania, in young persons, with Sulph. 8. One cure was effected in four days, the other in five.—Attomyr, page 477.

CASE 169.—An excitable brunette, aged 30, had suffered for many years with a violent, periodical headache, always occurring simultaneously with the monthly period, and characterized by a raging and painful hammering in the forehead and left temple, which was very much increased by mental emotions, or exertion. She had great irritability of all the senses, pulsations in every part of the body, chilliness of the body with glowing hot face, occasional bleeding from the nose, far sightedness, and roaring in the left ear, when she lay upon it; her stools were hard and difficult; her hair fell out profusely; she was irritable and inclined to anger.

Treatment.—Three doses of Sulph. 30, one dose every three days, followed after the lapse of four weeks by Sepia 30. She was entirely cured by this course of medication, and it seemed as if Sulph. was by far the most beneficial remedy.—Attomyr, p. 478.—Dr. Wurda.

VERATRUM ALBUM.

It acts upon the nerves of sensation as specifically as Nux v. does upon the nerves of motion; and acts upon the cerebral nerves much less decidedly than upon the great sympathetic, and spinal nerves of sensation. Veratrum and Veratrine excite and arouse the nerves of sensation, Aconite stupefies or paralyzes them.

On account of its specific action upon the abdominal organs and nerves and secondary action upon the head, it becomes a principal remedy in the true dyspeptic or sick-headache.

The indications for its use are numerous and important. It is useful in headaches attended with vomiting of green mucus; in those with pain in the small of the back, colic, and desire to vomit; in violent headache, attended with profuse flow of urine; aching pain in one side of the head, with pain in the stomach; severe headache, increased while the patient is walking, to such a degree that he staggers; drawing pain in the head, and in the small of the back; excessive headache, ceasing on the setting in of the menses. Headache with feeling as if the hairs were electrified, with tendency of them to stand on end.

In nervous headaches and nervous conditions attended with electric sensations; electric current in the nerves radiating in various directions; sensation as if boiling water were running down the back; electric current shooting to the nervous plexuses of the abdomen, breast and heart; pricking and tingling sensations in various parts, or burning and prickling sensations followed by electric emanations shooting in every direction; feeling as if cold air were blowing on several parts of the body, followed or not by sensation as if hot drops were poured on the limbs. Intense feeling of pain extending over the peripheral nerves, with drawing pains all along the spinal marrow, &c.

In headaches attended with burning, or a peculiar feeling of coldness in the stomach; with water-brash, disgust for food, nausea, colic and diarrhœa, irritation of the bladder, pains in the back, hips and knees, and increased flow of menses.

Headache with constant sickness at the stomach, with spinal irritation, constant twitchings of the limbs, diarrhœa, increased secretion of bile.

It cures headaches, and neuralgic pains which shoot to various parts, much more readily than it does fixed pains.

I have succeeded in curing several most obstinate and distressing headaches with Tinct. Verat., and with the 2d or 3d dilution of Tinct. Veratrine.

INDEX.

NOTICE.

To obtain the most rapid yet thorough and practical knowledge of the contents of this volume:

1st. Glance over the *Preface* and *Introduction;*

2d. Read carefully the remarks on the action of the different remedies against headache, in the *Synopsis*.

3d. Read the *General Remarks* before, and the *Reviews* and *Notes*, after the cases given in the body of the work.

4th. Look over the *Cases* both in the body of the work, and in the *Synopsis*.

5th. Finally, make use of the *General Review* and *Index*.

HOMŒOPATHIC MEDICINES.

Wm. Radde, 322 Broadway, New York, respectfully informs the Homœopathic Physicians, and the friends of the System, that he is the sole Agent for the Leipzig Central Homœopathic Pharmacy, and that he has always on hand a good assortment of the best Homœopathic Medicines, in complete sets or by single vials, in *Tinctures, Dilutions* and *Triturations;* also, *Pocket Cases of Medicines; Physicians' and Family Medicine Chests to Laurie's Domestic* (60 to 82 Remedies) —EPP'S (60 Remedies)—HERING'S (60 Remedies to 102).—*Small Pocket Cases* at $3, with Family Guide and 27 Remedies—*Cases* containing 415 vials, with Tinctures and Triturations for Physicians.—*Cases* with 260 Vials of Tinctures and Triturations to Jahr's New Manual, or Symptomen-Codex.—Physicians' *Pocket Cases*, with 60 Vials of Tinctures and Triturations.—*Cases* from 200 to 300 Vials, with low and high dilutions of medicated pellets.—*Cases* from 50 to 80 Vials of low and high dilutions, &c., &c. Homœopathic Chocolate. Refined Sugar of Milk, pure Globules, &c. *Arnica Tincture*, the best specific remedy for bruises, sprains, wounds, &c. *Arnica Plaster*, the best application for *Corns. Urtica urens* and Dr. Reisig's *Homœopathic Pain Extractor* are the best specific remedies for *Burns*. Also, Books, Pamphlets, and Standard Works on the System, in the English, French, and German languages.

HOMŒOPATHIC BOOKS.

JAHR'S NEW MANUAL OF HOMŒOPATHIC PRACTICE; edited, with Annotations, by A. Gerald Hull, M. D. From the last Paris edition. This is the fourth American edition of a very celebrated work, written in French by the eminent Homœopathic Professor Jahr, and it is considered the best practical compendium of this extraordinary science that has yet been composed. After a very judicious and instructive introduction, the work presents a Table of the Homœopathic Medicines, with their names in Latin, English and German; the order in which they are to be studied, with their most important distinctions, and clinical illustrations of their symptoms and effects upon the various organs and functions of the human system. The second volume embraces an elaborate Analysis of the indications in disease, of the medicines adapted to cure, and a Glossary of the technics used in the work, arranged so luminously as to form an admirable guide to every medical student The whole system is here displayed with a modesty of pretension, and a scrupulosity in statement, well calculated to bespeak candid investigation. This laborious work is indispensable to the students and practitioners of Homœopathy, and highly interesting to medical and scientific men of all classes. Complete Symptomatology and Repertory, 2 vols. bound, $6.

JAHR'S NEW MANUAL: originally published under the name of Symptomen-Codex. (Digest of Symptoms.) This work is intended to facilitate a comparison of the parallel symptoms of the various Homœopathic agents, thereby enabling the practitioner to discover the characteristic symptoms of each drug, and to determine with ease and correctness what remedy is most Homœopathic to the existing group of symptoms. Translated with important and extensive additions from various sources, by Charles Julius Hempel, M. D., assisted by James M. Quin, M. D., with revisions and clinical notes by John F. Gray, M. D.; contributions by Drs. A. Gerald Hull, George W. Cook, and Dr. B. F. Joslin of New-York; and Drs. C. Hering, J. Jeanes, C. Neidhard, W. Williamson, and J. Kitchen, of Philadelphia; with a Preface by Constantine Hering, M. D., 2 vols., bound $11

A

TREATISE ON APOPLEXY:

WITH AN APPENDIX

ON

SOFTENING OF THE BRAIN, AND PARALYSIS.

ON THE

NATURE AND CAUSES

OF

APOPLEXY.

APOPLEXY has generally been regarded as so simple and decided in its nature and required treatment, that any self-sufficient and semi-ignorant physician who knows how to bleed and purge, has been thought competent to understand and manage it. But the truth is, as COPELAND says: There are but few diseases which present a greater variety of modes of attack; or which arise from a greater number of affections both of the brain and its vessels, or of other and remote parts; or which differ so widely in the extent and severity of the injury done to the brain;—consequently there are but few diseases which require such precise and prompt, but varied, and comprehensive treatment. A glance at some of the names of the different admitted varieties of Apoplexy, will render this more evident than many words; we have:

(1.) Apoplexy from excess of blood in the whole system; the quantity of blood being absolutely greater than the organism requires for its proper nutrition and sustenance (PLETHORIC APOPLEXY).

(2.) Apoplexy from retention, or rush of blood to the head, without rupture of any blood-vessel, or excess of blood in the system (CONGESTIVE APOPLEXY).

(3.) Apoplexy from rupture of some blood-vessel, in, or about the brain, not necessarily caused by plethora or congestion, but frequently arising from brittleness, or other disease of the arteries of the brain (HÆMORRHAGIC APOPLEXY).

(4.) Apoplexy from debility, or other nervous disorder of the brain, or nervous system, and not necessarily accompanied with any disease of the blood, or blood-vessels (NERVOUS APOPLEXY).

(5.) From an increased quantity of watery fluid poured out suddenly upon, or in the brain (SEROUS APOPLEXY).

(6.) From primary disease, or enlargement of the heart (CARDIAC APOPLEXY).

(7.) From disease, or disorder of the liver, and retention of bile in the system, which are notoriously apt to cause heaviness of the system, and drowsiness (BILIOUS, OR HEPATIC APOPLEXY).

(8.) From Bright's, or other disease of the kidneys (NEPHRITIC, OR ALBUMINOUS APOPLEXY).

(9.) FEBRILE, OR INFLAMMATORY APOPLEXY.

(10.) From debility, or loss of blood (ASTHENIC, ATONIC, OR ANÆMIC APOPLEXY).

(11.) From indigestion, repletion, or other disorder of the stomach (GASTRIC APOPLEXY).

(12.) From convulsions in general, and epilepsy in particular (CONVULSIVE, OR SPASMODIC APOPLEXY).

(13.) From the effects of pregnancy (PUERPERAL APOPLEXY).

(14.) From injuries, blows on the head, &c. (TRAUMATIC APOPLEXY).

Many other varieties, and very many combinations of these forms of Apoplexy might easily be given, and I believe that not only all those above mentioned, but others, also, will be exemplified by the cases to follow in the body of this work; but sufficient has been done to give a fair view of the many different causes which are capable of producing Apoplexy, and to justify at the outset a protest against a *routine* treatment of all apoplectic conditions.

It must be equally evident that all cases of Apoplexy are not equally dangerous and fatal; some, will recover with little or no treatment, mainly by the recuperative powers of nature; others, will prove fatal in spite of all remedial means, either gentle, or heroic. But by far the most dangerous and frequent occurrence in Apoplexy, is the rupture of a blood-vessel in, or about the brain; and the result in recovery or death depends mainly upon the fact whether the artery which has given way be large or small, the quantity of blood which is poured in or upon the brain be great or trifling, and the laceration, contusion or compression of the brain be extensive or moderate. I repeat that the result in recovery, partial recovery, or death, does, or ought to depend, as much upon these circumstances, as upon the mode of treatment; although, it seems unfortunately, but too probable, that some of the milder cases are either allowed to progress into the severer forms by inefficient treatment, or else are treated so savagely and heroically as to be rendered fatal, when they would have terminated favorably with very gentle management.

WATSON candidly informs us: that "after a formal attack of Apoplexy, the results of allopathic treatment will be very uncertain; a large effusion of blood in, or upon the brain will prove fatal; a smaller amount of extravasation cannot be removed at all promptly by ordinary medical means; and that the best which the unfortunate patient can expect in too many cases, will be a long-continued or permanent palsy, a weakening of the mental powers, and sometimes a state nearly approaching to idiocy."

On the other hand, YELDHAM (see Homœopathy in Acute Diseases, p. 173) says: "It must not be supposed that Homœopathy, any more than Allopathy, pretends to cure every apoplectic patient; on the contrary, it is well known that there are many cases (as, for example, where, from the rupture of a vessel, a large quantity of blood is poured out, and presses on the brain) in which all medical treatment must, from a physical necessity, prove unavailing. In cases of this kind, the two systems, as far as relates to a *cure*, are on an equality." But while I admit this, I think it may be asserted positively that in the majority of these cases, the most prompt and heroic allopathic treatment does not, and cannot save life; and that the gentle, or so-called inefficient homœopathic treatment is not the cause of death.

But we are not obliged to deal in general assertions only: COPEMAN has collected 250 cases of Apoplexy treated allopathically, and many of them by the magnates of the profession, such as Morgagni, Portal, Abercrombie, Andral and others, and yet only sixty-eight recovered, seven escaped with their lives, and no less than 175 died. He says that this proves, not only, that the mortality from Apoplexy under old-school treatment is fearfully great, but that the proximate causes of the disease are either beyond the reach of medical art, or that the measures usually adopted in the dominant school are inapplicable, inefficient, or prejudicial.

In the New-York Hospital from 1847 to 1851, of thirty-five cases of Apoplexy, seventeen cases died, or about one-half; of seventeen cases reported by Dr. Huss, in the British and Foreign Medical Review (see Oct. No., 1846, p. 461), and treated allopathically, in 1842, eight cases proved fatal, or about one-half; in the preceding year, however, only four cases died out of fifteen, or about one-fourth.

On the other hand, we learn from the General Homœopathic Hospital Report, that of twenty-one cases of Apoplexy treated according to the views of Hahnemann, six died, or about one-third; four were not cured, or about one-fifth; and eleven recovered, or about one-half. These results are fully as favorable as those of the best, and much better than the general average of allopathic treatment; besides, in the following pages, upwards of sixty cases of recovery from Apoplexy under homœopathic treatment will be given. Still, the number which die under both modes of treatment, is certainly sufficiently great to render it but simply just, that each of the great contending parties should exercise great charity in judging of each other's practice. It seems equally true that in the present state of medical science, in at least one-fourth of all the cases of Apoplexy, every painful and cruel endeavor to save the patient's life should be instantly or quickly abandoned, and the physician's sole and earnest attention limited to soothing the fast-fleeting moments of the sufferer.

Premonitions of Apoplexy.

COPELAND has given the best *resumé* of the premonitory symptoms of Apoplexy, especially of the plethoric and congestive varieties. He says that, "The most common precursory symptoms are: a tendency to sleep at unaccustomed periods, a heavier sleep than usual, particularly if accompanied with profound, laborious or stertorous breathing; gritting of the teeth; nightmare; sudden jerks or starts of the body, when on the point of falling asleep; lethargic feelings and drowsiness, even during the waking hours; pains in different parts of the head; or general headache, with a sense of weight or fulness in the head; and pulsation of the arteries, especially if there also be a turgid appearance of the veins of the head and forehead, with lividity or redness of the countenance; slight or imperfect attacks of bleeding from the nose; loss of recollection, or an unusual serenity, or apathy of the mind; a disposition to shed tears; more especially if there also be torpor and numbness, or pricking of the extremities; partial or slight paralytic affections, marked by distortion of the mouth, drooping of the eyelids, imperfect utterance, or unsteady, or tremulous gait, and tripping on ascending, or descending stairs.

According to DAY, these premonitory symptoms require the utmost care, and caution on the part of the physician—for there are various and perfectly distinct conditions which may give rise to apparently similar head-symptoms; excess of blood and deficiency of blood; general debility; and an impure condition of the blood, from poor digestion, or imperfect action of the skin, liver, kidneys, or bowels, may all give rise to very similar symptoms. Anæmia, or deficiency of blood, may very easily be mistaken for hyperæmia, or excess of blood, and simple irritation of the brain may be mistaken for inflammation.

Headache, vertigo, or dizziness, singing in the ears, and throbbing of the arteries of the head may arise from either of the opposite states of excess, or deficiency of blood in the head. But, if excess of blood be present, the patient generally presents the appearance of rude health, is stout, short-necked, and even bull-necked; his face is flushed, he has headache, a tendency to doze, and dizziness which is increased by stooping, or looking upwards; nausea also is a common symptom of pressure on the brain.

When there is anæmia, or deficiency of blood in the whole system, and also in the brain, we usually observe the face to be pale, the heart's action quick and tumultuous, a tendency to faintness and dizziness, which are most felt on suddenly assuming the upright position. Still, the presence of headache, the feeling as if an iron band were around the forehead, with noises in the ears, throbbing in the head and neck, will be very apt to mislead the old-school physician, especially as it unfortunately happens that bleeding will give temporary relief. Aconite, and other depressing agents must be used most cautiously by the homœopathist, who fortunately has a strong prejudice in favor of the use of *China* in such states.

Again, aged persons are liable to a peculiar form of head-affection, depending for the most part on passive congestion, arising from want of tone in the vascular system. The compound infusion of horse-radish is much recommended in the old practice—*Carb. veg.*, in the new.

There is also a state of brain common in advanced life, characterised by alteration or diminution of the nervous energy, arising from general debility, over-exertion of the intellectual faculties, or long-continued anxiety, and distress of mind. Bleeding would most probably induce incurable paralysis, while Anacardium, Baryta, or other homœopathic remedies, may cause great relief.

A few more remarks may be made here, on other of the premonitory symptoms of Apoplexy. A flushed face, tendency to sleep, dizziness, nausea and headache, have already been alluded to; but sometimes unusual wakefulness points to an irritation of the brain, which may bring on Apoplexy, unless allayed by sedative treatment; a general incapacity for exertion, and an indescribable sensation of weight in the limbs may arise from fulness of blood about the head and spine, from a sluggish circulation, or from great debility; torpor, numbness, or a sense of creeping, crawling or formication, loss or perversion of feeling, so that everything touched feels like velvet, or felt, or itching in the limbs may arise from fulness or sluggishness of the blood, from a purely nervous affection, or from softening of the brain; slight paralytic affections, such as drooping of an eyelid, or distortion of the features, may arise from congestion of the brain, or slight apoplectic effusion, or from debility of the nerves of the part; double vision, difficulty of writing in a straight line, or of reading, the presence of motes or corruscations before the eyes, noises in the ears, or dulness of hearing, may be caused by excess or deficiency of blood in the head, by great debility of the nerves of the eyes or ears, or by indigestion; the substitution of one word for another, difficulty in pronouncing certain words, a sudden loss of memory, may all arise from weakness of the brain, a deficient flow of blood to it, or from the pressure of an excessive quantity of blood.

If the physician can constantly keep these distinctions and differences in his mind, he will rarely go wrong in his treatment; unless he be so slavishly wedded to system, that he will not follow the dictates of his own, and others' reason, and experience. But it unfortunately happens that in very many cases *no* premonitory symptoms precede an attack of Apoplexy. ROCHOUX even goes so far as to declare that in 69 cases in which he collected the histories, only 11 presented precursory symptoms; in such cases a fit of Apoplexy will, of course, set in without any warning, and the physician must treat the attack as best he may.

Prevention of Apoplexy.

The principal point generally dwelt on, is: to prevent too great fulness of blood in the head. This may arise either from too great a quantity thrown to it, by excessive action of the heart and arteries (Aconite); or, too great retention of blood in the brain and head, from retarded circulation (Conium, Carbo); or from diminished nervous energy (Nux, Plumbum).

HARTMANN says that in most cases we are undoubtedly

called upon to treat, or prevent nervous Apoplexy, because passive congestive-Apoplexy generally depends on nervous debility; and active congestive-Apoplexy upon nervous irritation of the brain, exciting increased flow of blood to it; or upon excitement of the sympathetic nerve, which presides over the circulation (Veratrum, Nux, Coffea). If there be a rupture of a small blood-vessel, Arnica, Veratrum, Millefolium, or Kreosote deserve attention.

We can prevent too much blood being made, by great care in diet and regimen. Watson gives the case of Dr. Adam Ferguson, of Edinburgh, who was a man of full habit, at one time corpulent and very ruddy, and, though by no means intemperate, lived fully. He had premonitions of Apoplexy, to which he paid no attention, and finally, in his 60th year, had a decided attack of Apoplexy, with paralysis. He recovered, and then became a strict Pythagorean in his diet, eating nothing but vegetables, and drinking only water and milk. He got rid of every paralytic symptom, became even robust and muscular, and died in full possession of his faculties, at the advanced age of 93; full thirty years after his first attack. Long after his 80th year his firm step, and ruddy cheek, contrasted agreeably and unexpectedly with his silver locks.

This course of diet is necessarily only suited against *true plethora*, or that state of the system in which an absolutely greater quantity of blood is made than the organism requires for its sustenance.

On the other hand, those who are pale and delicate, have lost much blood, or are reduced by chronic cough with profuse expectoration, by severe dyspepsia, or long-continued diarrhœa, or diabetes, or profuse flow of menses, or piles, &c., may require tonic diet, meat, even wine, China, Ferrum, &c. Still, if there be disease or brittleness of the blood-vessels—which may often be detected by the presence of a peculiar fulness or hardness of the pulse at the wrist—we should be very careful of stimulants.

Anything which is calculated to hurry the circulation

and increase the force of the heart's action, such as strong bodily exercise, anger, violent passion, loud and earnest talking, brisk or hurried walking, galloping on a hard horse, should be avoided; holding the breath, especially when some muscular effort is made, such as tugging at a tight boot, holding a high note in singing, in a violent paroxysm of coughing, or in straining at stool, are particularly dangerous; in all these acts blood is thrown violently to the head, the face may turn purple, the patient become giddy, the eyes bloodshot, and a fit of Apoplexy come on. Violent vomiting, sneezing, laughing, crying, singing, shouting, all have a somewhat similar effect. In short, a person liable to Apoplexy is obliged to exert such control over body and mind, that SOLLY categorically asserts, he must be content to live like a cabbage, to vegetate, merely exist, and barely live. Far better would it be for them to live like Dr. Adam Ferguson, already alluded to, whose mixture of original thinking with high moral feeling and extensive learning, his love of country, contempt of luxury, and especially the strong subjection of his passions and feelings to the dominion of his reason, made him, perhaps, the most striking example of the stoic philosopher which could be seen in modern days.—(WATSON.)

Dr. Fothergill thought it very unsafe for short-necked people to look backwards for any length of time, without turning the rest of the body, thus twisting the neck. He gives the case of a man seized with Apoplexy, while crossing a river in an open boat, keeping his eyes fixed upon a particular ship, until long after he had rowed past her.

Tight cravats are also injurious. A Swedish officer who was desirous that his men should look well in the face, caused them to wear tight stocks; in a short time quite a number of his regiment died of Apoplexy. The case of a boy is also given who had drawn his neckcloth remarkably tight, and was seized with Apoplexy, while exerting himself whipping a top.

Cold, is another frequent exciting cause of Apoplexy; it drives the blood from the surface, and accumulates it in the large vessels of the interior of the body. I have known several elderly persons, with a marked tendency to congestion of the head, attacked while dressing or undressing in a cold room, loitering about with their shoes and stockings off, and remaining partially, or very nearly undressed for a long time.

On the other hand, expansion of the blood may be caused by hot and stimulating food and drinks, large fires, crowded rooms, excessive heat of the sun, hot baths, &c. The whole mass of the blood becomes expanded, and cooling and refrigerating means are required.

This last state of the blood has been greatly overlooked by almost all writers on affections of the brain, although it was well known to the ancients. According to them, the so-called *Plethora ad volumen* depends upon an apparent quantitative increase of the blood from expansion, or increase of its volume, without actual increase of quantity. It was supposed to arise from vital turgor, nervous orgasm, or simple expansion of the blood from excessive heat. The best marked examples occur in sun-struck persons. SOLLY's friend, Dr. SAMUEL ROGERS, gives a most graphic description of this form of Apoplexy, as caused by great exposure to the heat of the sun. He says: "About 8 o'clock, a most melancholy scene commenced among the troops; men were seen to drop down and instantly expire; every hour added to our melancholy situation, for notwithstanding the utmost exertions of the physicians, the day ended with no less a loss than 18, and left us with 63 sick in the hospital. When warning of the attack was given to the patients, they usually complained of difficult breathing, with a sense of tightness and oppression about the chest, followed by giddiness, burning heat of the eyes, and a sense of great fulness about the head, in many amounting to excruciating pain, succeeded by loss of sense and motion, faltering of the tongue on attempting to speak, fulness of the eyes, dilated and fixed pupils, violent twitching of the muscles of the face, particularly those about the mouth, subsultus tendinum, and involuntary stools. Along with these symptoms the patient also had a strong, full, and frequent pulse, tremendous throbbing of the carotid and temporal arteries, flushed, swollen, and sometimes livid countenance, and throughout, a parched and burning skin."

Rogers says that "the violence, suddenness and urgency of the symptoms seemed to require immediate and profuse depletion; blood was accordingly abstracted from every assailable point, viz., the arm, jugular vein, and temporal artery; cold was applied to the head, and the feet were immersed in hot water; blisters were applied to the head, neck and legs; brisk purgatives were administered, and their operation assisted by purgative injections. In some cases, fifty, sixty, or even one hundred ounces of blood were taken, but the remedy was sometimes worse than the malady; in fact, two individuals became convulsed, and died shortly after they were bled, and after death it was found that although the heart was empty, the vessels of the head were loaded with blood. This clearly indicated that, whatever it was, that excited the heart's inordinate action, bloodletting would not subdue it, for as long as a drop of blood remained, it was sent to the head. How lucky it was for us (Dr. S. ROGERS), and truly so for our patients, that a most effectual remedy was found in the *cold affusion*. Just as one man had expired, as one might say, almost under the lancet, another was brought into the hospital; he was put into a bathing tub, and a constant stream of cold water poured on his head until he was relieved."—(SOLLY *on the Brain*, p. 392.)

Treatment of the Premonitions of Apoplexy.

I trust it has been made evident, that there is no more delicate, or momentous question in the practice of medicine, than that of the prevention, or primary treatment of attacks of Apoplexy; because, as we have seen, these seizures may arise from such different, or even opposite causes, that the very course of treatment, and regimen which is most conducive to safety in one case, has an opposite tendency in others.

If the patient be decidedly and undoubtedly plethoric, or full-blooded, a moderate bleeding may be allowed, if the symptoms be urgent, in order to reduce the whole quantity of blood to the healthy standard. This may avert danger, and certainly will not interfere with the action of the most delicate homœopathic remedies; but if the symptoms be not urgent, the excess of blood may be more slowly reduced by dietetic, and medical means. In deciding on the propriety of blood-letting, it is very important to be certain whether *true plethora* be present, or an absolutely greater quantity of blood than the organism requires for its sustenance, or can readily control the circulation of. If true plethora, or exceedingly active and dangerous congestion be *not* present, the physician should discard the *lancet;* but there can be no earthly objection to bathing the feet in simple hot water, or in hot pepper-, or mustard-water; the head and shoulders should be raised, the clothes all loosened, and cold applications made to the head. If the bowels be obstinately costive, or even moderately sluggish, some mild but efficient purgative, such as castor oil, may be given at once; or if the attack arise from the suppression of piles, or menses, Aloes should be preferred as a purgative. Aloes may also be given when there is bilious derangement, although as HARTMANN says, that Mercurius solubilis corresponds to every variety of Apoplexy, it may be allowable to give this in sufficient quantities to act on the liver and bowels, in appropriate cases. I say appropriate cases, because there are others, which are characterised by pallor of the patient, an inclination to dizziness with faintishness, palpitation, nervous tremors and timidity, in which all the symptoms are increased when the stomach is empty, or the bowels are freely moved, or from looking upwards, or resuming the upright position after stooping, or rising from bed, and in which all the above treatment would be injurious.

Aconite is regarded as the principal remedy when there is great heat and feverishness of the head and body (see article on Aconite); Bellad. or Stramonium, when there is great and active congestion to the head, with excessive restlessness, and more or less delirium; Opium, when there is a more passive- and venous-congestion, with much drowsiness, great constipation and some stupor; Cocculus, when nausea and giddiness constitute the prominent symptoms;

China, when there is beating in the head, with palpitation of the heart, dimness of sight, buzzing in the ears, heavy breathing, &c. Hartmann says that when the excessive use of coffee or wine causes an assemblage of symptoms much resembling those of Apoplexy, viz: fulness of blood about the head, bursting pain with commotion of the blood and throbbing of the arteries, constant uneasiness and heaviness of the limbs, languor and lassitude even from the least exertion, redness of the vessels of the eye, with sudden and frequently recurring paroxysms of loss of sight or darkness before the eyes with dizziness, obliging the patient to lie down, noises in the ears, &c., then Nux will remove many of the symptoms, especially if constipation also be present, but Belladonna may be required, and also to be assisted by several doses of Mercurius. Coffea has also been recommended, if the attack be of a nervous character, occurring in delicate and nervous persons, from great mental excitement, or from indigestion after a hearty meal, especially when the patient is excessively nervous, sad, sleepless from excessive bodily and mental excitement, with frequent flushes of heat to the face, dizziness, heaviness of the head, anxious restlessness of the whole body, sensitiveness of hearing, &c. Arnica has also been strongly recommended when symptoms of congestion to the head appear after a full or improper meal, especially if the head be hot, and the hands and feet cold. When spasmodic symptoms are prominent, Nux and Ignatia are the most homœopathic remedies. If suppression of perspiration has brought on the attack, Aconite and Opium should be thought of; if the urine be scanty, Cantharides and Digitalis; if the menses be scanty or suppressed, Pulsatilla and Stramonium, or Conium; while Ipecac. has been highly recommended in *Gastric* Apoplexy when the patient is restless, starts frequently, is irritable and inclined to vomit. Veratrum is particularly indicated, when the patient is pale, cold, and faint. The treatment of fully developed attacks of Apoplexy will be given minutely, when treating more especially of the different varieties of the disease.

TRUE, OR TYPICAL APOPLEXY,

With preceding plethora and congestion, followed by hemorrhage and paralysis.

The model type of Apoplexy occurs in persons with a robust body, ruddy complexion, who are hearty and stout by nature or good living, have too much blood in the whole system, and proportionately still more in the brain, or head. This is by far *not* the most frequent form of Apoplexy, although it has fixed the ideas of world about the nature and treatment of the disease.

Symptoms.—Such a plethoric, juicy and heavy man, apparently in good health, suddenly falls down deprived of all his senses, wholly unconscious of surrounding objects, his countenance livid, the vessels of the face and head turgid with blood, his breathing snoring or stertorous, his pulse full, slow, and intermitting, his limbs powerless. In the most violent cases, all the limbs are paralysed, but generally, the paralysis is confined to one-half of the body, in the form of hemiplegia; sometimes only a single limb is affected, and in this case the arm is much more frequently paralysed than the leg. The paralysis may be confined to the face, tongue, eyes, their lids, or other parts (see Hemorrhagic Apoplexy). From this state the patient may never rally, even under the most active allopathic, anti-phlogistic, and revulsive treatment; he often sinks without any change for the better in his symptoms, and dies in the course of forty-eight hours. This, Solly truly says, is an awful disease to suffer from, to witness, or to administer to; but death soon closes the scene, and the brain when examined after death, is found to have been more or less torn and destroyed by large masses, and clots of blood extravasated into and upon the brain. The case is *typical* because the extravasation of blood is so copious and severe that all the effects of extravasation are produced; all the centres of nervous power within the skull are either crushed, torn or compressed; or ploughed up by, and intimately mixed and intermingled with gore; while the neighborhood of large and rather large clots is converted into a more or less suffused, red, soft, and very moist, papescent mass consisting of comminuted and crushed brain-substance (SOLLY). Hence, the destruction of the brain is often so extensive that the patient cannot live by any possibility, except as a mere wreck of his former self; a burthen and a loathing to himself, an object of pity and the tenderest cares, perhaps, to his nearest and dearest relatives.

Typical Apoplexy is both *congestive*, i. e., an increased quantity of blood is thrown to, or retained in, or about the brain; and *hæmorrhagic*, i. e., more or less of blood has burst the bounds of its blood-vessels and been poured out, in or upon the brain. Too much blood was present in the system before the attack; too much blood has, perhaps, frequently flowed to the brain, but subsided without dangerous consequences; the blood-vessels of the brain have, doubtless, been frequently distended with blood before, but now the brain remains intensely crowded with blood, and one or more blood-vessels have given way, and are pouring out blood copiously upon the brain. The indication is, of course, to reduce as rapidly as possible the whole amount of blood in the system, at least to the natural standard, and especially to relieve the brain from its excess of blood, and stop the bleeding into, or upon its substance.

Plethora.

The principal points in typical Apoplexy, are: general plethora, or blood-fulness of the body, attended with great congestion to the head. Hence we propose to examine the subject of plethora more fully in this place. Watson says: in the adult state when the growth of the body has been completed, that blood may be made in greater abundance and more rich in the materials of nutrition than the wants of the body require, is not only conceivable, but true; full living and sedentary habits are causes likely to occasion general plethora, and they do occasion it; full diet, so long as the digestive powers are perfect, provides more chyle and conducts into the blood a larger quantity of its pabulum; a sedentary life precludes that freer circulation of the blood, and that more liberal expenditure of it through the skin, and by means of the other organs of secretion, which would occur under more active habits. Such persons are apt to become fat, the adipose tissue seeming to form a kind of safety-valve for the diversion of the superfluous blood; the muscular and fibrous tissues, however, suffer in their nutrition, because the imperfect respiration of heavy and sluggish persons does not form fibrin in sufficient quantity for their full development. Such persons naturally have turgid and florid cheeks, red lips, red mucous membranes, and not uncommonly ferretty eyes; their entire vascular system is preternaturally distended, and if you open a vein, you find that they bear a large abstraction of blood without fainting, and are even refreshed by it; while the blood drawn separates into a large, but not very firm mass of coagulum, with but little seren (WATSON).

The blood of the plethoric is also deficient in fibrin, and hence, decidedly inclined to hemorrhage. According to ANDRAL, in plethora and congestion of the brain, the fibrin of the blood is apt to *diminish* from $\frac{3}{1000}$ to $\frac{2}{1000}$; the quantity of blood globules to *increase* from $\frac{127}{1000}$ to $\frac{152}{1000}$; the solids of the serum to *increase* from $\frac{80}{1000}$ to $\frac{105}{1000}$, and the quantity of water or serum to *diminish* from $\frac{800}{1000}$ to $\frac{740}{1000}$. Hence the blood will be thicker, more sluggish in its action and less inclined to form a clot or coagulate, and even is disposed to exude from its vessels in the form of hemorrhage. The effect of this kind of blood upon the brain and other organs, is admirably described by BECQUEREL and RODIER; they say, that in true plethora or full-bloodedness, not only is the whole mass of the blood increased, but sudden accumulations of it in internal parts, frequently in the brain, are apt to occur, disturbing its functions, causing fits of insensibility, and sometimes even death itself. It is only too true, when blood already exists in too great abundance throughout the body, that it is apt to fall in excess upon any debilitated, or irritated organ. Above, we have referred almost exclusively to *true plethora* (PLETHORA ERA), or that state in which a greater quantity of blood is present than the organism requires for its healthy nutrition and sustenance. True plethora is necessarily universal, (plethora universalis) as contradistinguished from local or partial plethoras, (*plethora partialis*); it may also be not only venous, but also arterial in its character (*plethora venosa et arteriosa*); and of course, is widely distinguished from dyscratic-plethora, such as occurs in albuminuria, hydræmia, and other affections (*plethora cacochyma*). The principal causes of true plethora are: 1st, excessive production of blood, especially when associated with diminished consumption of it; this is particularly apt to be the case in true plethora, in which we have seen that the blood is deficient in fibrin, hence is less plastic, less inclined to assume a coagulable or solid form, consequently more disposed to remain as blood, rather than to be converted into any organized product. Arterial congestion and plethora are closely allied to the above state of things; the conveyed arterial blood is changed too slowly into venous, in consequence either of diminished nutrition of the tissues, or other causes, and consequently the arterial blood is only slowly and imperfectly driven from such parts.

Another form of plethora is the so-called *plethora ad vires*, in which the quantity of blood in the system, is relatively too great for its powers; this is apt to occur from nervous or mental exhaustion, long continued or extravagant grief, or anxiety, sudden fright, depressing mental emotions, &c. Of course the principal indication is not to remove blood, but to arouse and invigorate the nervous system.

The so-called *plethora ad volumen* has already been alluded to; but the fact that the blood in a dead body occupies only one-tenth part of the space which it occupies in the living one, may here be referred to in proof of the close connection which the volume of blood has with its life, or with its amount of orgasm, or vital turgor. The opposite of this state, or *collapse of the blood*, may be produced by depressing agents such as Digitalis, Prussic acid, Tobacco, deficient nervous energy, &c.; the pulse is then apt to be small, soft and frequent; the surface pale and cold, sensation and motion either deficient or extinct. In plethora ad volumen the pulse is apt to be full, large, slow, heavy and oppressed.

One other form may be mentioned, viz.: the *plethora ad spatium*, such as is apt to occur from diminution of the calibre of the blood-vessels, or after the loss of large and important limbs. (Stark.)

Although plethora is only one element of true or *typical* Apoplexy, particular attention has been paid to it here because the other elements, viz.: congestion, hæmorrhage, and paralysis will be treated of more fully under the heads of *Congestive, Hæmorrhagic, and Paralytic Apoplexy.*

Treatment of Typical Apoplexy. Ferrum is the most important homœopathic remedy against true plethora and Apoplexy. It is well known to increase the quantity of blood globules; but it is not so well known to diminish the quantity of fibrin in the blood. Simon found the fibrin to diminish from the normal standard of $\frac{3}{1000}$ as low as $\frac{1\cdot 3}{1000}$, after the use of sixty-four grains of iron in the course of seven weeks; Andral and Gavarret found it to lessen the quantity of fibrin in one case from the normal standard, to $\frac{2\cdot 5}{1000}$, in the course of four weeks; in another case from $\frac{3\cdot 5}{1000}$, or an excess above the normal mean, to $\frac{3}{1000}$, or the natural standard. Ferrum is also well known to diminish the quantity of water in the blood. Hence as far as the pathology of the disease is a guide, it is *a*, or even *the*, most homœopathic remedy to true arterial congestive plethora; while *Opium* is perhaps the most homœopathic remedy to true venous congestive plethora; in the former disease, the face of the patient is red and flushed, in the latter it is purplish, or livid.

Symptomatic indications for Ferrum. Active, sthenic congestion and hæmorrhage, with great vascular irritation. Rush of blood to the head, puffiness around the eyes, swelling of the veins and paralytic weakness. Headache from rush of blood to the head. Vertigo with disposition to fall forwards; staggering in walking; momentary shock in the brain, with giddiness; dizziness, dulness and confusion of the head;

hammering and throbbing headache, lasting for two, three or four days, and recurring every two or three weeks; drawing headache from the nape of the neck into the brain, with sense of hammering, and roaring in the head; undulating pain in the head; headache as if the brain were rent asunder; rush of blood to the head, with swelling of the veins and flushes of heat. Faint feeling in walking, with blackness before the eyes, roaring in the ears and head at every step, and sensation as if threatened with Apoplexy. Violent burning and pain in the head, with thirst. All the vessels of the brain turgid with blood, and six ounces of blood extravasated into the cerebellum (NOACK and TRINKS). Pain in the eyes, as if from excessive drowsiness. Darkness before the eyes, in the evening, with aching pain, and discharge of a few drops of blood from the nose. Heat and anxiety after meals, with drowsiness, gloominess and headache over the root of the nose. Dulness of, and pain in the head, violent eructations, and heat in the face. Tremor of the hands, cramps in the fingers, with numbness and insensibility. Numbness of the thigh, feeling as if the thighs had gone to sleep. Coldness of the feet, and such weakness that he is scarcely able to drag them along. Constant weariness and drowsiness in the day time; heavy sleep in the morning. Orgasm of blood in the day time, with heat in the hands, heat of the body and redness of the cheeks (NOACK and TRINKS).

It will be unnecessary to multiply remedies here for this form of Apoplexy; in due time and place all the others will be treated of.

SIMPLE, OR CONGESTIVE APOPLEXY,

With or without plethora, but with rush of blood to the head, and without the frequent occurrence of hæmorrhage or permanent paralysis.

The *symptoms* in this form greatly resemble those of true or typical Apoplexy, except that paralysis, or hemiplegia is generally wanting—it is often wanting entirely, or present only transiently when simple congestion is present, but it is thought to be very seldom absent when there is hæmorrhage. The patient falls down suddenly deprived of sense and motion, and lies like a person in a deep sleep; his face is generally flushed, or more frequently livid or purple, his breathing stertorous, his pulse full and not frequent, generally slower than the natural standard; sometimes slight convulsions of the limbs, or contractions of the muscles of one side of the body, and relaxation of those of the other are present. Of course, if the congestion be sufficiently great to cause unconsciousness, or paralyze parts of the brain, it may also cause greater paralysis of some parts or limbs, than of others;—still, as has already been said, paralysis is not commonly present. The patient may continue in a state of profound stupor for several days, or he may recover after some hours, especially if judiciously treated; a perfect recovery, however, rarely takes place after the attack has lasted over one or two days, although it does in some cases of several days duration.

In a larger proportion of this class of apoplectic cases, excessive injection of the vessels of the pia mater, and engorgement of the whole vascular system of the brain are the chief lesions. Under allopathic treatment the cases consisting of congestion solely, almost always recover; the patient may, indeed, survive numerous attacks of this form of Apoplexy, but there is always danger that a congestive stroke may be followed by one of a hæmorrhagic character; and even when this danger is escaped, the disease is apt to leave traces behind it, of an enfeebled condition of the memory and intellect; and it sometimes happens that a patient has numerous attacks, which reduce him at length to a state of mental imbecility, little short of idiocy. (WOOD.)

It is sometimes possible to make a distinction between Apoplexy from *active* congestion of the brain, and that from *passive;* in the former, there is often a full, strong, but sometimes slow pulse, with a red flushing of the face; in the latter the pulse is apt to be comparatively weak, or else natural, and the face has a livid hue. The symptoms of active congestion have already been sufficiently detailed among the precursory symptoms of Apoplexy; those of passive congestion are said to be a feeling of fulness, weight, and sometimes of *coldness* in the head; an actual diminution of temperature in this part is particularly apt to occur when the arterial blood conveyed to the brain is very slowly changed into venous blood. There is also apt to be a strong tendency to drowsiness and stupor, dizziness, faintness, impaired vision, motes before the eyes, forgetfulness of words or things, dulness of countenance, a livid or purplish hue of the lips and face, with paleness, and depression of the pulse, and breathing.

Congestive Apoplexy does not necessarily take place only from excess of blood in the whole system. WATSON says, even a deficiency in the whole mass of blood contained in, and circulating through the body does not protect many *parts* of the system from congestion, i. e., from having an undue share of blood sent to them. Far from it; local determinations of blood, especially to the head, *are very common* in persons in whom the mass of that fluid, and the proportion of its nutritive elements have been considerably diminished by nature, disease, or loss of blood. (ANÆMIC APOPLEXY.)

This remarkable tendency to an unequal distribution of the blood may thus be explained—a due supply of healthy blood is requisite for the steady and equable performance of the functions of the brain and nerves—when this supply is defective or uncertain, those functions become disorderly, irregular, and the flow of blood to the organs also becomes disordered and irregular. The circulation of the blood is more or less under control of the nervous system, as is seen in the flush of shame and anger, and the paleness of fear; hence persons endowed with great sensibility and irritability of the nervous system are very liable to partial, or irregular congestions.

ROKITANSKY takes somewhat different views of congestive Apoplexy from those ordinarily adopted. He says, it is a question of much importance, whether the frequent cases of sudden or unexpected death, in old-school practice, in previously healthy persons, in which the only, or the principal post-mortem appearance is a certain amount of congestion of the brain, are solely produced by this congestion, and are to be regarded as cases of paralysis of the brain from pressure, by the excess of blood?

(*a.*) He answers, that in a certain small number of cases, this congestion of the brain is the only morbid appearance in the body, and has reached a degree, which in the present state of our knowledge justifies the conclusion that the brain has been pressed upon, and paralyzed by it.

(*b.*) If, in a greater number of cases, moderate congestion of the brain is found associated with *congestion of the lungs*, it is scarcely possible to say which of these conditions was the primary, and which the secondary, or whether they did not arise simultaneously from the same source and cause, and which of them actually produced death. But as it is quite as common for congestion of the lungs to be the only morbid appearances in cases of sudden death, and as it is decidedly the more marked appearance in many cases in which congestion of the brain is also present, we may often conclude that the congestion of the brain is of secondary importance.

(*c.*) Besides cases of these two kinds, there is still a number of others, in which all that is discovered upon examining the body of persons dead under allopathic treatment, is so slight a congestion of the brain, that it would not be thought of, if any other morbid appearance presented itself. Such cases prove fatal only when there is a peculiar tendency of the brain to exhaustion, or paralysis. (NERVOUS APOPLEXY.)

Dr. NEISSER, of Berlin, has lately described a severe form of congestion of the brain, connected with dilatation of its arteries; he has termed it *Ectasis vasorum cerebri;* thinks it is most common in young persons of a plethoric habit, short neck, thick head, and stunted growth; that the disease most frequently attacks the basilar artery and its branches, which become simply and equally dilated along their whole length, and not in aneurismal pouches; the blood consequently moves more slowly along them.

Symptoms.—The patient is readily heated, complains of overflow of blood, and these symptoms recur continually in spite of the most energetic and methodical allopathic treatment. Finally the patient complains of vertigo, and a peculiar heaviness and dulness of the feet; he has neither pain, nor tingling, but walks with a tottering, uncertain step, staggering first to one side, then to the other, as if intoxicated; he often becomes so dizzy as to fall, especially towards evening, and in the dark; all the symptoms are aggravated at night, and remit in the morning; there are partial sweats on the head and face, and in some cases partial blindness. Dr. NEISSER found the most energetic antiphlogistic and revulsive treatment to be entirely inefficacious. Death, finally, generally occurred suddenly.

Treatment of Congestive Apoplexy. OPIUM is perhaps the most important homœopathic remedy; at least WOOD and BACHE say, that it in full doses reduces the frequency though not the force of the pulse, diminishes muscular power, and brings on languor and drowsiness which soon eventuate in a deep apoplectic sleep; the breathing is stertorous, there is a dark suffusion of the countenance, a full, slow and laboring pulse, an almost total insensibility to external impressions, and when a moment of consciousness has been obtained, a confused state of the intellect, and an irresistible disposition to sink back into comatose sleep are present. The pulse, though slow, is often full and powerful in its beat. But in the space of a few, say six or eight hours, a condition of genuine debility ensues; the patient will have a cool and clammy skin, cool extremities, a pallid countenance, a feeble, thread-like, scarcely perceptible pulse, a slow, interrupted, almost gasping respiration, and a torpor little short of absolute death-like insensibility.

It will be seen that Opium is homœopathic to some of the most formidable apoplectic conditions; even allopathic physicians need not, and do not fear to use it in some of the nervous and asthenic forms of the disorder, as it in moderate doses increases the force, fulness and frequency of the pulse, augments the temperature of the skin, invigorates the muscular system, quickens the senses, animates the spirits and gives new energy to the intellectual faculties, all followed by calmness, delightful placidity of mind, with quiet, but vague enjoyment.

It will be unnecessary to enter here into the minutiæ of the indications for the use of Opium in Apoplexy; but it may be well to notice some of the broader and more striking peculiarities. * According to CHRISTISON it is most homœopathic to congestive Apoplexy, or rather to turgescence of the vessels of the brain, and watery effusion into the ventricles, and on the surface of the brain. It is very rarely homœopathic to hæmorrhagic Apoplexy, at least CHRISTISON says that extravasation of blood is a very rare effect of Opium; but he gives one case in which several clots of blood were found in the substance of the brain, one of which in the anterior lobe, was an inch long; in a second case, the sinuses and veins of the brain were turgid, and a moderately thick layer of blood was effused over the arachnoid membrane; NOACK and TRINKS report RYL's case in which the veins of the neck were turgid with decomposed black blood, the sinuses of the head and all the cerebral vessels were distended with blood, while the ventricles of the brain contained a teaspoonful of a bright-red fluid; also COLIN's case in which extravasated blood was found in the brain, and the cerebral vessels were very much distended; LEROUX found in one case, about a teaspoonful of bright-red blood at the base of the brain, and the choroid vessels very much distended; JOURD found several clots of coagulated blood in the substance of the brain; in a child the sinuses of the dura mater were filled with dark coagulæ, and there was slight extravasation of blood on the surface of the posterior lobes, while all the internal vessels of the brain were turgid with blood, and there was effusion of serum at the base of the brain, and in the ventricles. Still it must be remembered that these cases, although they seem numerous, are in reality exceptional.

Opium is also homœopathic to the congestion of the lungs which so frequently attends congestive Apoplexy according to ROKITANSKY. CHRISTISON says that the lungs are sometimes found gorged with blood, as in many cases of Apoplexy; four cases are alluded to, in one of which they were so gorged with fluid blood that it ran out in a stream when they were cut.

It is also decidedly homœopathic to venous-plethora, and plethora ad volumen.

HÆMORRHAGIC APOPLEXY,

With or without previous congestion, or plethora, but followed by paralysis.

The type of this variety is the form so graphically described by ABERCROMBIE, and called the *gradually increasing*, or *Ingravescent Apoplexy*, by COPELAND. It depends upon the sudden rupture of a blood-vessel of considerable size, without any necessary previous disturbance of the circulation, such as fever, congestion, or plethora; the rupture probably arising from disease of the artery, at the part which gives way.

Symptoms.—The patient often experiences a severe shock in the head, or a sudden or violent pain in the brain at the moment when the blood-vessel gives way; sometimes attended with the feeling as if something were suddenly torn, or rent in the interior of the head; and very frequently accompanied with paleness, sickness, and vomiting. The pain in the head is sometimes so severe that the patient sinks down pale, faint and exhausted; or even experiences a severe shudder, or a slight convulsion. When the calibre of the ruptured vessel is smaller, the sudden attack of pain in the head is accompanied by slight and transient confusion only, and the patient does not fall down. In either case he commonly recovers in a short time from these symptoms, becomes quite sensible, and is able to walk; but the headache does not leave him, his pulse is apt to remain frequent and feeble, his face cadaverous and sunk, while his spirits are depressed, although he is quite conscious, and in full possession of his intellect. After this state has endured from a few minutes to several hours, or even more, the patient becomes heavy, forgetful, incoherent, and sinks into coma from which he never rouses again; or his skin acquires some heat, his pulse improves in strength, his face becomes flushed and his features turgid; the oppression then increases rapidly, he answers questions slowly and heavily, and at last sinks into a profound stupor and coma. (COPELAND and WATSON.)

This is the most fatal form of Apoplexy, and it is all-important to be fully aware of this, for, to an inexperienced eye these cases, at first, do not seem so terrible as those in which the patient falls down profoundly comatose from the commencement. The apparent amendment is fallacious, and apt to lead physicians and friends to indulge in hopes of recovery, soon to be dreadfully disappointed. A large quantity of blood is usually found extravasated in, or upon the brain.

The primary management of these cases is very difficult to the allopathic physician; the violent pain in the head, the faintness, sickness, vomiting, the paleness and ghastliness of the face, the weakness, frequency or irregularity of the pulse cannot be treated with bloodletting, and dare not be met with stimulants, although the preparations of Ammonia are generally relied upon. As by far the majority of patients soon rally from the first shock, and coagulation of blood with the formation of a clot is more apt to take place during the cold and faint stage, while fresh bleeding almost always occurs as soon as the circulation is restored, and reaction sets in, the physician should be bold enough not to be in too great a hurry to rally his patient. He should aid nature in forming a clot, and should first use styptic and blood-coagulating remedies, rather than stimulating ones. The principal astringents in use in old-school practice are: Acetic acid, Tannic acid, Elixir vitriol or Aromatic sulphuric acid, Alum, Catechu, Creosote, Chalk, Sulphate of Copper, Per-nitrate, and Muriate Tincture of Iron, Sulphate of Iron, Geranium maculatum, Logwood, Kino, Rhatany, Matico, Monesia, Acetate of Lead, Bistort, Oak bark, and Acetate of Zinc. Some of these, such as Plumbum, Cuprum, Ferrum, Zincum, &c., are more or less homœopathic to some of the symptoms and forms of Apoplexy. But Millefolium has the highest homœopathic reputation in controlling bleedings from various parts. I believe that the use of styptics against hæmorrhage of the brain has never before been so distinctly recommended as is here done, or will again be urged.

A glance at the principal effects of a great outpouring of blood in, or on the brain, will still more forcibly impress us with the importance of checking the bleeding as rapidly as possible.

ROKITANSKY says, that: Hæmorrhagic Apoplexy consists in the pouring out of blood into the substance, or upon the surface of the brain, and a proportionate laceration, breaking down, contusion and compression of its substance. There are various grades of this process:

(1.) A larger or smaller spot of white or grey cerebral substance becomes speckled or striped with a small number of dark red dots and streaks of extravasated blood (ecchymosis); the fibres of the brain are then generally separated, not entirely torn by the effusion of blood. The recovery of the patient should be perfect, although the symptoms may be severe, and some paralysis be present.

(2.) These minute extravasations may be more numerous, lie closer to one another, and some of them may have run together, so that some portions of the brain are uniformly suffused with red blood, are of a soft and pulpy consistence, and many of its fibres are broken into numerous shreds, and softened to a red pap. Recovery from this state of things is apt to be slow and imperfect.

(3.) In consequence of the continuance or recurrence of the bleeding, a single small extravasation may increase rapidly, or by degrees, from the size of a poppy seed, tearing and separating the surrounding brain, until a large clot and cavity are formed. It is this process which old-school physicians are so anxious to prevent by means of prompt and copious bloodletting; but as it is very generally caused and aggravated by the existence of hypertrophy of the left ventricle of the heart, it is also very important for them to use Aconite, Digitalis or Veratrum viride, to lessen the impulse of the circulation; and antiphlogistic styptics such as Acet. plumb., Alum, or Creosote to control the bleeding.

Hæmorrhage into the brain should be treated somewhat as the hæmorrhagies of other organs are treated—no old-school physician would attempt to control bleeding of the rectum, uterus, bowels, stomach, or lungs without the aid of remedies more or less styptic, as well as antiphlogistic. In point of fact simple antiphlogistic treatment is next to useless, if not injurious. COPEMAN says, when there is a rupture of a bloodvessel in the head, and consequent extravasation of blood has already taken place, then the mischief is done, the blood is effused, and the system has received a great shock, which bloodletting will aggravate, while it cannot remove the extravasated blood. But it may be said, that it will prevent farther extravasation by lessening the impetus of blood to the brain. But has it this effect? Do we not generally read that during the bleeding the pulse rose and became more free? and may there not be some truth in the proposition that extravasation is promoted, rather than counteracted, by the greater thinness of the blood and its diminished tendency to coagulate, induced by large bleedings?

When the clot is large, the portions of the brain around it are stretched and torn, the segment of the brain containing it is enlarged, swollen and more or less altered in form, it may be forced outwards against the dura mater and skull, and inwards towards the opposite half of the brain; the convolutions are driven close together, flattened, and diminished in size; the structures at the base of the brain are flattened; the opposite ventricle is narrowed, and its contents displaced; and when a cavity of this size and kind opens into the ventricle, the opposite hemisphere also shares in the compression and enlargement.

(*a.*) It is evident that hæmorrhagic Apoplexy may prove fatal at once, suddenly and primarily (*Apoplexie foudroyante*); or after short time, viz., in some hours, or a few days. Death results in such cases from the extensive destruction of the substance of the brain, and from pressure. This happens especially when there are large central cavities of the size of a hen's egg, or somewhat smaller.

Still more certainly fatal are larger extravasations which burst into the meshes of the pia mater without, or into the cavity of the ventricles within.

In certain parts of the brain, again, such as the Pons variolii, Medulla oblongata, or Corpora quadrigemina, a cavity which is not absolutely of inordinate size, may prove fatal, on account of the greater vital importance of these parts.

(*b.*) Apoplexy may prove fatal secondarily, after a shorter or longer interval of time, when reaction sets in, and the inflammation about the cavity and clot becomes excessive, or is followed by yellow softening of the brain.

(*c.*) The first effect of extensive Apoplexy is a permanent loss of a portion of the cerebral mass.

(*d.*) A very frequent, if not invariable consequence of this is a manifest Apoplexy of other parts of the brain, extending to considerable distances in the direction of those fibres which are included in the original apoplectic spot.

(*e.*) This Apoplexy, coupled with the subsequent diminution and closure of the apoplectic cavity, by the process of healing, gives rise to a corresponding amount of vacuum within the skull.

(*f.*) This atrophy of the brain, when it is not associated with œdema of the brain, is constantly combined with *Sclerosis*, i. e., induration, condensation, and leather-like toughness of the white substance; it gives rise to premature marasmus of the brain, and early failure of its powers.

(*g.*) The vacuum in the skull thus produced, leads to frequent congestions of the head, and consequent repetitions of apoplectic attacks, followed, or not, by acute or chronic œdema of the brain; finally a varicose state of the cerebral vessels occurs in the neighborhood of the apoplectic clots, cyst, or cicatrices.

Rokitansky, from whom all the above remarks have been borrowed, says that the hitherto unnoticed congestions, arising from the vacuum which attends atrophy of the brain, are of the utmost importance. These, especially when combined with brittleness of the blood-vessels, are without doubt the cause of the frequency of Apoplexy in advanced life, and especially of its frequent recurrence in some cases.

Hæmorrhagic Apoplexy is generally supposed to depend upon the relative, or proportionate thinness, fragility, or debility of the blood-vessels of the brain, as compared with the amount of blood circulating through the whole system, and especially of that which is thrown to the head by the action of a strong and vigorous heart, or active circulation. But it arises quite as frequently, from too great stress and pressure upon these fragile, thin, or weakened blood-vessels by a sluggish return of blood from the head into the general circulation; and also, from such an actual and absolute degree of attenuation, brittleness, or weakness of the blood-vessels, that they are not able to withstand the ordinary pressure of the circulation under the usual, and more especially from any extraordinary exertion of body or mind.

Under all circumstances hæmorrhagic Apoplexy will be most apt to occur in those localities where the blood-vessels of the brain and its membranes most abound. In the brain itself, the most vascular parts are: the Corpora striata, the Optic thalami, and their immediate neighbourhood; hence it is to be expected that hæmorrhagic Apoplexy will, and does frequently happen in those parts. Of 386 cases of Cerebral- and Spinal-hæmorrhage collected by ANDRAL, no less than 202 cases showed extravasation of blood in the hemispheres of the brain, on a level with these bodies, and at the same time in them; in sixty-one other instances the Corpora striata alone were involved; and the Optic thalami only, in thirty-five additional cases; amounting in all to 298 cases out of 386. Of the remaining eighty-eight cases, out of the 386; the Cerebellum was the seat of hæmorrhage in twenty-two, the Spinal marrow in eight, and all other parts of the brain in fifty-eight.

It would be very natural to draw the inference, that the most common and frequent symptoms and phenomena of hæmorrhagic Apoplexy arise from the mutilation of these organs. Loss of motion and sensation are the most common phenomena of hæmorrhagic Apoplexy, if we except more or less loss of consciousness; paralysis of motion is far more frequent than loss of sensation; paralysis of one side (Hemiplegia) is far more frequent than paralysis of both sides; paralysis of the arm is far more frequent than the same affection of the leg; and supposing the patient to recover wholly, or partially from hemiplegia, it is the *leg*, in nine cases out of ten, which recovers first and fastest, i. e., sooner and faster than the arm. In accordance with these pathological facts, we find: 1st, that hæmorrhage into one side of the brain is much more common, than into both sides; 2d, the Corpora striata are implanted on the *motor* tracts of the Crura cerebri, which descend into the pyramidal columns, and we have seen that extravasation of blood into the corpora striata is at least twice as frequent as with the optic thalami; accounting perhaps for the greater frequency of loss of motion in Apoplexy, than loss of sensation; 3d, the *sensory* tract of nerves may be traced upwards from the olivary columns until it spreads itself almost entirely through the substance of the thalamus; moreover, the optic nerves and the peduncles of the olfactive may be shewn to have a distinct connection with the thalami; the former by a direct passage of a portion of their root into these ganglia, and the latter through the medium of the Fornix; hence we may regard the thalami opticii as the chief focus of the sensory nerves, and more especially as *the* chief ganglionic centre of the nerves of common sensation, which ascend to it from the medulla oblongata and spinal cord; we have already seen that the optic thalami are the seat of hæmorrhage only one half as frequently as the corpora striata, and that loss of sensation occurs not nearly so frequently as loss of motion. Why paralysis of the arm is more frequent and obstinate than that of the leg, is still an enigma.

Apoplexy of the Corpus striatum. Solly says, he believes it to be invariable fact that extravasation of blood into this body is followed by paralysis; and consequently that there is no portion of the brain which pathology has so clearly indicated the function of, as the corpus striatum, in so far as its connection with the course, or production of voluntary motion is concerned. This fact was known as early as the times of Morgagni and Willis.

Apoplexy of the Optic thalami. Andral says: although sensation is perhaps more frequently affected by hæmorrhage into this part, than motion, still this body is not the only source or origin of sensation, for feeling may remain when it is diseased, and may be lost when other parts of the sensor tract are affected. Besides, we may add, that congestion of, or bleeding into one part may, and does cause sympathetic disorder and compression of more or less remote parts, attended with corresponding symptoms.

Apoplexy of the Medulla oblongata. The pouring out of blood into this part is more *suddenly* fatal than any other form of Apoplexy. This is the only variety that resembles, and is liable to be mistaken for death from disease of the heart. It fortunately is very rare, for the medulla oblongata is not very vascular, its blood-vessels are not very large, and they are well supported. Extravasation of blood takes place more frequently on its surface than into its substance, but this proves equally fatal, although not so very suddenly. The reason that this occurrence is so rapidly destructive to life, must be obvious to every physiologist; for, it is from this centre that the nerves of respiration, and the muscles which they supply with nervous energy receive their power of action. Apoplexy of the medulla oblongata may take place secondarily when blood is poured out primarily, either into the third ventricle, or from rupture of the vessels of the optic thalami, or corpora striata, and gradually finds its way down to the medulla oblongata. This is a very frequent termination of such cases under allopathic treatment. (Solly.)

Apoplexy of the Pons varolii. When the pouring out of blood takes place first in the pons varolii, and secondarily into the medulla oblongata the symptoms are so characteristic that the lesion may be easily recognized by the practitioner.

Extravasation into the Pons produces paralysis of one or both limbs, according to its extent, but after the first effect of the effusion is over, it does not affect the intellect, because the brain proper is left intact; but as the blood advances towards the medulla, the organs of respiration become affected; first the muscles of respiration are unnaturally and irregularly stimulated, and the sensibility of the respiratory passages abnormally exalted, until the stage of excitement is succeeded by one of paralysis of the organs of respiration, and the patient dies suffocated. (SOLLY.)

Apoplexy of the Crus cerebri. Extravasation into, or upon this organ, will produce paralysis of the limbs on the opposite side of the body, and often of the opposite eye, from its also affecting the optic eye. The intellect may remain clear as long as the brain itself is not involved. (SOLLY.)

Apoplexy of the white, or tubular substance of the brain. In these cases, after the first effect of the extravasation is passed, the intellect remains intact, or only slightly disturbed, while decided paralysis of the side opposite the clot is present.

Apoplexy of the Cerebellum. Disease of this part of the brain has, perhaps, excited more attention than its importance demands. GALL and SERRES have assumed that erections, or seminal emissions in man, and discharges, sometimes of blood from the female organs, are the distinguishing signs of Apoplexy of the cerebellum; but there is as much proof to the contrary as in favor of this assumption, although COPELAND suggests that effusion into that part more immediately connected with the medulla oblongata, occasions a partial asphyxia and stasis of blood in the lungs, and thus produces a state favorable to erections, &c. The cases of Apoplexy which take place during coitus, especially if there has been severe pain in the back of the head, followed by great vital depression, sickness or vomiting, convulsions, and general paralysis of sensation and motion, may with some certainty be predicted to depend upon disorder of the cerebellum.

Apoplexy of the cerebellum is said to cause a more serious lesion of the functions of respiration and circulation, and to be more dangerous than the same amount of disease in the brain itself. This seems quite probable, as it is in union with each segment of the great nervous centres upon which all the movements and sensations of the body depend, viz.: the antero-lateral columns of the cord, and the anterior pyramids and olivary bodies, supplying all the anatomical conditions necessary for the development of acts of sensation and volition. It has even been assumed that the cerebellum is the regulator of all the voluntary movements, and the source of sensibility. (COPELAND.)

Although Apoplexy of the cerebellum, like that of the brain itself, generally produces paralysis of the side of the body opposite to the seat of the injury, yet ANDRAL asserts that when hæmorrhage into the cerebellum occurs simultaneously with that of the brain, or a little time after it, but so that the blood is effused on the right into the cerebellum and on the left into the brain, or vice versa, then there will be paralysis only on the side of the body opposite to the hemisphere of the brain where the bleeding has taken place; i. e., on the same side as the extravasation of blood into the cerebellum. It is most interesting and extraordinary that the movements of the limbs of the right side should be abolished when there is an effusion of blood into the left side of the brain, while the effusion which takes place simultaneously into the right side of the cerebellum should no longer possess the power of paralyzing the limbs of the left side.

Ventricular Apoplexy. The symptoms of this form are not positively known, but the bleeding has been traced by MORGAGNI, DE HAEN, and HUFELAND, to rupture of the vessels of the choroid plexus, in many of those cases in which the extravasation is confined to the ventricles of the brain, without being preceded by laceration of the surrounding cerebral substance.

Aneurismal Apoplexy. COPELAND says that small aneurisms in various parts of the cerebral vessels may form, and by their rupture occasion hæmorrhagic Apoplexy. SERRES relates cases in which rupture of an aneurism occurred in the basilar artery, and in one of the small arteries of the circle of Willis. Numerous other cases have been observed by Blane, Hodgson, Morgagni, Lieutaud and others, but especially by Bouillaud and Bright. COPEMAN, too, cites six or eight cases, one of which, viz.: case 102, occurred in a patient only 19 years of age; case 32, aged only 21; case 43, aged 30; and case 2, aged 35. These ages are certainly younger than those in which aneurism is thought to be most common.

Arterial Apoplexy. An immense number of cases of hæmorrhagic Apoplexy arise from disease of the arteries of the brain, without aneurism; in fact COPELAND asserts that the most common causes of hæmorrhage in the gradually increasing, or ingravescent Apoplexy, are: ossification, earthy, and atheromatous deposits in various places on the arteries, and a peculiar brittleness, or friability of the vessels of the brain. COPEMAN gives but few cases of this kind occurring in young persons; still case 120 in his book happened in a person aged only 20 years; case 202, aged 35; cases 12 and 34, aged 40; case 80, aged 42; cases 109 and 119, aged 45; and case 190, aged 46. Six other cases happened in persons between 50 and 60 years of age; five cases between 60 and 70 years.

Meningeal Apoplexy. This variety has been studied minutely and curiously by several physicians, especially by PRUSS and HEWETT. Pain in the head is said always to accompany it, and when the effusion of blood takes place slowly, the pain experienced is excessive; it is excruciating, there being blood enough poured out to irritate the membranes of the brain and arouse their sensibility to the uttermost, but not enough to smother or paralyze the organs whose office it is to receive impressions, and recognize pain. At times this extreme suffering lasts for some or many days, but generally coma comes on rapidly, and relieves the patient. (SOLLY).

Another of the most important occasional characteristics of meningeal Apoplexy is the *intermission* of the symptoms, and the consequent masking of the disease. HEWETT had a case in the person of a lady, aged 65, who after having suffered for several days with great mental excitement, was suddenly seized with violent pain confined to the right eyebrow, which lasted for two or three hours, and then disappeared. This pain continued for several days to recur twice in the 24 hours, presenting all the characters of brow-ague, and it was apparently relieved by quinine, but was succeeded by a train of low symptoms, accompanied by a brown tongue, wandering and impairment of the intellectual faculties, terminating in coma. This lady died in twelve days, without having had any paralysis, or contractions of the limbs; a large quantity of blood was found extravasated into the cavity of the arachnoid.

According to DAY the premonitory symptoms of Apoplexy, such as headache, drowsiness, numbness, vertigo, &c., may or may not occur; premonitions were only present in eighteen cases out of forty-one recorded by BONDEL. Occasionally the attacks set in so rapidly and severely as to merit the expressive term of the French writers, *Apoplexie foudroyante.*

PRUSS has endeavored to establish the diagnosis between *sub-*, and *intra-*arachnoid Apoplexies. In the former, the bleeding, even if considerable, is followed by no paralysis of motion or sensation, when the blood is poured out by exhalation, or from rupture of a vein; but when an artery is ruptured, paralysis sometimes occurs, owing to the greater impulse and shock with which the blood escapes. In *intra-*arachnoid Apoplexy paralysis of motion is very common, while paralysis of sensation is more rare.

In *sub-*arachnoid Apoplexy there is never a *sudden* loss of consciousness, whereas, in the latter there is.

In the *sub-*arachnoid variety there is somnolence and coma, without headache, fever, dryness of the tongue, or delirium; in the latter, all these symptoms are very apt to be present.

In the former we are apt to find neither convulsions, contraction or rigidity of the limbs; in the *intra-*arachnoid variety we generally have at least one of these phenomena.

Sudden loss of consciousness and paralysis do not occur so frequently in meningeal Apoplexy, as in Apoplexy of the brain;

deviation of the mouth to one side, is also much less frequent; while both forms of meningeal Apoplexy frequently assume an *intermittent* character, which is very rare in ordinary Apoplexy.

It is sometimes impossible to distinguish it from softening of the brain. The duration of *sub*-arachnoid Apoplexy does not often exceed eight days; while the *intra*-arachnoid variety may last for a month or longer, and then occasionally terminate in recovery.

Treatment of Hæmorrhagic Apoplexy.

(Atheroma.)

The preventive treatment of a very large number of cases of hæmorrhagic Apoplexy will consist in the prevention of that disease of the arteries which leads to the formation and deposition of atheroma, and to ossification of the arteries. According to ROKITANSKY atheroma is formed, and poured out from the walls of the internal coat of the arteries; at first it resembles coagulated albumen; although it is generally associated with an arterial crasis of the blood, still, it is not the product of inflammation of the arteries; it is rarely associated with tubercular disease of other organs; but is frequently coexistent with an excessive formation of fat in the whole body. Chemically, atheroma has been found to consist of a great number of cholesterine crystals, some oil globules, and of large, small, and very small molecules consisting of albumen, and salts of lime; this atheromatous mass often thickens and is transformed into a moist, soft, mortar-like substance, and finally into a granular, rough, stalactite-like lime concretion; another transformation of the deposit is ossification of parts of the walls of the arteries, which is very frequently preceded, and associated with fatty degeneration of the fibrous coat of the arteries.

The homœopathic treatment of atheroma has not yet been pointed out; if there be a preceding arterial crasis, Ferrum, China, Natrum muriat., Manganese, &c., would be homœopathic; if there be a strong tendency to the development of adipose tissue, Calc. c., Antim. crud., Kali c., Kali hydriod., &c., will be most indicated, although CHAMBERS (see work on Corpulence) gives most striking results from the free use of Liquor potassæ in excessive corpulence. When atheromatous deposits are fairly formed upon the arteries, we must get rid of them as best we may; we have already seen that they consist mainly of cholesterine crystals; *cholesterine* is a white, crystallizable, fatty substance, somewhat like spermaceti, free from taste and odor, and composed almost entirely of carbon and hydrogen; it may be obtained by a chemical process of no great complexity from the serum of the blood, and is conjectured by some physiologists to be altered *Serolin*, or the natural non-saponifiable fat of the serum; one of its most striking characteristics is, that it is not affected by a solution of Caustic potash, and that concentrated Nitric, Muriatic, and Arsenious acid exert no chemical effect upon it. On the other hand, WAGNER found that four parts of *soap* solved in water would dissolve one part of cholesterine; according to SIMON it dissolves so freely in heated Holz-geist or *Naphtha*, that the solution appears crystalline when it cools; ether, the fatty oils, and turpentine also dissolve it; but, the latter only in a moderate degree; while it requires twelve parts of cold ether, to solve one part of cholesterine. As cholesterine exists in the normal brain and nerves in considerable quantities, and is a principal constituent of atheroma, we may readily infer that the arteries of the brain would often be found in an atheromatous condition. Again, CARPENTER has suggested that one of the principal sources of bile is the continual waste of nervous matter, which in some respect so nearly approximates to bile in its composition, that it is asserted by FREMY, that the peculiar acids of the brain may easily be detected in the liver; hence we may infer, the frequent practical connection of bilious derangements, with Apoplexy and atheroma. For want of better remedies against atheroma, it may be justifiable to use the chemical ones, above pointed out, viz.: Naphtha, Ether, Sapon. commun., some of the fatty and volatile oils, and Terebinth. Turpentine is homœopathic to some of the symptoms of Apoplexy, especially when attended with urinary troubles, and there is sudden dizziness with dimness of sight, stupefaction and deep sleep, from which the patient awakes confused and languid, and with reeling; when there is dull headache with colic, aching pains in the whole head, going and coming, and attended with vomiting; heavy oppressive pain over the left eye; tearing headache on the right side for nine days, &c. If there were any provings on the healthy, with the other remedies, doubtless one or more of them could be shown to be homœopathic to some of the varieties of Apoplexy.

The albuminous condition of athemora in its first stages, may be treated with Merc. corr., Nitric acid, or Kali hydroid.; the fatty degeneration of the fibrous coat of the arteries may be treated by, 1st, Calc., Caps., or Ferrum; or 2d, by Ant. crud., Cuprum, Lycopod., Puls., Sulph., or other remedies. The calcareous and ossific deposits on the arteries, may be treated with Calc. c., Calc. phos., Silex, or especially by the Silicate of Potash, which was found so useful by Ure against the earthy, and tophaceous deposits of gout.

When an absolute rupture of one of the arteries of the brain has taken place, after, or in connection with the ordinary symptomatic treatment, we must also depend much upon styptic, or anti-hæmorrhagic remedies. This has already been alluded to before; among the strictly homœopathic remedies, Arnica, Millefolium, Ferrum acet., Plumbum, Acidum sulph., and others deserve most attention.

FEBRILE AND INFLAMMATORY APOPLEXY.

Apoplexy with bleeding into, or upon the brain may occur in consequence of an exudation from the capillary vessels, owing to a febrile excitement and inflammatory congestion. This mode of hæmorrhage is indicated, apart from the febrile symptoms, by the gradual accession of the signs of Apoplexy; if a blood-vessel had been ruptured, the fit would be more sudden and instantaneous. In fact, in some of these cases the brain being already excited, resists the oppressive effect of the effused fluid longer than it would in its natural condition; so that at first the symptoms of compression are not in proportion to the amount of the effusion.

In febrile and inflammatory Apoplexy we always have increased heat of skin, and a febrile pulse; while Apoplexy from hæmorrhage is characterized by a slow pulse and diminished temperature. One of the most common causes of this form of Apoplexy, is extension of rheumatism of the muscles of the nape to the membranes of the brain; the muscles of the neck will then be found to be tense, swollen, and so tender to the touch that if but slightly pressed the patient's countenance expresses pain, he will often be roused from his unconscious state, and mutter loudly some unintelligible words; he will hold his neck in a constrained position, and if we attempt to move his head or neck there is an expression of pain on the countenance, and the head returns at once to its unnatural position. (NEISSER.)

The treatment of febrile and inflammatory Apoplexy is so well known that it requires but few words to indicate it. Aconite, Belladonna, Bryonia, and Tart. emetic, are the most important remedies.

SEROUS APOPLEXY.

WATSON says, that a moderate quantity of serous fluid poured out rapidly during life will certainly occasion a degree of pressure adequate to the production of fatal coma—but how the serum comes to be so effused, it is not always so easy to say—yet there is one condition of the blood-vessels of the brain which, when it can be proved to exist in a given case, is sufficient to account for the effusion. Any real or virtual retardation of the blood in the cerebral veins would lead to what is tatamount to dropsy, there, as well as in any other part of the body.

SOLLY assumes that serous Apoplexy is always more or less dependent on general debility, with local vascular excitement, and congestion of an asthenic character—for instance, a man of intemperate habits gets a blow upon the head causing concussion; if this is judiciously treated, he will recover in the course of a few days—but if he be bled largely from the arm, and purged freely the result will almost certainly be serous Apoplexy. But the most unequivocal cases of asthenic serous Apoplexy are those which occur from suppression of urine, the result of disease of the kidneys. Convulsions, and apoplectic coma are among the most common fatal terminations of Bright's disease of the kidneys, especially in pregnant women. Whenever a pregnant woman has a bloated, or tumid state of the hands and face, the urine should always be tested for albumen; if this be present, and a peculiar and intense pain in the forehead set in, especially if accompanied with a severe pain in the stomach, and vomiting of bile, puerperal convulsions and Apoplexy will almost certainly set in.

The attacks may perhaps be prevented by the timely use of Merc. corros., Nitric acid, Cantharides, or Kali hydroid.; but if there be a great deficiency of urea in the urine, Colchicum will also be required. If an attack fairly set in, Venesection and Opium are the most reliable remedies; with them, only forty-two mothers were lost out of 152 cases, or rather more than one-fourth; without them almost all die, except the cases of purely hysterical, or epileptic convulsions and Apoplexy. It is not a little singular that the majority of cases of puerperal convulsions and Apoplexy occur in primaparæ; thus, of thirty-six cases related by Dr. Merriman, twenty-eight were with first children; of Dr. Ramsbotham's more than two-thirds were with first children; and of Dr. Collins' thirty cases, twenty-nine were with first children. The majority of those women who suffer thus with their first child, are not particularly liable to a recurrence with their other children.

Copeman gives several cases of serous Apoplexy especially when attended with more or less general dropsy, and Bright's disease of the kidneys, viz.: cases 57, 61, 63, 64, 65, 66, 87, 101, 205, 229 and some others. Case 229 of Copeman's collection deserves to be reprinted here. A hearty woman, aged 30, but somewhat dropsical, and near the full period of gestation, fell down suddenly; she instantly became insensible, with stertorous breathing, a hard vibrating pulse, and violent convulsions, which recurred paroxysmally. Delivery of the child occurred in a few hours, but the symptoms of Apoplexy remained unabated, until thirty drops of laudanum were given. The next morning the insensibility, stertorous breathing and convulsions returned, and remained after an injection, which had a proper effect, had been administered; then twenty drops of laudanum were ordered every ten hours, until the symptoms should abate. At the end of the third day manifest advantage had been gained over the disease; in four days recovery appeared certain, and it happened accordingly. (KIRKLAND.)

I claim the credit of being the first to point out a truly homœopathic, and specifically curative remedy, viz.: *Mercurius corrosivus*, against one variety of Bright's disease of the kidneys (see Homœopathic Examiner, new series, vol. 1, p. 285), as long ago as the year 1846. Besides the successful cases there recorded, I have heard of numerous other fortunate recoveries, both in our public allopathic medical institutions, and in private practice. It is well to add that ROKITANSKY distinguishes no less than eight different varieties of Bright's disease; hence we require at least eight different remedies to cure all these varieties, and doubtless several more will be necessary to meet all the peculiarities of some cases. Of course Mercurius corrosivus will not cure all cases of Bright's disease; some require Cantharides, others Nitric acid, or Hydriodate of Potash, or Copaiba; while remedies for the remaining varieties have yet to be discovered. Marsh Marigold will probably cure some cases. (PETERS.)

NERVOUS APOPLEXY.

WOOD says it is now generally admitted by old-school authorities that death may occur, even after, and perhaps in consequence of the most active treatment, with all the phenomena of Apoplexy, without leaving any observable lesion in the brain. Such cases are denominated by some, *nervous* Apoplexy. He says they are rare, but the probability seems to him, to be, either that some *slight* phenomena of congestion have been overlooked, or that some of the blood-vessels of the brain have been violently distended, sufficient to press upon and paralyze the action of some of the nervous centres essential to life, but have become emptied of blood before death, after the mischief has been produced.

In fact, in hæmorrhagic and congestive Apoplexies the symptoms are owing to distension, or compression and consequent paralysis of some portions of the brain. This paralytic state of the brain may occur quite independently of any congestive trouble, and give rise to all the symptoms of Apoplexy.

Copeland says, that the circulation of the brain is chiefly under the dominion of that portion of the sympathetic nerve which is ramified on its blood-vessels, and that an exhausted or morbidly depressed state of the influence which these nerves exert on the circulation and manifestations of the brain, particularly in dilating or congesting the capillaries and disposing to their rupture, is the principal cause of, and often constitutes the whole of the apoplectic seizure. From this it may be inferred that the proximate cause of a large proportion of the cases of Apoplexy, not excepting even those which are attended with retarded circulation and hæmorrhage is here imputed primarily to the weakened condition of that part of the sympathetic nerve which supplies the blood-vessels of the brain, and the brain itself.

Hence, the most important indication of treatment is to give tone and vigor to these nerves. Nux, Veratrum, Quinine, Arnica, &c., should be more useful than bloodletting. Hufeland, in particular, considered Apoplexy frequently to proceed from that state of the nervous power which he considered defective.

Cooke (see Burrows, p. 79) says, the opinion that Apoplexy is caused by an obstruction of the passage of the nervous fluid into the organs of sense and motion has been the favorite hypothesis of physiologists, and seems more satisfactory than any other to explain the manner in which the exciting causes act in producing the symptoms of the disease. (Ibid. p. 80.)

ABERCROMBIE says, it is an important fact that Apoplexy has, by extensive observation, been ascertained to be fatal (under allopathic treatment) without any morbid appearance in the brain, or with appearances so slight as to be altogether inadequate to account for the disease. There is a modification of Apoplexy, depending on a cause of a temporary nature, without any real injury done to the substance of the brain; and that the condition upon which this attack depends may be speedily removed, or it may be fatal without leaving any morbid appearance on the brain. BURSERIUS relates instances of the kind, and quotes Vallisnieri, of Modena, who asserts that in several bodies of persons who had died of Apoplexy, to the great amazement of the dissectors, not the smallest injury was discoverable either in the membranes of the brain, or in the cortical or medullary part, or in the ventricles, or in the vessels, or in any other part of the head. WILLIS, NICOLAI and KORTUN, have seen such cases, and finally such distinguished pathologists as GRISOLLE and LOUIS have met with them. Grisolle has reported a case in which the brain was examined into its most minute parts, and VALLEIX saw in the service of Louis, a patient who after having succumbed in consequence of an attack of Apoplexy, attended with complete loss of consciousness and hemiplegia, did not present a single visible cerebral lesion, although the examination was most minute. Such cases as these should lead the dominant school to be more charitable and just in their judgments of homœopathic physicians. If such a case should by chance happen to a homœopathist, there would be no end of the contumely and reproach which would be heaped upon him, and his mode of practice; but the very numerous fatal cases of this kind which happen under allopathic treatment, are very cavalierly ignored, or forgotten.

CARDIAC APOPLEXY,

Or Apoplexy connected with, or arising from preceding Organic disease of the heart.

In every case of threatened or happened Apoplexy, it should be regarded as imperatively necessary for the physician not only to examine the pulse carefully, but also to investigate the condition and action of the heart. According to BURROWES, "simple hypertrophy of the left ventricle of the heart will cause an increased activity in the general circulation; the blood will be thrown to the head with more than usual force, and there will be a more rapid transit of the blood through the arteries of the brain. But, after a time, this constantly increased force of the left ventricle will have the effect of dilating the cerebral arteries, and thus of overcoming the healthy elasticity of their tunics. Congestions of the brain will now ensue, and the coats of the dilated vessels no longer protect the surrounding substance of the brain from the inordinate momentum of the blood propelled from the heart. Apoplectic coma is now very likely to occur from some sudden accidental increase of pressure of blood on the brain, or from rupture of an artery, and pouring out of blood into the brain.

Hence, enlargement of the left ventricle of the heart must be admitted as a powerful predisposing, or even exciting cause of Apoplexy, and sudden paralysis. In 132 cases of Apoplexy collected by various authors, the heart was found diseased in no less than eighty-four instances, or sixty-three per cent. Andral, in twenty-five cases, found the heart diseased in fifteen; Clendinning, in fifteen cases, out of twenty-eight; Hope, in twenty-seven cases, out of thirty-nine; Burrowes, in twenty-three cases, out of thirty-four; Guillemin, in four cases out of six; Rochoux, in four cases out of fourteen.

But, simple enlargement is not the only disease of the heart apt to cause Apoplexy; in Andral's fifteen cases, there was valvular disease in eleven cases; in Burrow's twenty-three cases, there was valvular disease in sixteen.

A careful examination of the state of the heart of an apoplectic patient is much more necessary for the safety of one under allopathic treatment, than under the homœopathic. For if the Mitral valve be diseased, and allow of regurgitation from the left ventricle, then the small and irregular pulse so generally attending that state of the valves, will probably dissuade the allopathist from that free abstraction of blood, which the state of the brain seems to require, according to his mode of treatment. Again, if in another case of Apoplexy or paralysis, the Aortic valves be found diseased to the extent of not only obstructing the onward current of blood, but also of allowing regurgitation into the ventricles, there will probably be associated with this lesion, considerable enlargement of the left ventricle. Then we will find a full and vibrating, or thrilling pulse, but a pulse of increased action without real power, and hence a deceptive pulse; and one which, if it be regarded without reference to the disease of the heart, would tempt the physician to a more copious abstraction of blood than will be called for by the general symptoms. (Burrowes.)

It will be unnecessary to enter here upon the treatment of those affections of the heart which are attended with Apoplexy, because the treatment of Organic affections of the heart has been given minutely and completely by the translator in the Homœopathic Examiner, vol. 2, (new series, 1847), and reprinted, both in Hull's Laurie's (Appendix), and in Hull's Laurie (new edition, 1853,) all published by Wm. Radde.

BILIOUS APOPLEXY.

Budd (see Treatise on Diseases of the Liver,) has made quite a large collection of fatal cases of jaundice, followed by delirium, coma, paralysis or convulsions. Rokitansky, however, was the first to call attention to this formidable disorder, under the name of acute yellow softening of the liver; owing to his researches, the disease can now be readily detected during life; its course is acute, there is extreme pain in the region of the liver, which organ rapidly becomes extremely soft, and diminished in size; this diminution of size can easily be recognized by means of careful percussion, and this diagnostic sign is of very great importance, as in most other diseases in which jaundice occurs, the liver is generally enlarged. The prognosis in severe jaundice with decided diminution of the size of the liver, is much more serious than when the liver is enlarged. Until quite lately this form of disease was regarded as almost necessarily fatal, but now the patient may often be saved, even after he has fallen into a state bordering on apoplectic coma, the patient being unable to speak, with slow pulse, dilated pupils, and almost total loss of sensation and voluntary motion.

Among the remedies homœopathic to Apoplexy, Cuprum aceticum, and Phosphorus are also decidedly homœopathic to profound bilious derangement and jaundice. According to Christison, Cuprum is homœopathic to violent headache with vomiting, cutting pains in the bowels, cramps in the legs, and pains in the thighs; he also mentions six or eight cases in which it proved homœopathic to jaundice; and others, in which it was found homœopathic to convulsions, palsy, coma, and insensibility; others, again, in which the patient was insensible, with the jaws locked, the muscles rigid and frequently convulsed, the breathing interrupted, and the pulse small and slow; one case in which there was convulsions and loss of consciousness followed by extraordinarily paralytic weakness of the arms and legs, and attended with congestion of the surface of the brain.

Christison also gives a case in which Phosphorus proved homœopathic to spasms, delirium and palsy of the left hand, the limbs being neuralgic, the intellect clouded, and the breathing stertorous, while the whole of the skin was generally yellow.

GASTRIC APOPLEXY.

A very large number of cases of Apoplexy occur after a full meal; a person predisposed to Apoplexy, either from plethora, or disease of the arteries of the brain, but especially when both are present, is very apt to be attacked with Apoplexy, after a full meal. This is best illustrated by a case.

A colored woman, aged about 50, and somewhat corpulent, after a hearty meal of meat, peas and rice, fell down in a state of insensibility, and soon expired. As soon as the skull was opened, a considerable collection of blood was found about the base of the brain, and large clots were discovered in its substance; the arteries of the brain were rigid, much dilated, and studded over with numerous points of ossification; the bleeding had taken place in consequence of a rupture of some of these arteries. On examining the stomach, that organ was found impacted with peas, rice, hominy and other articles of the individual's repast, to a degree to which it would scarcely be possible to believe could be borne without extreme suffering, and an extensive embarrassment of the functions of the whole of the associated organs. It was so distended as to encroach upon the intestines, compress the aorta, and the vessels given off by it in the epigastric region, press upon the plexus of nerves behind the stomach, and finally, force up the diaphragm upon the lungs so as to interrupt their play, and thus embarrass the function of respiration, thereby interrupting the passage of blood through them, and consequently impeding its return from the head. The blood being thus confined on the one hand to the vessels of the brain, by these causes, and driven upon it, on the other hand, by the pressure sustained by the aorta, which prevented the distribution of the usual quantity of blood to the lower part of the body, it is not to be wondered at, when the fragile state of the coats of the arteries of the brain is considered, that they should have been unable to sustain the pressure thus suddenly thrown upon them, and that they gave way under its influence. (COPEMAN.)

The above is a fair exposition of one cause of a very large

number of cases of Apoplexy. The frequency of this occurrence has given rise to the dispute among physicians as to the propriety of administering emetics in Apoplexy, or not. COPEMAN says, that the practice of giving emetics when the attack has succeeded a full meal, has not only been safe, but effectual; case 36 in his book, recovered from Apoplexy excited by eating cucumbers and whortleberries, after the action of an emetic; also case 37; case 26, after vomiting some pints of fœtid bile; case 90, recovered after spontaneous vomiting set in. On the other hand, WATSON says, that the treatment of Apoplexy with emetics is an extremely hazardous measure, which is almost sure to do harm if there is already any extravasation of blood. He merely mentions the practice to protest against it.

Still, an overloaded stomach must be relieved from its excessive and often disgusting contents; we have seen that it exerts an exceedingly injurious pressure upon various important organs, and obstructs the return circulation from the head; it must be manifestly the height of folly to put infinitesimal and delicate doses in a foul stomach; hence, if emetics are injurious, what are we to do? The bowels may evidently be fully emptied, thus leaving more room in the abdomen; the whole quantity of blood may be reduced, if the patient be decidedly plethoric, and then the stomach may probably be evacuated, with safety and benefit; after the stomach has been thoroughly cleansed and purified, infinitesimal doses may be used.

Dr. W. HERING (see Brit. Jour. of Hom., July, 1852, p. 377) gives eight instances of apoplectic attacks arising from excessive or improper feeding; in three cases, free vomiting was induced with great relief to the patient; in three other cases, large draughts of hot water were used to relax the pyloric orifice of the stomach, and allow the offending substances to pass out of the stomach into the bowels, and be carried off by spontaneous diarrhœa.

This may not be an improper place to speak of the use of cathartics in Apoplexy. WATSON says, that "purgatives are of signal service; they empty the intestines, which are sometimes loaded, and which by distending the abdomen have perhaps occasioned undue pressure against the diaphragm, embarrassed the breathing, and through it the circulation in the brain; another very important purpose of hard purging, is the producing of copious watery discharges from the bowels, whereby the blood-vessels are drained, and the tendency of blood to the head especially relieved."

I am sorry to say that in my experience, purging has had no such good effects; in at least four cases of Apoplexy, previously treated by allopathic physicians and in several by myself, I have seen decided purging produce not only no good effect upon the patient, but render his condition one of great misery and filth to those around him, all the evacuations being necessarily passed in the bed, while the necessary attentions in cleansing and moving the patient have certainly aggravated a state which requires the utmost repose and quiet. Copeman even gives two cases, viz.: cases 193 and 194, in which hypercatharsis seemed to bring on Apoplexy.

"A foreman of a mill, strong and stout, was under the care of a physician for disorder of the liver, which was treated by mercury; this produced a hypercatharsis so prodigious that he nearly became bereft of all power, and all pulse; he rallied partially, but in twelve hours presented all the symptoms of cerebral Apoplexy; he was lethargic and flushed; notwithstanding the usual treatment, he went on into all the degrees of Apoplexy, and died in twelve hours more.

A stout, unwieldy lady, aged 70, in her usual health in the morning, had taken a purgative, which produced a hypercatharsis; after the evacuations she was struck with Apoplexy. Copeman exclaims: Emptied vessels, with great debility, yet the blood determined fatally to the head!"

West gives the case of a child attacked with diarrhœa, producing great exhaustion; and while suffering from this affection, he suddenly became comatose, cold and almost pulseless, and his breathing became so slow that he inspired only four or five times in a minute. In this state he lay for twenty-four hours, and then died quietly. Nearly six ounces of dark coagulated blood were found in the cavity of the arachnoid. (See Lectures on Diseases of Infancy and Childhood, p. 54.)

INFANTILE APOPLEXY.

Alois Bednar, of the Vienna Foundling Hospital, met with thirty-seven cases of hæmorrhage into the pia mater in the course of three years; viz.: twenty-two times in boys, and fifteen times in girls. In the same space of time, he met with Apoplexy of the arachnoid, only fifteen times, viz.: in seven cases in boys, and in eight, in girls. Of the thirty-seven cases of Apoplexy of the pia mater, the bleeding was extensive in three cases only; of the fifteen cases of arachnoid Apoplexy the disease was extensive in all but three cases. Bednar also met with sixteen cases of bleeding into the substance of the brain, viz.: eleven times in boys, and only five times in girls.

The principal symptoms of bleeding into the cavity of the arachnoid membrane are: distension and pulsation of the anterior fontanelle, dimness of the cornea, clonic cramps, rigidity or paralysis of the limbs, sopor, coolness and blueness of the skin, slow beating of the heart and slow respiration. The age of the child, the recency of birth, and the course of the disease will aid the diagnosis.

According to West all periods of childhood are not equally exposed to this accident, but it is oftenest met with immediately after birth. The head of the infant has been subjected to severe, and long-continued pressure; immediately on its birth the course of the circulation is altogether changed, and should any difficulty occur in the establishment of the new function of respiration, a long time will elapse before the blood flows freely through its unaccustomed channels. The tumid scalp and livid face of many a still-born child point to one of its most important causes, since they are but the external signs of that extreme congestion of the vessels within the skull, that has at length ended in a fatal effusion of blood on the surface of the brain.

There will be reason to fear that this occurrence has taken

place, if an infant when born, were to present great lividity of the surface, and especially of the face; and if the heart were to beat feebly, and at long intervals, although the pulsations of the cord were slow, or faint, or had altogether ceased. Death may take place without any effort at respiration being made, the beatings of the heart growing feebler and fewer till they entirely cease; but at other times the child breathes irregularly, imperfectly, and at long intervals. The hands are generally clenched, and spasmodic twitchings are of frequent occurrence about the face; or these twitchings may be more general, and more severe, and may amount almost to an attack of convulsions. (WEST.)

Bleeding within in the skull in the new born infant takes place almost under the same circumstances that bleeding into the tissue of the scalp, or extravasation of blood between the bone and pericranium takes place (*Cephalhæmatoma*).

Infantile Apoplexy, though at no time so frequent as immediately after birth, may occur at any subsequent period of childhood, either under the influence of causes which favor congestion of the brain, or even independently of any cause that we can discover.

WEST, LEGENDRE, RILLIET and BARTHEZ, all concur in representing its symptoms as exceedingly obscure; paralysis was observed only twice in twenty-six cases of hæmorrhage into the cavity of the arachnoid, owing probably to the pressure exerted on the brain being generally diffused over its surface, and being nowhere very considerable; just enough, perhaps, to cause general dulness and torpor. On the other hand, the sudden occurrence of violent convulsions, and their frequent return, alternating with spasmodic contraction of the fingers and toes in the intervals appear, to WEST, to be the most frequent indications of effusion of blood upon the surface of the brain.

Both BEDNAR and WEST lay some stress upon hæmorrhage into the brain, in children, being connected with an altered state of the blood, and with disease or enlargement of the liver; bilious symptoms are often present, the region of the liver is often tender to touch, and the liver itself is sometimes found enlarged. WEST has met with only two instances of distinct extravasation of blood into the substance of the brain in older children; one was in a little girl, aged 11 months; the other also in a girl, but aged 11 years.

SECONDARY EFFECTS OF APOPLEXY.

Having made some remarks about the nature and treatment of the principal varieties of Apoplexy, it may not be out of place to refer to the precautions and remedies necessary for the after-effects of the disorder.

A principal precaution is to prevent the patient from making any exertion for some time after the first effects of the attack have passed off. A very large number of lives have been lost from want of attention to this. In Copeman's 18th case, the patient, after being successfully treated, so that he became conscious, knew his friends and was able to walk with assistance from one bed to another, soon relapsed after this exertion, and finally died. In case 21, the patient had recovered sufficiently to walk across his room, when he cried out suddenly with pain in the head, fell down insensible, and died in thirty minutes. It will be useless to multiply cases to this effect; BURROWES (see on Disorders of the Cerebral circulation, p. 146) has an excellent chapter on, and very instructive cases illustrative of the bad effects of premature exertions of body or mind after Apoplexy.

In other cases, two or three days after the emergence from coma, we often observe the patient's face to become flushed, the scalp hot, a frowning or knitting of the brows, slight squinting, and complaint of pain on one side of the head. This pain is usually referred to the side opposite to the palsied limbs; and if the patient be deprived of the power of expressing his sensations, his uneasiness is often indicated by the occasional movement of the sound hand to the forehead; at the same time the paralysed arm is perhaps observed to be occasionally drawn up to the face, or across the chest. This latter movement taking place after the fit, often gives rise to the hope that the paralysis is not so complete as it was at first supposed to be; but such movements are involuntary, and arise from commencing irritation and inflammation in the substance of the brain immediately around the extravasated blood. At the same time, the circulation becomes more active, the patient is thirsty, and is sometimes troubled with an oppressive heat of the skin. These symptoms, which are indicative of inflammatory action commencing around the clot of blood in the brain, should be met by the application of cold to the head, restricted diet, extreme quiet in the sick-room, and the use of Aconite, and other antiphlogistic means and remedies.

Simultaneously with the above-described train of symptoms, or soon after their appearance, the paralysed limbs are not uncommonly affected with involuntary movements, which usually consist of spasmodic contractions. The patient will also, most probably, complain of severe pains in the palsied limbs, of burning heat in them, so that he will long to plunge them into cold water; the integuments of these limbs often feel hot, and are red and swollen. These pains in the paralysed limbs often constitute a most striking feature in the after progress of a case of Apoplexy. At each visit of the medical attendant, the patient piteously demands something to alleviate his sufferings, which greatly interfere with his night's rest. These wearing pains are not confined to the integuments, but appear to pervade the deeper-seated parts, so that the periosteum of the bone of a palsied limb will become swollen and painful. In some cases these pains have appeared to be attributable to the continuance of irritation from the clot upon the brain; in others, there is no evidence of irritation of the brain, but this painful state of the limbs seems to depend upon returning functions in the nerves, and partly upon the capillary circulation in the tissues of the limb not being duly regulated by the nervous system. These pains in palsied limbs are very analogous to those which are experienced in a part when the circulation and animal temperature are returning to it after it has been benumbed by cold. Almost all local applications except Aconite are useless. It will sometimes happen that the redness and heat will subside, but the neuralgia remains. These cases are very distressing to witness, on account of the constant suffering which we cannot remove by allopathic treatment; nevertheless, after the lapse of some time, weeks or months in different cases, the pains gradually disappear (BURROWES). Aconite, Nux and Veratrum are important homœopathic remedies against the irritative, inflammatory, spasmodic and neuralgic affections, although Creosote, Phosphorus, Colocynth, Spigelia, and Ranunculus bulbosus may also be required.

Another most important point in the after-treatment of hæmorrhagic Apoplexy is to aid nature in the removal of the clot; old-school physicians generally depend upon the use of mercury, given so as to act as a purgative, and to slightly affect the gums, but not allowing it to produce salivation, which is always very distressing to the patient, whose powers of mastication and swallowing are already impaired by his disease. Kali hydriodicum would probably effect this object more promptly than Mercury, and might at the same time relieve the pains and swelling about the periosteum and bones, and consequent neuralgic pains. Arnica and Baryta also deserve attention. (J. C. PETERS.)

ON THE

HOMŒOPATHIC TREATMENT

OF

APOPLEXY.

RÜCKERT has furnished twenty-four cases of Apoplexy, treated and cured by means of homœopathic remedies. I have added about thirty additional cases from BLACK, SIMPSON, DUNSFORD, MALAISE, BEAUVAIS and others. I have also thought it advisable to include the cases of *Congestive vertigo*, collected by RÜCKERT, and those instances of "*Affections of the Speech*," which seem to depend upon some disorder in, or of the brain; they are so closely allied to Apoplexy, or its premonitions, that I trust no excuse will be necessary for this liberty.

RÜCKERT truly says, that quite favorable results have been obtained in these formidable disorders by homœopathic treatment. He also assumes, that these not very numerous cases prove that, whenever life can be saved at all, it can be saved without the aid of exhausting bloodletting, and quotes SCHUBERT, who asserts that whenever he bled his apoplectic patients, their disease and recovery progressed more slowly than when he omitted it. SCHUBERT only found bloodletting useful when decided plethora, or full-bloodedness was present; but always found homœopathic remedies useful, and even indispensable.

Of RÜCKERT's cases he has assumed that fourteen cases were instances of *sanguineous Apoplexy*, while nine cases are assumed to be examples of *nervous Apoplexy*.

The remedies treated of by RÜCKERT, are: Aconite, Arnica, Baryta, Belladonna, Cocculus, Crotalus, Ipecac., Hyosciamus, Laurocerasus, Nux vomica, Opium and Phosphorus.

Numerous notes and several additional articles have been added. (PETERS.)

1. ACONITE.

GENERAL REMARKS.—(*a*). [Fortunately, both old and new school physicians agree about the utility of Aconite, in the treatment of congestive and inflammatory affections of the brain, although they entertain almost diametrically opposite views about the general action of this remedy. Dr. FLEMING, *President of the Royal Medical Society of Edinburgh*, thinks that it exerts a purely sedative action upon, and diminishes the flow of arterial blood to the brain, acting in the same way as excessive loss of blood, between which and the action of Aconite, he says there exists a very strong analogy. On page 30, he draws the inference that it is an advisable antiphlogistic in Apoplexy, inflammation of the brain, or in any disease in which the circulation of the brain is excited, because it exerts a direct, sedative influence upon the vascular system, reducing more or less, according to the dose administered, the strength, volume and frequency of the pulse. He asserts that the pulse often falls to 60 per minute, and in some cases sinks to 48, 40 and even 36. On page 36 he draws the inference that Aconite is a powerful antiphlogistic, and that it is calculated to be of great value in all cases where there is an inordinate activity of the circulation. (*See Inquiry into the Physiological and Medicinal Properties of Aconitum napellus. London*, 1845.)

A majority of the most able old-school writers on the Materia Medica, viz.: PEREIRA, WOOD and BACHE, TAYLOR, CHRISTISON, NELIGAN and others, now agree with these views of FLEMING; but it should not be forgotten that HAHNEMANN pointed out the use of Aconite in congestive and inflammatory affections full fifty years ago.

Many old-school writers now compare the action of Aconite on the circulation to that of Digitalis, Tobacco, Colchicum, and Veratrum viride, excepting that Aconite has also been found to act specifically on the skin, causing ready and profuse perspiration, while Digitalis acts more decidedly on the kidneys, causing a free flow of limpid urine; Tobacco acts more decidedly on the stomach and muscular system, causing great nausea and muscular debility, while Colchicum not only diminishes the action of the heart, but causes profuse flow of bile from the liver, and an increased excretion of urea from the blood and kidneys. Hence of late, various uses and combinations of these remedies have been proposed, in the dominant school, in congestive, comatose, febrile and inflammatory affections. Colchicum has been more particularly recommended in cases of Apoplexy arising from or connected with bilious derangements, jaundice, or deficient secretion of bile; but still more, especially by Dr. McLagan, of Edinburgh, in all cases of coma and Apoplexy connected with suppression of urine, presence of albumen and deficiency of urea in the urinary secretion; in all cases in which albumen and urea appear to be vicarious, and where coma supervenes evidently from the accumulation of urea in the blood, viz.: in all cases of Bright's disease of the kidneys, and dropsy dependent thereon. The use of small or moderate doses of Aconite, Digitalis and Colchicum, promises ere long to usurp the place of profuse bloodletting, active purging, and other savage treatment in the dominant school.] (Peters.)

(*b*). According to Kreussler, Aconite is decidedly indicated against sanguineous Apoplexy, and almost every other remedy must yield the priority to this, which generally affords the most speedy relief. Hence, he always gives it, even in cases in which he is somewhat undecided about the proper treatment, without being fearful if it does not afford relief, of not being able to make up the lost time by some other remedy; still, he only waits a quarter of an hour for signs of improvement, which in the majority of cases become evident in the course of a few minutes.

It is most indicated in the Apoplexies of persons who present the appearance of the apoplectic habit, or constitution;

who have previously suffered with disease which can be traced to some affection of the vascular system; or who have been attacked with Apoplexy in consequence of the suppression of accustomed hæmorrhages. In these cases the head is apt to be hot, the carotids to beat violently, the skin to be warm, the pulse full, strong, hard, or labored, but not intermitting.

(*c*). [Of all the narcotic remedies, Aconite is most homœopathic to Apoplexy, as proven by the case of a young man who had incautiously chewed some seeds of this plant; he was shortly afterwards seized with a sense of numbness of the face, soon followed by complete Apoplexy, complicated with paralysis, from which he recovered with great difficulty, and with palsy of one side, with which he is still affected, now upwards of twelve months from the time of the attack.] *Dict. Prat. Med.*, p. 92. (PETERS.)

(*d*). Aconite is most homœopathic, when Apoplexy is attended with paralysis of *sensation*, rather than of motion; according to TAYLOR, (see Medical Jurisprudence, p. 225,) it proved homœopathic in one case to tremors of the muscles, a pricking sensation over the whole body, unconsciousness, followed by confusion of sight and intense headache, the skin being cold and clammy, the pulse slow and irregular, the breathing short and hurried. Also in another case, with: a sensation of swelling of the face, a general feeling of *numbness and creeping* of the skin, restlessness, dimness of sight and stupor, almost amounting to insensibility, arising from exhaustion, however, rather than from congestion; followed by speechlessness, frothing at the nose and mouth, clenching of the hands and jaws; the patient appearing occasionally as if dead, and then again reviving; cramps and *tingling* in the flesh succeeded, and he did not entirely recover for five weeks. Sir BENJAMIN BRODIE found Aconite homœopathic to staggering, excessive weakness, slow and laborious respiration, with slight convulsive twitches. CHRISTISON found it homœopathic to a gradually-increasing paralysis of the muscles, which terminates in immobility of the chest and diaphragm, and consequent asphyxia. PEREIRA thought it most homœopathic to an extraordinary *diminution of common sensation*, evidenced by insensibility to pinching and pricking, there being a total absence of stupor. Dr. FLEMING found it most homœopathic to weakness and staggering, gradually increasing paralysis of the voluntary muscles, slowly increasing insensibility of the surface of the body, more or less blindness from excessive weakness of the eyes, with great contraction of the pupils, excessive languor of the pulse, and convulsive twitches. FLEMING also infers decidedly, that Aconite is more homœopathic to *nervous* paralysis and Apoplexy, than to sanguineous Apoplexy, as it does not occasion vascularity of any membrane to which it is applied; even the lips and tongue while burning and tingling from its topical action, do not show the least sign of redness or inflammation, and hence this peculiar effect is decidedly a *nervous* phenomenon. FLEMING also found it homœopathic to warmth in the stomach, nausea, *numbness and tingling* in the lips and cheeks, extending more or less over the rest of the body, diminution of the force and frequency of the pulse, which sometimes sinks to 40 in the minute, great muscular weakness, confusion of sight or absolute blindness. In very severe cases, there may be a sense of impending death, sometimes a slight delirium, and a want of power to execute what the will directs, but without any loss of consciousness. The warmth of the skin to which Aconite is homœopathic, is a purely *nervous warmth*, being unattended with any elevation of temperature, vascularity of the skin, or acceleration of the pulse. It does not cause any true hypnotic effect, but merely drowsiness from excessive exhaustion, debility, or languor; but by inducing serenity or deadening pain it may also predispose to sleep.

According to FLEMING, it is homœopathic to extreme depression of the circulation; also to an overwhelming depression of the nervous system, so severe that it may prove fatal in a few seconds, without arresting the action of the heart; and finally to asphyxia, or arrestment of respiration, the result of a paralysis gradually pervading the whole muscular system, respiratory as well as voluntary.

Fleming also assumes that the least variable symptoms to which it is homœopathic, are: *numbness*, burning, and *tingling* in the mouth, throat and stomach; then sickness, vomiting and pain in the pit of the stomach; next general *numbness, prickling, and impaired sensibility of the skin*, impaired or annihilated sight; deafness and vertigo; also frothing at the mouth, constriction of the throat, *false sensations of weight, and enlargement in various parts of the body;* great muscular weakness and tremor, loss of voice, laborious breathing; distressing sense of sinking and impending death; small, feeble, irregular, and gradually vanishing pulse; cold, clammy sweats; pale and bloodless features, together with a perfect possession of the mental faculties, and no tendency to stupor or drowsiness. Slight spasmodic twitches of the muscles may be present, and probably depend, as Dr. Fleming suggests, on venous congestion, the result of incomplete asphyxia. Stupor and apoplectic insensibility do not always preclude the use of Aconite, when they arise from the same kind of venous congestion above alluded to, but there is every reason to believe that it is more homœopathic to extreme nervous depression and faintness, than to the stupor and coma, for which they are often mistaken.

Pereira found Aconite homœopathic to burning and *numbness* in the lips, mouth and throat, extending to the stomach, and followed by vomiting; when the extremities became cold, the lips blue, the eyes glaring and the head covered with cold sweat; provided there was no spasm or convulsion, but some tremor; no delirium, stupor or loss of consciousness, but violent headache. In another case he found it homœopathic to such weakness and stiffness of the limbs that the patient was unable to stand; could utter only unintelligible sounds, but had no spasms or convulsions. He experienced a *strange sensation of numbness* in the hands, arms, legs, diminution of sensibility over the whole skin, especially of the face and throat, where the sense of touch was almost extinguished; some dimness of vision, giddiness, and at times an approach to loss of consciousness, but no delirium, sleepiness or deafness.

In another case, Mr. SHERVIN found Aconite homœopathic to sensation of swelling of the face and contraction of the throat; the patient was nearly blind, and excessively feeble, but did not lose her consciousness; although her eyes were fixed and protruded, the pupils *contracted*, the jaws stiff, face livid, whole body cold, pulse imperceptible, heart's action feeble and fluttering, and breathing short and laborious, yet she was at all times so sensible, as to be able to speak about her condition. PEREIRA, and PERRIN, of Bordeaux, found it homœopathic to pungent pains in the limbs, cold sweating, anxiety, extreme general prostration, great slowness and irregularity of the pulse, convulsions and congestion of the whole venous system.

BALLARDINI found it homœopathic to great injection of the pia mater and arachnoid membranes (*congestive Apoplexy*); much serous effusion under the arachnoid, and in the base of the skull (*serous Apoplexy*); and to considerable engorgement of the lungs with blood (*pulmonary Apoplexy*). In PEREIRA's case it proved homœopathic to venous congestion of the head and chest; the lungs in particular being much gorged with blood. PALLAS, when the lungs were dense, dark and gorged with blood, and the vessels of the brain turgid.

Of all the symptoms of Apoplexy, Aconite is most homœopathic to great and general muscular debility and paralysis; slowness of the pulse and failure of the circulation; excessive numbness and tingling; and to the severe pains in the bones, periosteum, and paralyzed parts which sometimes follow an attack of Apoplexy (see page 190).

Aconite-general muscular debility, and paralysis.

AETIUS and AVICENNA report, swooning and sinking together of the legs; RICHARD, great weakness; paralysis of one arm and leg; MATTHIOLUS, great powerlessness, paralysis of left arm and thigh, so that all power of moving them was lost, but left hand could be moved a little; recovery of the use of the left side, but then the right became paralyzed; this paralysis was transient and affected each side alternately, thus when the patient could lift the right arm, he could not move the left, and vice versa, but finally he recovered the control of both arms. BACON noticed such exhaustion of the strength that the patient was obliged to lie down; weakness and unsteadiness of the joints, especially of the knees; BALDRIANI: rapid prostration of strength in ten cases, with an unusual degree of exhaustion. SHERVIN: failure of the legs to such an extent that the patient fell down and had to be carried to bed. PEREIRA: trembling of the limbs, swooning. DEVAY: trembling of the legs so as to produce a peculiar, staggering gait. PEREIRA: excessive trembling, great weakness, yet with ability to walk until a few minutes before death, in one patient; while in another, the muscular debility was so great, that standing was impracticable; in animals it weakens the muscular system so much as to cause staggering in walking. HAHNEMANN: weakness and instability of the ligaments of all the joints, unsteadiness of the knees, paralysis of the rectum and bladder, transient paralysis of the tongue, loss of power in the thighs, which prevents walking, paralytic weakness of the thighs and legs, with staggering and fear of falling; in fact, many signs of paralysis of the lower portion of the spinal marrow, and of the pelvic nerves. AHNER: feeling of paralysis in the right forearm and hand while writing, disappearing after more active exercise of the limb, to return again when at rest. HORNBURG: immediate trembling of the arms and hands. RÜCKERT: trembling of the hands, great lassitude of the limbs, while walking; forty drops of the tincture produced such heaviness and weakness of the limbs, in a stout peasant girl that she was forced to lie down. ARNETH: lameness and weakness of the left shoulder-joint, weakness of the knees, so that he could not stand straight, nor walk without his knees giving way (from forty drops of the tincture). BOHM: (from twenty drops), walking and talking tired him quickly; he felt lassitude and feebleness. GERSTEL: (from ten drops), unusual but transient weakness of the legs; (from forty drops) persistent weakness of the feet, when going up stairs; (from fifty drops) lassitude of the feet. MASCHAUER: (from fifteen drops) great lassitude; (from twenty drops) great general lassitude; (from ten drops night and morning) feverish lassitude; (from twenty drops) lassitude with chilliness; (from fifty drops) palpitation, with slow pulse, and such sudden loss of strength that he was unable to stand up; (from sixty drops) excessive relaxation. REISINGER: (from one hundred and twenty drops) *leaden heaviness of the feet, while sitting or standing;* (from one hundred and forty drops) *tottering of the legs and leaden heaviness of the feet,* so that he can scarcely move; (from two hundred drops) leaden heaviness and relaxation of the limbs; (from one hundred and sixty drops) extreme relaxation of the limbs, *tottering of the knees,* general debility, so that he was unfit to attend to his business; anxious trembling. Trembling of the limbs. General relaxation. Relaxation of the arms and thighs. Relaxation and lassitude of all the limbs. Sudden prostration of strength. Paralytic stiffness of the outside of the right arm. *Lassitude of the feet,* especially while at rest. The feet refuse their office. *Trembling of the legs.* Sensation as if the ligaments of the joints had given away. DIERBACH: extraordinary sensation of weakness and lassitude.

Aconite-failure of the circulation, has already been sufficiently alluded to. (See page 193.)

Aconite-numbness and tingling.

BRODIE: singular numbness of the lips. CHRISTISON: numbness and prickling from chewing a single seed; tingling in the jaws, extending subsequently over the whole body. DUNGLISON: one or two grains of Aconitine to a drachm of alcohol or lard, if rubbed for a minute or two on the skin, causes heat and prickling, followed by a sense of numbness and constriction, as if a heavy weight were laid upon it, or as if the skin were drawn together by the powerful and involuntary contraction of the muscles beneath; this lasts from two to twelve hours or more. DIERBACH: the leaves, roots and seeds if chewed, occasion a violent burning in the tongue and lips which lasts for many hours, and is attended with a peculiar feeling of numbness. VOGT: large doses excite a peculiar sensation of numbness and heaviness in the stomach, pharynx, tongue and neck. BACON: Tingling heat in the tongue and jaws, which gradually extended farther, until it involved the whole body, especially the extremities. SHERVIN: piercing and prickling in the arms and fingers, then numbness in the shoulders, tongue and mouth, finally in the thighs and feet. DEVAY: Insensibility of the palms of the hands, so that deep pricks with a needle were not felt. PEREIRA: burning and numbness of the lips, mouth, and throat; in another case: some burning and numbness of the lips, mouth and throat; curious sensations of numbness in the hands, arms, legs; sensibility of the body was greatly impaired, so that face and throat were almost insensible to touch. TAYLOR: burning in mouth, throat, œsophagus, and stomach, general feeling of numbness and creeping in the skin, tingling in the flesh. PEREIRA: Aconite destroys common sensation, without causing stupor: a dog under its influence will sometimes follow his owner around the room, recognize him by wagging his tail, and yet be totally insensible to pinching, pricking with needles, &c.; in ten minutes a dog has been rendered insensible to the pains caused by the introduction of pins into his legs, paws, body, tail, nose, &c. HAHNEMANN: Pricking sensation upon the tongue, and throat; crawling sensation in the fingers, cheeks, and chest; scrabbling in the chest as if from bugs; crawling and itching of the skin. HOMBURG: Crawling and pricking on the left side of the head, as if caused by a hair brush; crawling in the fingers, even while writing. GERSTEL: (from twenty drops) Prickling and biting in the eyelids; crawling in the cheeks; pains in the left side, especially in the thigh and arm, which pass over into numbness; minute piercing, drawing, and prickling in the left upper and lower jaw, in the right molar teeth, in both shin-bones and arms, and especially in the left side of the nape. Prickling, pricking-burning sensations in the skin in various parts of the body, attended at times with a sense of heaviness, numbness, or swelling. REISINGER: (from five drops) slight crawling with sense of warmth in the left fingers; (60 drops) prickling and burning upon the tongue; (80 drops) numbness from the sacrum down to the legs, while sitting or standing; it seemed as if his feet fell asleep, or as if an attractive power held them fast to the earth; this feeling disappeared instantaneously while walking, but returned again as soon as he stood still, or sat down; falling asleep of the right foot, while walking; a sense of boiling and simmering through the body, as if the hands and feet would fall asleep; (160 drops) a kind of numbness spread itself from the teeth, over the jawbones to the external angle of the eye, and then almost over the whole body; (from 108 drops) numbness of the lower limbs, especially of the feet, even while walking, so that he was often obliged to stand still, in order to get rid of this unpleasant sensation by moving his feet to-and-fro. WATZKE: sensations not unlike those produced by a pretty large electro-magnetic apparatus; prickling in the forehead, back, sides of the chest, fingers, backs of the hands, and other parts of the body, as if he stood upon the isolating stool of an electrical machine, and sparks were drawn from him. Tickling in various parts of the muscles, especially of the forearms, as if one held the conductors of an electrical apparatus in the hands. ZLATAROVITCH: Over the whole body a peculiar sensation, comparable with that felt when steam falls rapidly upon one in a steam-bath, and one feels the drops upon the skin; crawling over the scalp; falling asleep of the feet; crawling and creeping (from 150 drops) over the whole body, attended with a troublesome rather than a violent chilly sensation, first in one place, then in another, but most marked in the arms and legs; formication in the scalp, down the back, and over the arms and thighs; *numbness of the fingers and toes;* (from 170 drops) creeping and crawling in the skin, over the whole body, and at the roots of the hair; a constant crawling and creeping, especially in the right leg, with the sensation at times, as if the cuticle were separated from the true skin by a thin layer; (from 200 drops) chilliness and formication, especially between the shoulders and down the back, increased by motion; numbness and coldness of the fingers and toes; *the scalp feels as if swollen and numb;* creeping and crawling again over the whole skin; creeping and biting over the whole skin, first here then there, as if from fleas.

Aconite-nervous, and -rheumatic pains.

VOGT (see Materia Medica) says: After great restlessness comes relaxation, diminution of pulse and heart-beats, the head becomes confused, and often very painful, the face puffed up and livid, while pains set in, in the limbs, *especially pains in the bones and joints.* SOBERNHEIM (see Materia Medica) says: It causes painful sensations in the bones and joints, which disappear after the breaking out of a profuse sweat and abundant flow of urine, and adds that it differs from Conium by its more prominent action on the fibrous system, as is evident from the bone- and joint-pains which it causes. HARNISCH: It causes painfulness and trembling of the limbs, especially of the legs, and the patient suffers from the most violent pains in the bones and joints. KÜTTNER: General painfulness of all the joints not unfrequently arises, after the use of large doses of Aconite. CLAUDIUS RICHARD's case of poisoning, is probably the source of the above old-school writer's information, he says when the delirium passed away, the patient complained of pain in the stomach and head, in the jaws, chest, and here and there in the joints; after the lapse of seven hours, *all his joints were painful.* MATTHIOLUS, noticed such violent pains in the jaws, that the patient held fast to them in the fear that they would drop off. PEREIRA: trembling and formication in the limbs, attended with piercing pains. HAHNEMANN: aching compressing pain in the sides of the chest; pain as if bruised in the sacro-lumbar joint; *rheumatic pain in the nape, only felt when moving the head;* drawing piercing pain in the bones of the forearm, piercing pain in the right side. AHNER: violent piercing, boring pain for two hours along the whole left side of the spine down to the sacrum, so much increased by inspiration, that it repeatedly forced tears from him (rheumatism of the spinal muscles or ligaments). DR. GERSTEL says that the most of the pains experienced by AHNER, were of a piercing-boring character, which points to an affection of the periosteum, or of the fibrous aponeuroses of the muscles; the rending and drawing pains are probably seated in the muscles themselves. WAHLE: burning, biting pain in the right side of the spine; aching pains to the left of the cervical vertebræ. ARNETH: (from 40 drops of tincture); pain and sense of shortening in both tendo-achilles lasting for twenty days, preventing the free use of the feet, and depending according to Dr. Gerstel, upon a slight inflammation of the tendons. GERSTEL: (from eight drops,) Bruised feeling in the nape, when moved, especially in the evening and at night; (from 10 drops) pain in the nape again; (from 16 drops) same pain in the nape again); (from 40 drops) pain in the nape during the whole day; sensation of swelling of the whole body, especially of the left side, attended with various pains, such as bruised feeling in the muscles, bruised or aching sensation in the bones, first in one, then in another rib, then in the left arm; pain in the bones around the ear; constant penetrating piercing about the left wrist; constant pressing pain in the left shoulder, in connection with a drawing, and *numb feeling in the left side of the occiput*, and in the posterior surface of the left arm, followed at a later period by a bruised feeling in these parts, especially in the arm (from 40 drops); drawing pain in the right side of the nape. WACHTE: (from 20 drops) bruised pain in the sacrum; stiffness, with bruised pain in the left side of the neck, extending beyond the left shoulder-joint to a portion of the back, aggravated when in bed, and lying down, relieved in the free air, and by motion, lasting three days, alternating at times with similar feelings in the arms and legs, then suddenly returning to its original seat in the back, (this reminds one of wandering rheumatism, or spinal irritation). WURSTL, it is a little remarkable, although predisposed to rheumatic affections, experienced none while using Aconite, though he took it in divided doses, for six months. The homœopathicity of Aconite to numbness, paralysis, and the severe pains which often attend apoplexy has been made abundantly evident. PETERS.

CASE 1.—A maiden, aged 20, of blooming health but apoplectic habit, being extremely plethoric, although subject to profuse menstruation, was attacked with Apoplexy after sudden fright and vexation.

Symptoms.—She fell down in a death-like state; her breathing was slow and stertorous; her face andbody corpse-like, marbled with livid and violet spots; her pulse could not be felt; her heart beat slowly and tremblingly; her pupils were insensible to light; urine was passed involuntarily, and her limbs were cold and stiff.

Treatment and result.—Aconite, 1st dilut., cold applications to the head, and dry, warm clothes to the body and limbs. After taking five doses of Aconite, 1st dilut., one dose every quarter of an hour, she gave signs of life; then Aconite was given every one, or one and a half hour, and at the end of eight hours life and consciousness were restored, but the whole left side was paralyzed, the left arm and foot being cold and incapable of making the slightest movement; her speech was stuttering; her tongue was drawn to the right side, when it was put out; she was deaf in the left ear, and had roaring noises in it, and in the whole head; the lips of the left side scarcely moved in breathing; the breasts were cold to touch, and retained the impression of the finger.

One drop of Aconite, 3d dilut., was now given every two hours, and in the course of thirty hours her whole condition was improved, with the exception of the loud roaring in the head, and the paralysis of the limbs.

Opium, 1st dilut., was given in drop doses every six hours, and on the fourth day of the disease the congestion of blood to the head was relieved, her speech could be understood, the tongue could be put out in a straight line, and she began to move her limbs. Opium 6, one dose every twelve hours, enabled her to leave her bed on the sixth day. Arnica 3, one drop daily, removed a remaining swelling of the left foot and paralytic weakness of the knee, in the course of ten days. —Gen. Hom. Journal, vol. 1, p. 66. (STURM.)

CASE 2.—A robust man, aged 64, with short neck and broad shoulders, much given to excesses with wine and women, was attacked with sanguineous Apoplexy, with all the signs of departing life.

After the use of Aconite, 1st dilut., one drop every hour, signs of returning animation ensued; then Aconite 3, every three hours, and cold applications to the head were used with such good effect, that in twelve hours consciousness was entirely restored, with warmth of the body, mobility of the upper limbs, but paralysis of the *lower*, and also of the bladder and rectum. He complained of great pain in the loins and back. Nux vom., 6th dilut., followed by the 15th dilut., repeated every twelve or twenty-four hours, restored him perfectly in ten days.—Ibid., p. 67. (STURM.)

CASE 3.*—A lady of full habit of body, laboring under well-marked enlargement of the heart, was very subject to congestion of the head; for this she had always been cupped and purged, and such attacks were apt to occur three or four times a year. She derived some benefit from my prescriptions, as regarded the heart; but when one of these attacks threatened her, her confidence was much shaken, and with difficulty her scruples in favor of cupping were overcome. The attacks came on with sensation of great fulness and heat in the back of the head, giddiness, stiffness of the nape of the neck, roaring noises in the ears, flushing of the face, and full, bounding pulse.

Treatment.—Aconite, 3d dilut., for a few hours, followed by Belladonna, speedily gave relief; in some attacks Lachesis was more useful than Bellad.—Brit. Jour. Hom., vol. 5, p. 49. Dr. BLACK.

CASE 4.*—A commercial traveller, aged 35, with short neck and stout body, had returned the night before from one of his circuits, and had for some days previously indulged in eating and drinking too much, although not habitually intemperate. His breathing was so stertorous through the night as to alarm his wife; he was unable to stand or sit up, his eyes were prominent, his face turgid, and of a sub-purple color;

he complained of great fulness in his head, of dimness of sight, and giddiness; his pulse was slow and labored, he was aroused with difficulty to answer a few questions, his breathing was oppressed, in fact an apoplectic seizure seemed most imminent. I bared his left arm to look at his veins, it being my opinion that he must lose blood; but I then observed on his wrist an immense malignant carbuncle, very much raised above the surface, blue and turgid. The sight of this made me pause; the carbuncle, according to allopathic treatment, required generous diet, bark, &c., while the threatened Apoplexy demanded the lancet; I gave him Aconite, 3d dilut., a dose every hour, and in a few hours I was sure that the danger was over, for his eyes were less fixed and prominent, his face had a more natural expression, the breathing was greatly relieved, and the pulse more free. The Aconite was continued with directions to take it only every two hours, if he should improve much. The next day the danger of Apoplexy had passed away, but the tumor on the wrist seemed gangrenous, and a deep slough was to be expected. He took Aconite and Lachesis, 7th dilution, alternately every two hours; on the second day his pulse and breathing were natural, he had slept calmly, the carbuncle had improved, as it had shrunk considerably, and was now of a pale brown color. On the seventh day he was able to go out, as there was only a healthy-looking circular sore of the size of a shilling on his wrist, and that healed perfectly in a few days more.—Brit. Jour. Hom., vol. 5, p. 50. Dr. CHAPMAN.

CASE 5.*—A lady, aged 30, in delicate health, from strong mental excitement was suddenly seized with dizziness, and confusion of thought, but shortly afterwards recovered so far, as to be able to converse; in the course of two hours more, however, she fell into a state of stupor, which gradually became confirmed, and in which she continued for nearly a fortnight, during which period she frequently had severe convulsive paroxysms, which affected only the left side of the body, the right being completely paralyzed. I had almost relinquished hope in this case, but homœopathy triumphed over the disease, although the constitution of the patient was exceedingly delicate.

Treatment and result.—Under the use of Aconite, Bellad., Ipecac. and Cocculus, the patient gradually recovered her faculties; and although the paralyzed limbs were not immediately restored, yet in about three months afterwards almost every trace of this most serious illness had disappeared.—DUNSFORD, p. 108.

CASE 6.*—W. D., aged 31, stout built, florid complexion, works at a furnace, but is very temperate; has been liable to dizziness off and on for years, and has been bled for it; has now been suffering for a month, and is forced to leave his work.

Symptoms.—He complains of a hard, thumping, plunging pain in the head, attended with dizziness and swimming; he is worse on lying down, when everything seems to run around, and he sees sparks flying before his eyes; his sleep is disturbed and unrefreshing; his appetite very bad; pulse not much accelerated.

Treatment and result.—Aconite 2, directly, and repeated three times a day; followed by Bellad. 12, in 6 hours. On the third day he was better, but still felt badly when lying down, especially on waking from sleep; his pain was now chiefly in the back of his head. Took Bryonia, three times a day, and in three days more was much improved, had slept soundly for three nights, no dizziness or swimming, eye-sight clearer, but still felt very weak, and had no appetite. China 3, once a day; in two days more felt stronger, appetite was good and head seemed right; was quite restored in three days more.—YELDHAM, p. 176.

CASE 7.—A man, aged 40, light blond, but with much color; healthy, but formerly accustomed to be bled, had not been bled for four years.

Symptoms.—Had suffered for four weeks with attacks of general heat, with redness of the face, perspiration, and violent dizziness, so that he was obliged to sit down; lasting for two hours at a time. Latterly, he has had two such attacks, attended with vomiting, and great weakness; his walk was unsteady and slow.

Treatment.—After taking six doses of Aconite, 3d dilut., one drop night and morning, he was entirely restored.—Gen. Hom. Jour., vol. 32, p. 228. Dr. LEMKE.

CASE 8.—A young man of apoplectic habit, suffered from frequently-returning attacks of dizziness, with roaring in the head; he was often affected with transient loss of consciousness, and was obliged to hold on to something to prevent his falling.

Aconite, 3d dilut., one drop per dose, daily, cured him entirely.—Hygea, vol. 5, p. 102. Dr. SCHROEN.

CASE 9.—A lady, aged 43, was attacked with vertigo, after a fright, recurring whenever she attempted to rise, with great anxiety, and feeling as if she would die, so that she was obliged to lie down again. After the fright she had a feeling of turning in the stomach, ascending up into the head, and attended with trembling, faintness, and dizziness.

Treatment.—Aconite, 15th dilut., followed by two doses of Opium, 9th dilut., relieved her entirely.—Annals, vol. 1, p. 72. BETHMANN.

Dose. The 1st dilution was used successfully in two instances; the 2d dilution in one case; the 3d dilution, in six instances; the 15th in one case, while Dr. Kreussler prefers the 15th or 18th. The very high dilutions do not seem to have been trusted to in any case, of so severe a disease as Apoplexy. NOACK prefers 1 or 2 drop doses of the 2d dilution every half, one, two, or four hours. In very acute and severe cases, 3 or 5 drops of the tincture, or of any of the above dilutions which may be preferred, may be put in a tumbler half full of water, and a dessert- or tablespoonful given every five, ten, or fifteen minutes in very urgent cases, or every half, one, or two hours, in less dangerous attacks. Or, six globules may be dissolved in a wine-glassful of water, and one teaspoonful given as often as above recommended; or two or three globules may be given dry upon the tongue, at the same intervals of time. It is rarely used in chronic cases. PETERS.

2. AGARICUS.*

GENERAL REMARKS.—[Dr. BLACK suggests Agaricus as homœopathic to some varieties of Apoplexy, because the proving of *Agaricus muscarius*, by HAHNEMANN shows symptoms approaching to those of complete Apoplexy.

A man who ate of Agaricus campanulatus, mistaking it for A. campestris, was suddenly seized ten minutes after commencing his repast, with dimness of vision, giddiness, debility, trembling, and loss of recollection. In a short time he recovered so far as to be able to go in search of assistance; but he had hardly walked 250 yards when his memory again failed him, and he lost his way. His countenance expressed anxiety, he reeled about, and could hardly articulate; his pulse was slow and feeble; he soon became so drowsy that he could be kept awake only by constant dragging; an emetic was administered and the stupor gradually went off.—Brit. Jour. Hom., vol. 5, p. 54.

A remarkable set of cases of pure narcotism has been related by Dr. PEDDIE. In half an hour after eating *Agaricus procerus*, an elderly man, and a boy of 13, were attacked with giddiness, and staggering as if they were intoxicated; in an hour they became insensible, the man indeed so much so, that for some time he could not be roused by any means; when sensibility was in some degree restored by means of emetics and powerful stimulants, occasional convulsive spasms ensued, and afterwards furious delirium, attended with frantic cries and vehement resistance to remedies, all followed by a state like delirium tremens. The pupils were at first much *contracted*, afterwards considerably dilated as sensibility returned; and in the boy, contracted while he lay torpid, but dilated when he was roused. In neither instance was pain felt at any time. Another boy, who took a small quantity only, had no other symptoms but giddiness. drowsiness, and debility.

A singular form of the narcotic effects occurred in the case of a boy of 14, who had eaten of the *Agaricus panterinus*, near

Bologna. In the course of two hours he was seized with delirium, a maniacal disposition to rove, and some convulsive movements; ere long these symptoms were succeeded by a state resembling coma in every way, except that he looked as if he understood what was going on, and in point of fact, he really did so.

The *Amanita citrina* caused vomiting, followed by deep sopor, in a lady, servant, and one child; her other children became profoundly lethargic, and comatose.

The effects of the small mouse-colored, conical fungus, called *paddock stool*, or *Hypophyllum sanguineum*, are still more peculiar; it is homœopathic to convulsions, as well as sopor; in a family of six persons, four of whom were children, it caused pain in the pit of the stomach, a sense of impending suffocation, and violent efforts to vomit; which symptoms did not commence, in any case, under twelve hours after partaking of it, in one not till twenty hours, and in another, not till thirty hours. One child had acute pain in the belly, which soon swelled enormously; afterwards he fell into a lethargic sleep, but continned to cry; in twenty-four hours the limb became affected with permanent spasms, and convulsive fits, followed by a tetanic state. Another child, aged 10 years, had convulsions of still greater violence. The mother had frequent bloody stools, and vomiting, her skin became *yellow*, the muscles of the abdomen were contracted so spasmodically, that the navel was drawn towards the spine; profound lethargy, and general coldness supervened. A third child had trembling, delirium, and convulsions. The father had a severe attack of dysentery for three days, and remained speechless for five days.

A striking circumstance, in relation to the effects of these fungi, is the great durability of the symptoms; even the purely narcotic effects have been known to last over two days; a deep lethargy may prevail for fifty-two hours.

In five cases, mushrooms produced a kind of tertian fever and the formation of abcesses, which discharged a thin, ill conditioned pus, and passed rapidly into spreading gangrene.

Pathological appearances: Lividity of the body, very great fluidity of the blood, abdomen distended with fetid air, excessive enlargement of the liver, congestion of the lungs, vessels of the brain very turgid.

The *Agaricus muscarius* is homœopathic to enormous distension of the sinuses of the dura mater, as well as the arteries with blood; scarlet color of the arachnoid and pia mater; excessive engorgement of the vessels of the membrame between the convolutions of the brain, together with the Plexus choroides; redness of the substance of the brain; clot of blood as big as a bean in the cerebellum. Christison. P.

Dose. No cases of Apoplexy treated with Agaricus have yet been reported. Noack prefers 1 or 2 drop doses of the 2d or 3d dilution, repeated as often as occasion requires. The same doses as those directed for Aconite, may be used. It is most serviceable in acute cases, or in acute aggravations of chronic attacks. Peters.

3. ARNICA MONTANA.

General Remarks.—[This remedy, too, is beginning to find some favor in the dominant school, in the treatment of apoplexy, or its consequences. It has long been supposed to possess the power of promoting absorption of extravasated blood—Sobernheim asserts that it facilitates the circulation of the lymph, increases the absorbent powers of the whole lymphatic and venous systems—hence its well-known efficacy in extravasations of blood from mechanical injuries, viz.: from falls, blows, concussions, and rupture of blood-vessels; for these reasons it has also received the name of *Fall-Kraut*, and was admitted as an ingredient of the Thea Helvetica, or Thé Suisse of the French Codex, for wounds, bruises, &c. Tabernæmontanus, once physician to the Churfurst Von Plalz, says that in olden times it was customary, in Saxony, for persons who had fallen, or injured themselves, to use this remedy; it also came into use in the town of Danzig, but as it did not grow in that neighborhood, it was imported in casks from Lower Saxony.

Besides its absorbing powers, the root of Arnica, from its

Tannin-like properties, is supposed to exert an astringent action upon asthenic and profusely-secreting mucous membranes, and to check passive hæmorrhages, such as asthenic dysenteries, scorbutic, septic, and petechial fluxes.

As an absorbent remedy, it was used, and highly recommended in *Arachnoiditis infantum*, by the celebrated GOLIS, of Vienna—he had the head of the child bathed with Arnica, when signs of effusion, or of a sub-paralytic state of the brain came on—and regarded it as a main remedy in concussions of the brain or spinal marrow, in sanguineous, or sero-lymphatic exhudations from contusions, falls, blows, concussions, &c.

It must prove as useful in the apoplexies of debilitated persons, as it has often done in the stupor and coma of typhus and typhoid fevers. VOGT recommends it in asthenic fevers, attended with indifference to everything, dejection of spirit, sleepiness, dull unconcerned look, or when there is sopor, or even stupor and other signs of a suppressed, sunken, torpid, or paralytic state of the nervous system. Also in typhus fever, when blue or brownish petechiæ are present, oppression and sluggishness of the vascular system, torpid state of the nerves, and when the skin is cool, thick and flabby. SOBERNHEIM also recommends it strongly in typhus fever, when there is great prostration, dulness of the senses, typhous hebetude of the brain, with muttering delirium and sopor; tongue trembling, cracked and black, the look inexpressive, and the eyes staring —in typho-septic affections, when attended with colliquative hæmorrhages, passive sweats, decubitus and septic meteorism. The following are the celebrated STOLL's indications for the use of Arnica in fevers—great weakness, slow pulse, dry tongue, or coated with much sordes, especially if the patient be dull and sleepy, hears badly, has a slight delirium, and a miliary eruption, or petechiæ show themselves.

In addition to all this, the careful use of Nux-vomica has been found useful in both schools, in some of the torpid and paralytic states which follow apoplexy—too frequently the incautious use of Nux and Strychnine in the hands of old school physicians, causes great irritation and mischief, but fortunately, according to A. T. Thompson, the flowers of Arnica contain a small portion of Igasaures strychnion, and experiments upon, and accidents to the healthy, have proved that some of the effects of Arnica are similar to those of Nux-vomica and Strychnine—and hence it is much more safe in the earlier stages of paralysis from apoplexy, than these remedies; it promotes the absorption of the apoplectic clot, which Nux and Strychnine do not, and acts, perhaps, quite as powerfully, and certainly much more safely than Mercury, in promoting absorption of effused blood, and serum; it tends to check hæmorrhage, while Mercury dissolves the blood, and perhaps favoring increased bleeding.

Again, Arnica has been admitted, and decreed to act like the nervines, exciting and giving strength in certain regions of the nervous system; and used to obviate the incautious, and too hasty use of stimulants in apoplexy with great depression.

Of course it cannot now be a matter of surprise, that Arnica should have been found useful in some forms of apoplexy and paralysis. The oil of Arnica is said to have done wonders in the hands of Schneider in old apoplexies, even after several attacks had occurred; when a new attack was about setting in, he gave ten drops of Oleum arnicæ at once, with admirable effects. Another old physician kept at bay upwards of thirty attacks of apoplexy; a priest who had had no less than four attacks of nervous or congestive apoplexy, prevented all recurrence for six years. It has been particularly recommended against the congestions of the head, and threatened apoplexies, which so often attend the cessation of the menses in women.

Notwithstanding all this, it will be very easy to prove from the distinguished old-school writers on the Materia Medica, from whom the above observations have been obtained, viz.: from Dierbach, Sobernheim, Vogt, Ables, Mitscherlich and others, that Arnica, is more or less homœopathic to some of the symptoms, or forms of apoplexy. Dierbach says it not unfrequently causes a sensation of formication, and a prickling, piercing, spasmodic feeling, which may be compared with that produced by slight electric shocks—also headache and vertigo. SOBERNHEIM says it may produce hebetude and heaviness of the head, formication, anxiety, flow of blood to internal parts. VOGT says it may affect the whole organism, especially the brain and spinal marrow, and cause vertigo, stupefaction and hebetude of the head, glittering before the eyes, roaring in the ears, anxiety, pusillanimity, oppression at the pit of the stomach, and inability to hold ourself upright; at a later period it may cause increased action of the pulse, violent congestion, especially to the head and chest, formication, prickling, and piercing sensations, with trembling, and subsultus.] PETERS.

CASE 10.—A man, aged 72, after having complained of dizziness, fell suddenly to the ground, struck with apoplexy; he was inconscious, his jaw dropped, the limbs on the *left* side were perfectly paralyzed, and without feeling; he stammered inarticulate and incomprehensible words; and pointed to his head with his right hand; his pulse was strong and full, intermitting every seventh beat; and his face was flushed.

Treatment.—After taking 2 doses of Arnica, he was able, in the course of twelve hours, to speak more plainly, could move his jaw, swallow better, his consciousness returned, and he felt a creeping or crawling in the paralyzed limbs; the redness of his face had disappeared. Nux-vomica, was now given for fulness and torpor of the bowels, and heaviness of the head; on the following morning his bowels were relieved, his head more clear, speech more sonorous, and he began to move his paralyzed limbs.

Archiv, vol. 14, part 1, p. 128. Dr. SCHULER.

CASE 11.—A man, aged 53, of medium stature, with a short neck, otherwise healthy, but fond of whiskey, had had an apoplectic attack for which he had been bled. After the lapse of several days, he remained in the following state:

Symptoms.—He awoke at night in order to swallow much fluid which had accumulated in his mouth; followed by shivering, stretching and yawning, recurrring every half hour, without his being conscious of it; during the day he complained of aching in the forehead, roaring in the ears, vertigo, sparks before the eyes, and illusion that some one attempted to put something into his mouth; his limbs felt as if bruised; his legs were cold; cold shiverings ran through his body; his pulse was moderately strong, labored, beating 60 per minute, and at times irregular. He had an outbreak of nettlerash, with itching, and burning upon the skin.

Treatment and result.—One dose of Arnica 30, 2 drops, repeated on the second day, relieved him entirely by the third day. Five months after he had a similar attack, followed by eructations at night, hiccough, with rumbling and rattling in the bowels; attacks of rigidity, with dull, staring look, and loss of consciousness for one hour, followed by coughing, with cold sweats, and bad odor of the breathing. Such attacks recurred several times, but in a slighter degree. On the next day he had aching in the forehead, eructations, thirst, and nettlerash as before; his pulse was small and slow. He took Arnica 1, 1 dose of 1 drop, and all his symptoms ceased, and did not return again.—Hygea, vol. 8, p. 149. Dr. Käsemann.

CASE 12.—A Teacher, aged 37, had had an attack of apoplexy five years before, since which time he had been annoyed with great forgetfulness; he forgot his train of thought, and whatever he read escaped his memory very quickly.

Several doses of Arnica 3, cured him entirely.—Hygea, vol. 8, p. 34. Käsemann.

CASE 13.—Dr. Frank refers to sixteen cases of Paralysis and Apoplexy, arising from mental emotions, and mechanical causes, occurring in patients of various ages and sexes, most of whom had been treated fruitlessly with bloodletting cured by drinking of an infusion of Arnica, half or one ounce of the flowers, to one pound of water, aided by the alternate or subsequent use of Extract of Aconite. Attomyr.

Dose. In Rückert's cases the 3d and 30th dilutions were used. Noack prefers 1 or 2 drop doses of the pure tincture, or of the 1st or 2d dilution, repeated every one, two, four, six, or eight hours, according to the urgency of the case. If preferred, globules may be dissolved and given as directed for Aconite; or given dry upon the tongue, in the same quantities, and at the same intervals of time, as there recommended. Arnica is useful against the first shock of apoplexy, before reaction has taken place; also after the first force of the disease has been moderated by Aconite and other remedies; and finally in the latter stages of the disease, to promote absorption of the clot, and to remove paralysis. PETERS.

4. BARYTA.

GENERAL REMARKS: [Baryta has been supposed to possess a peculiar curative relation to dulness of intellect, softening and other morbid states of the brain, either when preceding, or following an attack of Apoplexy. Also against the almost idiotic condition which follows Apoplexy. According to NEUMANN, the Muriate of Baryta is an admirable curative remedy against many affections of the brain, and irritations of the cerebellum, or Apoplexy of this latter organ, when the sexual inclination is very much increased. Many old-school writers assume that it is a liquefacient or absorbent remedy; assert that it improves the appetite, increases the flow of urine and perspiration, and causes looseness of the bowels; that with no other more obvious symptoms than these, glandular swellings, enlargements, indurations, thickenings, &c., will become softer and smaller, and finally disappear; and hence the inference has been drawn, that it might also liquefy and dissolve apoplectic clots, and finally absorb or remove the softened mass.

It is very easy to prove, from the same authorities, that it is more or less homœopathic to some of the varieties, or at least symptoms of Apoplexy. PEREIRA found the Carbonate of Baryta homœopathic to dimness of sight, double vision, ringing in the ears, pain in the head with throbbing, and palpitation of the heart. He also says that it is homœopathic to decided staggering, great muscular weakness, almost amounting to paralysis, with trembling; also to pain in the head with deafness. It is suited to some of the after-effects of apoplexy, viz., when a febrile state sets in, with dryness of the tongue, giddiness, debility, and some pains in the legs and knees, with cramps in the calves of the legs.

CHRISTISON adds his testimony to the homœopathicity of Baryta to brain-affections; he says that its remote effects are indicated by narcotic symptoms, and that this narcotic action is more decided and invariable in its occurrence, than in the case of any of the other metallic remedies. GMELIN noticed that it causes strong signs of action upon the brain, spine and voluntary muscles. BLAKE and CAMPBELL found it homœopathic to languor, slow respiration and feeble pulse, to excessive muscular debility, amounting to absolute paraplegia of the limbs, lasting twenty-four hours, and then gradually going off. Campbell always found it homœopathic to congestion of the brain and its membranes, and in one case the Baryta post-mortem appearances were precisely those of ordinary congestive Apoplexy; it is most indicated when there is thick, dark blood in the vessels of the dura mater, in those of the brain and cerebellum; and when the falciform and lateral sinuses, the plexus choroidei, and the ventricles of the brain are filled with blood.

NOACK (see Jahr's Symptomen-Codex, translated by Chas. J. Hempel) says, Baryta is particularly suitable for aged persons with mental or physical debility; in Marasmus Senilis marked by childish, thoughtless manners; in disorders of old persons characterized by groaning and murmuring, fixed pupils, dim and reddened eyes, circumscribed dark redness of the cheeks, cold hands with blue spots on them, weak pulse which may be either quick or slow, frequent micturition, constipation, and weakness which obliges one to walk, or sit very much bent over. In the apoplectic affections of drunkards, when the mouth is distorted, the tongue paralyzed, the voice hoarse or indistinct, with partial paralysis of one or the other arm, but the consciousness remains pretty clear. In the Apoplexies of old people and drunkards, and in organic affections, and tubercles of the brain. Noack also gives an admirable description of the despondency, pusillanimity, weakness of mind and irresoluteness to which Baryta carb., is so homœopathic. It should not be forgotten when the patient is troubled with forgetfulness, dulness, gloominess and heaviness of the head, with drowsiness; and with vertigo, headache and nausea.

The specific action of Baryta upon the cerebellum, as conjectured by NEUMANN, is fully borne out by a reference to the Materia Medica Pura. It is homœopathic to pressure in the brain below the vertex, extending towards the back of the head, most severe on waking from sleep, and attended with stiffness of the nape of the neck, probably from pressure on the twelfth pair of nerves; also to dull aching pain in the right side of the back of the head, extending from the bones of the neck obliquely to the side of the head, and recurring regularly at 4 o'clock, P.M., for several days in succession; sense of weight in the whole back of the head, close to the nape of the neck, with tension; sudden and intensely-painful drawing pain, extending from the back of the head across the right ear, as far as the lower jaw; tearing pain in the left side of the occiput; rheumatic pains in the back bone of the head, with swelling of the glands of the nape, so as to compress the blood-vessels; tearing pains, shooting deep into the brain behind the right ear. Dull stitches in the left side of the head from the occiput to the forehead. Pain with feeling of fulness and distension, commencing in the left side of the head, traversing the whole left side of the occiput, and terminating in the bones of the neck. Throbbing in the occiput, the impulse of which is felt as far as the forehead. Considerable rush of blood to the head, so that the blood seems to stagnate in it, and circulate slowly; whizzing in the head as if from boiling water; heaviness and heat in the head.

Slowness of the pulse is very common in Apoplexy, and BLAKE found Baryta homœopathic to depressed arterial action; two grains, injected into the veins, completely arrested the heart's contractions in twelve seconds.

In one case it was found homœopathic to dimness of vision, followed by double vision, ringing in the ears, pain in the head, throbbing in the temples, and violent palpitations; the skin was hot and dry, the face flushed, pulse 80, full and hard; sleeplessness from pain in the head and ringing in the ears, followed by profuse perspiration; then cramps in all the limbs, with a sense of weight in them, and soreness to the touch; severe pain in the head, with great and long-continued palpitations.

WILSON also found it homœopathic to severe headache, throbbing in the temples, frequent and long-continued palpitations, abnormal vision, ringing in the ears, cramps, pain, sense of weight, and numbness in the limbs.

In another case it proved homœopathic to twitching of the muscles of the face, and convulsive jerking of the hands and feet. It is also decidedly homœopathic to Apoplexy, arising from, or attended with great disturbance, or inflammation of the stomach and bowels; to brain affections from inflammation of the peritoneal coat of the stomach; from ulceration of the stomach, especially when the ulcer assumes the perforating form; and when the colon is contracted throughout its whole extent, so that its calibre is more than one-third less than that of the small intestines in their natural state.—PETERS.]

(*b*.) According to KREUSSLER, Baryta carb. 30, is indispensable in the apoplectic affections of old, cachectic persons, of scrofulous constitution, especially when gouty derangements are also present.—Kreussler's Therapeutics, p. 129.

CASE 14.—An old man, aged 84, remained in the following state, on the third day after an attack of Apoplexy.

Symptoms.—He sat crooked and helpless, unable to speak an intelligible word, or to put out his tongue; he was unable to think clearly; his manners were childish and thoughtless; he was drowsy, but his sleep was disturbed, and attended with groaning and muttering; his pupils were sluggish, his eyes dull and somewhat reddened; there was a circumscribed, dark redness upon his cheeks, his hands were cold and mottled with blue spots; his pulse was weak, and rather quick; he was troubled with frequent urination, and constipation.

Treatment.—Baryta acet., 1st and 2d dilut., restored him after 3 doses had been taken.—Hufeland's Journal. Dr. Messerschmid.

CASE 15.—An aged drunkard was attacked with Apoplexy, after taking cold.

Symptoms.—Speechlessness, with paralysis of the tongue; the mouth was drawn to one side; the *right* arm could not be moved by any exertion of the will, although he seemed conscious.

Treatment.—Baryta, 30, effected a cure in the course of forty-eight hours.—Archiv, vol. 15, part 1, p. 103. Dr. Gross.

CASE 16.—Hartmann thinks that Baryta is the principal remedy in paralysis of old people, especially when it remains after an apoplectic fit, and refers to a case in which it did more good than Causticum or Stannum. (See Hartmann's Acute and Chronic Diseases, translated by Dr. C. J. Hempel, vol. 4, p. 7.)

Dose. Messerschmid preferred the 1st and 2d dilut.; Gross and Hartmann, the 30th. Noack advises grain-doses of the 1st, 2d, or 3d trituration to be given dry upon the tongue, once or twice a day in chronic cases; or 1 or 2 drop doses of the 1st, 2d, or 3d dilutions. If preferred, 2 or 3 globules may be given, per dose, dry upon the tongue; or 5 globules may be dissolved in a wineglassful of water, and 1 or 2 teaspoonfuls given at a time. Baryta carbonica is only suitable in chronic, or sub-acute, or slow cases; while Baryta acetica and muriatica may be used in acute cases, and given in doses as large, and as frequently repeated as those recommended for Aconite. Peters.

5. BELLADONNA.

General Remarks.—[It proved homœopathic in a case with vertigo, faintness, and dimness of sight in a lady, so that she had to keep her bed all the next day—for thirty or forty hours she could not lift her head from her pillow without experiencing a strange and disagreeable sensation. In another case, with slight delirium and great vertigo.

Johnson says it is one of the most effectual remedies in reducing morbid sensibility of parts, and morbid contractility of the muscular fibres, and may be used when there is irritation, with rigidity; hence it may prove homœopathic in the pains and stiffness of the limbs which follow attacks of Apoplexy, and especially in the painful disorders about the head and face. BAILEY, of Harwich, England, published an octavo volume, some years ago, on this point.

It proved homœopathic in the cases of two boys; at first they could not speak, but laughed immoderately and kept grasping at imaginary objects; afterwards their silence was changed into immoderate and incoherent loquacity, with constant bodily motion; they were laughing and talking alternately; their extremities were in violent almost constant motion; eyes fixed; pupils dilated and insensible to light; jaws firmly locked; respiration loud and croupal; face swollen and red; in four hours their breathing became loud and stertorous; face turgid and swelled; skin cold; pulse weak; and there was an occasional strong inclination to sleep. Next day there was a loud croupy cough; and they were not sensible to surrounding objects for three days; they were quite blind, and candles held to their eyes produced no effect, nor did they seem at all conscious of the light.

Old-school writers, GRAVES especially, have recommended Bellad. in cerebral affections when the pupil is *contracted*, which is one of the most alarming symptoms in these affections;—pin-hole pupil is a fatal sign in Apoplexy and typhus.

In Apoplexy with *quick* pulse; LEURET in seventeen cases of epilepsy found Bellad. to quicken the pulse from the second day of treatment, and to continue to do this for three or four, or ten or even twenty days. It is homœopathic when the pulse is quick, and pupil dilated. Another of the most frequent and durable of the effects of Bellad. was a very marked development of the papillæ of the tongue.

PEREIRA says Atropin is homœopatic to vomiting, dilatation of the pupil, and stupor. One-tenth of a grain caused difficulty of swallowing, dilatation of pupils, and headache.

FLOURENS thinks it acts specifically on the tubercula quadrigemina.

BAILEY found it homœopathic to dilatation of the pupils,

obscurity of vision, absolute blindness, amaurosis, visual illusions, suffused eyes, singing in the ears, numbness of the face, confusion of the head, giddiness and delirium; all of which symptoms may be combined with, or followed by stupor. These symptoms are usually preceded by a febrile condition, with redness and swelling of the face, hurried and small pulse.

DIERBACH says it is peculiarly homœopathic to violent congestions to the head, redness and swelling of the face, and inclination to sleep, which may pass over into deep sopor and coma, but be interrupted by delirium.

It is indicated in paralysis of the sphincters, when the fæces and urine pass off involuntarily.

VOGT says ROGNETTA exercised considerable ingenuity when he indulged in the opinion that Bell. was an antiphlogistic remedy, and placed it in the same category with blood-letting.

VOGT also asserts that in the first degree of Belladonna-action we observe a more active motion of the blood, quicker, fuller, and harder pulse, greater flow of blood to the skin and head, whence the face seems more reddened, and the skin, especially that of the head, hotter. After a while the increased arterial action ceases, and greater venosity supplies its place, soon followed by increased secretion from skin and kidneys; the throat also becomes moist, and mucus is ejected from the bronchiæ, and genitaliæ.

Bellad. is homœopathic when there is a violent and convulsive change of arterial into venous blood, while Aconite, Digitalis, Hyosciamus, Prussic acid, &c., do this without previous orgasm and excitement of the vascular system.

It is homœopathic when there is fever, dryness of the throat, glimmering before the eyes, with flocculi and sparks, even actual blindness, with dilated pupils, dulness of feeling, and roaring in the ears; when the eyelids droop and sink with heaviness, are half closed, and the patient is sleepy; or when the eyes are widely open, and the look is fixed and fiery; when there is a feeling of heaviness in the head, staggering, confusion, and drunkenness, which may gradually pass over into a perfect loss of consciousness. The pulse from the first is more frequent, fuller, and harder; the skin becomes hot, red and itching; the face swollen and very red; the lips dark, blood red; the eyes red and protruding. Everywhere there is greater vital turgor, and excited arterial action; breathing is quicker and shorter; the limbs rather stiff, and tongue rigid.

After the lapse of twelve hours the arterial storm ceases, and great venosity becomes evident; the redness of the face becomes livid, the veins everywhere seem to be filled, the muscles are more relaxed, confusion and stupefaction of brain ensue. Finally profuse sweat and urination restore the balance of the system. But headache, vertigo, imperfect vision, general lassitude, continued inclination to sweat, burning and itching of the skin remain.

The third degree of action of Belladonna-action is marked by paralysis of the nerves and decomposition of the blood, the patient becomes soporose and paralytic; blue spots and petechiæ form on the skin; and decomposed, dissolved, brown and stinking blood exudes from the various openings of the body. With the exception of Stramonium, it causes a more constant and far more violent action on the circulation than the other narcotics; the brain is at first not only quickened and excited, but forcibly excited, and rendered delirious; still the collective action of Bellad. does not represent a pure inflammatory fever, but a *Febris inflammatoria nervosa.* VOGT.

SCHNUCKER, SELLE, and EVENS, have cured paralysis after Apoplexy with it. PETERS.]

(*c.*) Dr. BLACK advises Belladonna in Apoplexy, in the stage of excitement, when the face is flushed, head hot, eyes suffused and glistening, with hallucinations of sight, dilated pupils, throbbing of the carotids, incoherence, tremors, and convulsions, followed by coma; especially when the disease has not progressed beyond general congestion of the brain and its membranes.—Brit. Journ. Hom., vol. 5, p. 53.

(*d.*) [According to CHRISTISON, Bellad. is homœopathic to apoplectic symptoms, with dilatation of the pupil, also to blindness, even when this is a very obstinate symptom, sometimes remaining after the affection of the brain has disappeared; it was homœopathic in two cases in which the eyes were insensible to the brightest light for three days; and in general, when the dilated state of the pupils continues long after the other symptoms have departed; the pupil is not only dilated in all cases, but likewise for the most part insensible, and the eyeballs are often red, and prominent.

It is generally supposed that delirium with dilated pupils, generally precedes Belladonna-coma, but sometimes the relation of the delirium to the coma is reversed, as in a case related by Mr. Clayton, where sopor came on first, and delirium ensued in six hours; but sometimes delirium again returns when the stupor goes off; still the most frequent order of the symptoms is dryness of the throat and delirium, soon followed by drowsiness and stupor; this succeeding, stupor may remain for nearly two days, and the departure of the stupor be attended with a return of delirium for some hours longer; Sage has related a case in which the patient was comatose for thirty hours.

In Belladonna-apoplexy convulsions are rare, and when present, slight; in one case there were convulsive twitches of the face and extremities; in another case the muscles of the face were somewhat convulsed; there is also, at times, more or less locked-jaw, or subsultus tendinum, and occasionally much abrupt agitation of the extremities, but well-marked convulsions, or paralysis do not appear to be ever present.

From Christison's remarks we may also infer that Belladonna will prove homœopathic to some of the severest, and most hopeless stages of Apoplexy, viz.: when there is aphthous inflammation of the throat and mouth, great swelling of the belly, when the body is almost putrid, even before the patient is fairly dead, when the skin is covered with dark vesicles, the brain soft, the blood-vessels of the head gorged, and the blood everywhere fluid, flowing profusely from the mouth, nose and eyes. Peters.]

(*e.*) *Belladonna-Apoplexy.*

ATTOMYR (*see Primordien einer Naturgeschichte der Krankheiten, p.* 487) has given so accurate a delineation of this disorder, in all its nuances, degrees, and stages, that we give it, even if at the risk of being considered tedious.

Premonitions of Belladonna-apoplexy. Vertigo. Vertigo, as if objects staggered to and fro. Turning in the head, vertigo with nausea, as after rapid turning in a circle, or after the morning sleep, which succeeds a night-debauch. Turning in the head, accompanied with a similar turning in the pit of the stomach; after getting up, these sensations increased while walking, to such a degree, that he could no longer distinguish anything, and everything disappeared from before his eyes. Vertigo, as if everything turned around in a circle. Dulness, and turning in the head, relieved in the open air, aggravated in the room. Attacks of dizziness, both while at rest, and when in motion. Vertigo, and trembling of the hands so that he could not accomplish anything with them. While walking he staggered, was obliged to hold on to the wall, complained of oppression and dizziness, and often speak irrationally like a drunken person. Attacks of dizziness and dulness of the senses, lasting for several minutes.

Stupidity. Intoxication. Feeling as if intoxicated immediately after a meal. The slightest quantity of beer caused immediate intoxication. Confusion of the head, and feeling of intoxication, with swelling and redness of the face, as if one had been drinking wine. The whole head seems confused and empty for many days. Cloudiness of the brain, as in intoxication. Mistiness of the forehead, as if an oppressive mist moved to and fro, especially under the frontal bone. His senses deceive him. Reverie, he sat as if in a dream. Loss of consciousness. Dull fulness of the head, increased by motion. Stupefaction. Head feels as heavy as if he would fall asleep, and he is indisposed to any exertion.

Disinclined to all mental labor. Relaxation of body and mind. Stupidity.

Loss of memory. Great weakness of memory, he forgets immediately what he intended to do, and cannot remember anything.

The blood rushes to the head, when one stoops, and one becomes heavy and dizzy. Congestion of blood to the head, without internal heat in the brain. When one bends his head backwards, it seems as if the blood rushed into it. Swelling of the external veins of the head. The veins of the limbs are distended, and the arteries of the neck beat so violently, that when he opens his mouth the lower jaw is constantly forced against the upper, so that a slight chattering of the teeth ensues; attended with a warmth, and a sensation of warmth in the whole body, especially in the head. Beating of the arteries of the head, and of the whole body, early in the morning, on awaking. Excessive heat of the whole body, with especially frequent and more violent beatings of the temporal artery, with dulness of the head, all followed by profuse perspiration. Great heat of the body, especially of the head, so that the face becomes very red, from time to time, occurring daily after dinner. Frequently, excessive paleness of the face is converted immediately into redness, with coldness of the cheeks, and hotness of the forehead. Unusual redness of the face. Great heat and redness of the face, not followed by perspiration. Great heat and redness of the face, with icy-coldness of the limbs. Glowing-redness of the face, with violent, and inexpressible pains in the head. Heat and redness of the head only. Congestion of blood to the head, with redness of the cheeks. Heat and redness of the whole face, as if he had been drinking. Dark redness of the face.

The whites of the eyes are streaked with red, early in the morning, with aching pains in them. Dimness, darkness and blackness before the eyes. Dulness of sight, with trembling in all the limbs. Darkness before the eyes, as if from a mist.

Roaring in the ears. Noises in the ears, and dizziness, with dull pain in the abdomen. Deafness, as if a skin were stretched before the ears. Difficulty of hearing.

Immediate bleeding of the nose. Epistaxis early in the morning, and at night.

Violent gritting of the teeth. Gritting of the teeth, with frequent flow of spittle from the mouth.

Sensation in the morning, as if the tongue were asleep, numb, dead, and covered with fur. Trembling of the tongue. *Stammering weakness of the organs of speech, with clearness of the intellect, and dilatation of the pupils.*

Attacks of nausea in the forenoon. Frequent nausea and retching. Vomiting, dizziness and flushes of heat. Excessive vomiting, [from pressure on the brain].

Trembling in all the limbs, inability to walk, swelling of the veins of the whole body, and unpleasant irritation in the throat, all lasting for several days. Trembling and tired feeling of the limbs. Lassitude of the limbs. In the evening he is so tired he can scarcely walk. Sluggishness of all the limbs, and disinclination to work. *Disinclination, and disgust for all labor and motion.* Weakness of the body. Loss of strength. General debility. Frequently recurring, transient paroxysms of great weakness, in which everything seems so heavy, and presses downwards as if he must sink together. Fainting fits.

Sleepiness. Persistent dulness and drowsiness. Frightful, and vividly-remembered dreams.

Attack of Belladonna-Apoplexy.

He lay without sense or consciousness. Extreme stupefaction of all the senses. Unconsciousness. Perfect unconsciousness, so that he does not recognize anything. Loss of sensation. Apoplectic condition. He lay motionless for four days, without taking any nourishment. Lethargic, apoplectic state; he lay night and day without moving a limb; when griping pains set in, he opened his eyes, but did not utter a sound.

Noise and rattling in the air-tubes. Difficult respiration. Violent, short, frequent and anxious drawing in of the breath. At times he breathed, at others the last gasp seemed to have escaped him; recurring in paroxysms, four times in the course of fifteen minutes.

During his drowsy stupefaction he opened his eyes, looked wildly about him, and then relapsed into a heavy slumber, with rattling in the throat. Choking attacks of snoring, during inspiration, while asleep.

Largeness, fulness and slowness of the pulse. Very small, quick pulse. Largeness of the pulse, which is ten beats too frequent. Strong and quick pulse.

Widely-opened eyes. Contracted pupils. *Dilated pupils.* Dilated and immovable pupils. Excessively-dilated pupils. Protrusion of the eyes, and enlargement of the pupils. Fixedness of the eyes. Staring look. The eyes are staring and sparkling. Glistening, and glassy appearance of the eyes, with widely dilated pupils.

Spasmodic motions of the lips. The right angle of the mouth is drawn outwards. Distortion of the mouth from spasm (Risus Sardonus).

Bloody foam before the mouth.

Stuttering speech; he stutters as if intoxicated.

Difficulty of swallowing; painless inability to swallow.

Involuntary discharge of fæces; paralysis of the sphincter ani. Small, sudden and involuntary stools. Suppression of stools and urine, with profuse perspiration.

Difficulty in urinating. Suppression of urine. Retention of urine, which only passes off in drops. Involuntary discharge of urine. Paralysis of the neck of the bladder. He cannot retain his urine.

Paralysis of the right arm. Heaviness and paralysis of the upper limbs, but most decided in the left arm. Paralysis of the feet. Paralysis of the right arm, and right leg. The left side, especially the left arm and thigh, are quite paralyzed.

Cold sweat on the forehead.

CASE 17.—A plethoric man, aged 60, of short stature, was found early in the morning, lying by the side of his bed, in a fit of Apoplexy.

Symptoms.—He lay immovable, stretched out as if dead,

and stiff; frothing at the mouth, snoring, and groaning; he was unconscious, the upper eye-lids were paralyzed, his pupils dilated and immovable; his face was swollen, and somewhat reddened; he had twitchings and jerkings; the carotids beat violently; his lower jaw was dropped, and much spittle ran from his mouth; his lips quivered; he had incessant snoring respiration, with frequent groaning; slow, deep respiration, increased warmth of the body; skin soft, but not moist; pulse full, strong, somewhat hard, bounding, and quickened.

Treatment and result.—A small venesection, followed by Ipec. 6, 1 drop, every two hours; in a quarter of an hour, great restlessness set in, he tossed from side to side, grasped about with his hands, opened his eyes, had frequent twitchings of the facial muscles, and gritted his teeth; his pulse became quicker, and his skin moist; vomiting of mucous and bilious substances set in, followed by a loose stool, and discharge of urine.

After the lapse of eight hours, he was in a state of coma-vigil, and unconscious; when loudly spoken to, he mumbled and stammered, looked at the person who spoke, and then closed his eyes again; his pupils were dilated, his face pale, but bloated, and twitching; at times he chewed and gritted his teeth slowly, then his jaw dropped again; tough spittle flowed from his mouth; he groaned and snored incessantly, and grasped, at times, at the somewhat swollen genitalia; his breathing was slow and deep; skin dry; pulse full, regular, and somewhat quickened. He took 1 drop of Bellad. 30, and in the course of twelve hours his improvement had progressed so far, that his consciousness had returned, he could speak, and all immediate danger was over. A kind of mental derangement, which remained after the apoplectic attack required farther treatment, before full recovery ensued.—Archiv, vol. 6, part 3, p. 104. Dr. SCHUBERT.

CASE 18.—A woman, aged 45, was attacked with Apoplexy, and suffered with the following

Symptoms: Loss of motion and sensation on the right side of the body; inability to speak, loss of sight and smell;

mouth drawn towards the ear; consciousness undisturbed; convulsive motions of the face and left arm; difficulty in swallowing; increased flow of saliva; thirst; bloating of the face; redness and protrusion of the eyes; constipation.

Treatment.—Bellad. 24, removed the whole attack.—Dr. Bigel, vol. 2, p. 97.

CASE 19.—A powerful girl, aged 19, fell down unconscious, after an attack of vertigo and anxiety.

Symptoms.—She lay stupefied; with dilated pupils, reddened, and somewhat mottled face; eyes reddened; she could neither speak nor swallow; made signs of having pain from the root of the tongue to the pit of the stomach, and in the left leg; she ejected every kind of fluid from her mouth with force; her pulse was hard; and she had not improved any for two days.

Treatment.—In two hours after taking Bellad. 30, she made signs that she could swallow; in five hours she could speak, the redness of her face had disappeared, and she commenced to move the left leg. In three days she was perfectly restored. Archiv, vol. 5, part 1, p. 165. Dr. Baudiss.

CASE 20.—A man, aged 60, of apoplectic habit, and asthmatic, fell suddenly to the ground in a fit of Apoplexy, after an attack of dizziness. He lay in a soporose state, unconscious and speechless, with much rattling upon the chest.

Treatment.—Two doses of Bellad. removed the stupor, and rattle in his breathing, after it had induced perspiration. Rhus and Cocculus cured the paralysis of motion and sensation in the course of fourteen days.—Archiv, vol. 14, part 3, p. 129. Dr. Schuler.

CASE 21.—A priest, aged 33, of lymphatic temperament, and unusually corpulent, had three apoplectic attacks in the course of one month, followed by paralysis of the right side.

Symptoms.—Dejection of mind, with uneasiness about his condition; confusion of thought; he was affected by the slightest movement; heaviness of the head, as if it would fall off; fulness, especially in the forehead, with dizziness; anxious feeling in the stomach, which ascended to the head; dulness of the head, as if he were intoxicated; noises and beating in the head; sleepiness during the day; paleness and bloating of the face; dilatation of the pupils, intolerance of light, squinting of the right eye, with lachrymation, and constant winking. Paralysis of motion and sensation of the *right* side of the face, with a sense of crawling and pulling; his mouth was greatly drawn to the *left;* his food fell out of his mouth; he chewed with great difficulty, could not hold a cigar between his lips, bit his tongue while eating, and swallowed with difficulty. His speech was tedious and difficult; he had much thirst; his mouth was pasty; he had no appetite; his abdomen was much distended, chest oppressed, and breathing difficult. He had troublesome constipation, with internal piles. Stiffness of the joints of his legs, and weakness of the whole right side.

Treatment and result.—One globule of Bellad. 2000, followed in a few hours by tearing pains in the shoulder, as if the head were drawn backwards; his head became more clear, and on the next day he was entirely restored.—Genl. Hom. Jour., vol. 34, p. 152. Dr. NUÑEZ.

CASE 22.—Capt. S., aged 72, short, stout and plethoric, was attacked suddenly with the following

Symptoms: Redness and bloating of the face; redness and lachrymation of the eyes, with complete paralysis of the lids; dilatation of the pupils; face drawn to the *right* side; violent shaking only caused him to mumble a little; clean spittle flowed over the drooping lower lip, out of the distorted mouth; his tongue was thick, and projected beyond the lower lip; his inspirations were snoring, his expirations blowing; he was in a constant slumber; the arteries of the neck and face beat violently; his pulse full and slow, and urine passed involuntarily.

Treatment and result.—1 drop of Bellad. 15, to be given immediately, was followed by such improvement in twelve hours, that he could move his tongue and open his eyes; his face was less red, and pulse not so tense; he could move the limbs of the right side, but could not close, or grasp with his *left* hand. During the next day he slept much, and spoke irrationally; for which he received *Opium* 10, 1 drop every three hours; in the evening he was able to walk about the room. He then took one dose of Bellad. every second day, until the fourteenth day. Despondency, loss of memory, and difficulty in speaking, were entirely removed by Anacardium, Baryta, and Rhus.—Gen. Hom. Jour., vol. 8, p. 68. Dr. ELWERT.

CASE 23.—A lady, aged 61, was attacked with vertigo and confusion of the head. In the course of a few hours she had an unusual snoring and blowing out air through the lips; her face was red and bloated; her mouth somewhat drawn to the *right;* lips and *left* side in alternate convulsive motion; she had fits of yawning, entire unconsciousness, *paralysis of the left* half the body, and violent throbbing of the carotids; her pulse was full and slow; urine was passed involuntarily; her pupils did not contract when exposed to light; she made no sound, except a kind of groaning noise; her hands were cold.

Treatment and result.—Several drops of Bellad. 2, were mixed in water, and a teaspoonful given every half hour, at first; afterwards, a drop of the pure Tincture was occasionally put between the lips. The above condition of things persisted for two days, and the same treatment was continued; then she groaned more frequently, seemed to hear when she was loudly spoken to, and could swallow some food; she lay on her back, unable to alter her position, but could move the limbs of the right side. On the fourth day, her consciousness returned; her stuttering speech could be comprehended; she knew not what had happened to her; complained of weakness, especially of the left side, which she could move, however; and could take nourishment, although swallowing was difficult.

The remainder of the disease was removed by Bellad. 3, Nux-vom. 3, and Rhus 2. Dr. ELWERT, p. 40.

CASE 24.*—HARTMANN (see Acute and Chronic Diseases, translated by Chas. J. Hempel, M. D., vol 4, p. 6,) reports a case of Apoplexy in a weakly, emaciated woman, aged 80, suffering with dropsy of the legs. The arms and head dropped suddenly; her mouth was drawn to one side; she could not speak; her breathing was short and rattling; skin cool; pulse small, weak, and scarcely to be felt; all her secretions were suppressed; she was entirely unconscious; and food dropped, or poured out of her mouth again from inability to swallow.

Treatment.—Bellad. improved her condition very much. The remaining paralysis was removed by Stannum, Causticum, and Baryta, after the œdema had been cured.

CASE 25.*—A man-cook, aged 40, having received a repulse in the presence of his master, from his betrothed, which he took much to heart, was attacked on his return to the kitchen with vertigo, but still continued to do his work, although his sight became much obscured, and he went staggering around the room, scarcely knowing what he was about; at length he fell senseless to the ground. He was carried to bed in an insensible state; his face was swollen, and of a reddish yellow color; his eyes red and fixed, pupils dilated; he gave no signs of hearing; from time to time he had violent convulsive movements in his arms, particularly in the right; breathing very slow; pulse slow and hard; forehead very hot.

Treatment.—Bellad. 20, 9 pellets dissolved in an ounce of water, a spoonful every half hour; in two hours the convulsive movements were less frequent and violent, his face less flushed, he gave signs of hearing, and put his hand to his head. In the course of the night he fell into a general perspiration, and on the following day he replied in a distinct voice when spoken to, opened his eyes and looked about with an unsettled and frightened air, and wished to be carried into his own room, where in fact he then lay. His sight was obscured, his eyes moved spasmodically, and were rolled upwards, always with a profound sigh; he complained much of severe pain and weight in the head, especially in the forehead; his face was still much flushed; tongue yellowish-white; mouth slimy, with a bitter taste, loss of appetite and great thirst; bowels constipated; urine red and clear; pulse freer, and less hard. *Ignatia* 20, 12 pellets in solution, a spoonful every half hour. In the evening, *Bellad.* was repeated; he perspired again, and more copiously during the night, and on the following morning he could see better, recognized his room and the bystanders; his eyes were less red, but the rolling motion upwards recurred occasionally, always accompanied with sighing; pulse febrile, but skin almost natural. *Ignatia* at longer intervals; and on the fourth day he was nearly well, although some bilious symptoms required *Chamomilla.*—Brit. Jour. Hom., vol. 4, p. 370. Dr. LADELCI.

CASE 26.*—A lady, aged 23, had a good confinement, four days after which the lochia ceased, and fever with pain in the bowels set in. Her allopathic physician prescribed injections of Assafœtida. On the 9th day, headache came on, increased steadily, became constant and often intolerable; her physician diagnosed neuralgia, and gave Castoreum, without benefit. By the 12th day the disease had assumed a serious aspect; the patient lay on her back motionless; her features were spasmodically disturbed and expressed much suffering; she was very weak, entirely unconscious, her tongue was almost immovable, and she cried out distractedly at long intervals; her right arm and leg were paralyzed. She passed urine involuntarily; her abdomen was soft, and she was constipated. Her physician now leeched and bled her on account of congestion and irritation of the brain, but she became more heated, convulsions of the left arm occurred, her pulse became thread-like, her face pale, and she lay as if dead. Dr. RAMPAL was now called in consultation and advised *Belladonna*, but the other physician would not consent and gave more Assafœtida; the next day she was still worse, and Bellad. was given, ¼ grain of the extract, in six ounces of water, a spoonful at night; the night was more tranquil and some color returned to the face; in the morning two-spoonfuls were given within four hours, and in the evening the patient moved the right leg several times, noticed a little, and put out her tongue; that evening and the next morning she got another spoonful of the medicine, and the improvement went on, so that on the 17th day she could move her arms and legs; on the 18th, she ate with appetite, and soon recoveredly completely.—Brit. Jour. Hom., vol. 8, p. 281. Dr. Rampal.

CASE 27.*—A man, aged 42, of sanguine-choleric temperament, who had suffered for a long time with his head, and with pains in his limbs, was seized with an attack of apoplexy one afternoon, in the midst of most violent pains in his head; he was left paralyzed on the whole of the *right* side.

Symptoms. He was unable to speak; his mouth was drawn to one side; at times the sound *left* side was agitated with convulsive movements; the saliva flowed constantly from his mouth; he had some hiccough; his pulse was full and hard; eyes red and prominent; his face flushed; thirst excessive; he had been constipated for four days; but he retained his consciousness, understood his situation, and felt that his great misfortune had reduced his beloved family to a very distressing situation.

Treatment and result.—He took two pellets of Bellad. 30, and a quarter of an hour had scarcely elapsed before a change was observed in his state; the pain in his head became less violent; the redness of his face less decided; the convulsive movements less severe, and in half an hour after, he fell into a pleasant sleep, which lasted two hours, and from which he awoke in a slight perspiration; he was able to speak in a brief, comprehensible manner; sensation and motion had returned in a slight degree to the paralyzed parts, and in twenty-four hours more the paralysis had entirely disappeared; some pain and heaviness in the head persisted for a few days after.

Beauvais' Clinique Homœopathique, vol. 1, p. 276. Dr. Bethmann.

CASE 28.*—A printer, aged 36, fell while at dinner, with an attack of apoplexy, followed by paralysis of the whole *left* side; when his arms or legs were raised, they fell heavily like inert masses; his face was red, his eyes brilliant, and full of tears; he had not entirely lost consciousness, but was unable to speak a word; his tongue was drawn to one side; and his pulse was full and strong.

Treatment and result.—Bellad. 30, 1 drop. In the evening the paralysis had entirely disappeared; his speech had returned, but his *voice* was stammering; his pulse was frequent, but soft. The same prescription was repeated, and by the next day he was out of danger.—Malaise' Clinique Homœopathique, p. 1.

CASE 29.*—A woman, aged 38, of violent temper, but pale and delicate, had suffered for several years with *Congestive vertigo.*

Symptoms.—The attacks occurred several times a day, generally in the morning, after stooping; were attended with flimmering before the eyes, and dimness of vision; she was obliged to lay hold of something to prevent her falling, on account of staggering and pitching about; afterwards she felt exhausted in body, and mind.

She also was annoyed with aching pain in the forehead over the eyes, increased by bodily exercise, and attended with throbbing in the head, and heat in the face. She had but little appetite, an aversion for meat-diet, with nausea and inclination to vomit. In the forenoon she had flushes of heat, attacks of unconsciousness, and aching, and pulsation in the epigastrium after eating, and while walking. She was costive, with bearing down upon the uterus; also had a chronic cough, and shortness of breath.

Treatment.—After nine doses of Bellad. 15, one drop per dose, the vertigo and headache had entirely disappeared. Nux., Sulph., and Stramon., removed the remaining symptoms. Genl. Hom. Jour., vol. 19, p. 313. Dr. ELWERT.

CASE 30.*—A boy, aged 15, who had suffered for a year with attacks of vertigo and transient fits of unconsciousness, was cured by Bellad. 4, one dose every day, for four weeks. Genl. Hom. Jour., vol, 19, p. 314. Dr. ELWERT.

CASE 31.*—A girl, aged 13, had suffered for several years, with attacks of turning-dizziness attended with anxiety, pressing headache, and staggering about, occurring several times every week. She was entirely cured by Bellad. 5, 30 drops in 2 drachms of Alcohol, 10 drops to be taken every other day.—Gen. Hom. Jour., vol. 19, p. 313. Dr. ELWERT.

CASE 32.*—A lady, aged 48, was subject to vertigo on rising from her seat, so that all objects seemed to stagger to and fro; she was also apt to fall down, and to vomit mucus.

Symptoms.—The attacks of vertigo were preceded by a putrid taste in the mouth, nausea, and at times by bilious and mucous vomits; occasionally, she was dizzy at night; the vertigo was increased whenever she lessened the quantity of meat she ate; she had a disgust for milk; and was every now and then troubled with diarrhœa, or acrid leucorrhœa. She often awoke at night in alarm; her sleep was disturbed before midnight, and during the day she was anxious, unhappy, and irritable.

Treatment and result.—She was somewhat relieved by Bellad. 10, but still the dizziness and loss of memory remained; whenever she sat bent forwards heaviness in the back of the head came on; near objects were seen indistinctly: she had pain in the urethra while urinating; her urine was turbid with mucus, and an acrid leucorrhœa was increased; her stools were still loose; and she had a frequent inclination to doze. *Conium* 10, then cured her almost entirely, although Lycopod. was required for the vertigo when stooping, the flatulent distension, and the stools which had now become too hard.—Annals, vol. 1, p. 231. Dr. SCHRETER.

CASE 33.*—A man, aged 26, of large and robust constitution, had suffered for three days with turning vertigo, and dimness of sight after rising up from sitting or lying, from moving the head or eyes, and from rising up from stooping. He also complained of lassitude in his limbs, with trembling of them while walking, of fulness in the head and pain in the chest.

Treatment.—Four doses of Bellad. 9, were given, one drop per dose, every six hours, with decided improvement: then four doses of Bellad. 12, 1 drop per dose, every six hours, cured him entirely.—Gen. Hom. Jour., vol. 44, p. 47. Dr. HAUSTEIN.

CASE 34.*—The patient, aged 34, suffered with numbness and weakness of the left side; paralytic drooping of the eyelids: lachrymation and squinting of the left eye: double vision; distortion of the mouth. The head was dull and confused; the tongue coated; appetite poor; pulse rather tense; sleep restless.

Treatment.—*Bellad.* was administered in repeated doses of the pure Tincture, for four weeks. For the obstinate remains of the Paralysis, Rhus 1st dilut., was given every forty-eight hours, for four weeks more, when the patient was entirely restored.—Dr. ELWERT, (Homœopathy and Allopathy in the Balance, p. 42).

Dose. Of the eighteen cases treated by Bellad., three were treated with the pure Tincture, which effected a cure in one case where the 18th dilution had failed; the 1st, 2d, 3d, 4th, 5th, 9th, 20th, 24th, and 2000th dilution, were each successful in one case; the 15th in two cases, and the 30th dilution in six cases. In four cases, single doses of the 15th, 24th, and 30th dilution, sufficed to effect a cure; in other cases the doses were repeated as frequently as every half hour, and from four to five, or even nine or ten doses were required. In six cases, favorable results ensued in the course of two hours; in three cases, after the lapse of ten or twelve hours; in others, in the course of a few days. NOACK prefers one or two drop doses of the 1st, 2d, 3d, 6th, or 12th dilution, repeated every two, three, four, six, eight, or twelve hours, in acute and severe attacks. In very severe cases, they may be given every five, ten, or fifteen minutes, or every half, or one hour. If preferred, from 3 to 6 pellets may be dissolved in a wineglassful of water, and a teaspoonful given as often as above directed. PETERS.

6. BLOOD-LETTING.

Even if it be admitted that allopathic physicians bleed too much in apoplectic attacks, it is generally supposed that homœopathic physicians bleed too little—if the strength and vascular condition of the patient permit of it, or seem to require it, it seems very certain that bleeding will not interfere with the action of homœopathic remedies—and it is even supposed that in some apoplectic and congestive affections of the brain, the pressure upon it and the nervous system may be so great, that they are as it were benumbed, and unable to respond to the action of any remedy until the pressure be relieved by blood-letting—hence I will endeavor to state as fairly as possible the advantages and disadvantages of blood-letting in apoplexy.

Wood, the latest American writer on the theory and practice of medicine, says: "If the strength of the pulse admit, blood should be drawn from the arm—but bleeding is not to be indiscriminately resorted to, or pushed to an unlimited extent; much injury has probably been done in this disease by excessive bleeding; if nature have already accomplished a great reduction of the heart's impulse, if the pulse at the wrist be small and feeble, no advantage is to be derived from the further loss of blood. It should be remembered that in the hæmorrhagic and serous cases of Apoplexy, the disease is not over when the effusion is suppressed; the brain has sustained a great shock, and a long series of actions will be necessary to repair the mischief done; it is bad practice to destroy all the resources of the system which may be necessary to sustain this course of action, by an inconsiderate and exclusive obedience to the first indication, viz., that of arresting effusion, or correcting congestion. The practitioner should be guided by the strength of the pulse whether he shall bleed or not."—Vol. 2, p. 628.

Solly says, "blood-letting is the most dangerous remedial agent in some cases of Apoplexy. Many a valuable life has been saved by the prompt and free use of the lancet; but *more* have been hastened into eternity by its indiscriminate employment. At one time this opinion of the imperative necessity of blood-letting in Apoplexy was almost universal, but it has lately been much modified; the deservedly-high reputation of

Abercrombie gave too much value to the use of the lancet in Apoplexy. Watson, he says, advises after *one* full, and sufficient bleeding from the arm, to abstain from farther use of the lancet; the disease itself is most depressing, and in its treatment we must not consider the present moment simply, but we must also look to the future. Solly is convinced that large abstraction of blood gives rise to serous effusion, or dropsy of the brain. He also quotes Dr. Holland, who asks, "Is not depletion by bleeding, a practice still too general and indiscriminate in affections of the brain"—he believes that the soundest medical experience will warrant this opinion. Watson says, that he does not mean altogether to praise the modern (allopathic) practice in apoplexy; for it is often one of mere routine—this routine may be most proper in many cases; unnecessary in others, and pernicious in some, but there are persons who seem to think that they have not done their patient justice if any part of the usual active intermeddling has been omitted—they think that the patient must be copiously bled, cupped or leeched, blistered, and thoroughly dosed with calomel, senna and croton oil, and mustard poultices must be applied to the legs, &c.

Burrows says: until a very recent period, repeated and copious blood-lettings and active purgatives were the principal, if not the only remedies recommended to be employed in all Apoplexies by authors held in the highest esteem. Several, however, of the present day have pointed out many circumstances which would cause such profuse expenditure of the vital fluid in the treatment of apoplexy to be highly prejudicial—Burrows says that his experience leads him fully to concur in reprobating the indiscriminate use of the lancet in these cerebral affections. He also adds that: the principles of treatment of apoplexy recommended by so eminent and experienced a physician as Dr. Abercrombie, have, he doubts not, misled many into the abuse of the lancet. They have been afraid to abstain from blood-letting, since that remedy has been declared to be almost a panacea by this writer. Several modern writers have alluded to states of the brain simulating congestions of its vessels, and where depletion would only aggravate the symptoms.

But the most formidable antagonist in the old school against blood-letting is Copeman. He asks, "Could things be worse under any plan of treatment, or would the mortality be greater without any treatment at all. Surely there is a complete justification for leaving the well-beaten allopathic track that has hitherto been trodden with so little satisfaction, and endeavoring to find out a path that might lead us to more encouraging prospect. Of 155 cases, 129 were bled and only 26 were not; of the 129 who where bled only 51 recovered and 78 died; of the 26 who were not bled, 18 were cured and 8 died.—See p. 6.

"From these facts," Copeman infers, that "bleeding generally speaking, is so ineffectual a means of preventing the fatal termination of Apoplexy, that it scarcely deserves the name of a remedy for this disease. That bleeding in the foot was the most successful mode of abstracting blood, but that the treatment without loss of blood was attended with most success; and that the mortality of the disease increased in proportion to the extent to which bleeding was carried; the more copious the loss of blood, the more fatal the disease." (*See Collection of Cases of Apoplexy, by Edward Copeman*, p. 7.)

Copland says, that during his own experience he has often had cause to regret that apoplectic and other sudden seizures had been treated by blood-letting by the first medical man who had seen the patient. For many hundred years an idea has been entertained by medical practitioners that active practice was good practice: that blood-letting was the best part of active practice; and that this constituted the chief and greatest part of a medical reputation. They could not perceive the fact that blood-letting could be injurious in any of these cases; and they fully believed that patients died notwithstanding the bleeding, and not in consequence of it. Now matters have somewhat amended with the progress and diffusion of medical knowledge; but there still remains much to reform even in this, and other practical measures. The number of cases collected by COPEMAN might have been easily very much increased, and especially in support of the views which he has espoused, and which had been fully insisted upon by myself (COPLAND) and others long before he wrote." (*See Copland on Palsy and Apoplexy*, p. 275.)

We have already seen that ABERCROMBIE was most enthusiastically in favor of free blood-letting in Apoplexy, and that he carried his prejudices and practice in this respect so far as even to be blamed by his fellow allopathic practitioners therefore. It would almost necessarily be supposed that ABERCROMBIE was unusually successful in his treatment; it would hardly be guessed that a celebrated physician could carry his opinions and practice out in spite of the repeated and abundant ill success. In COPEMAN's work we find 28 cases of Apoplexy reported by ABERCROMBIE, no less than 24 of which terminated fatally; in 4 of these fatal cases "all the usual allopathic remedies were employed in the most active manner without the least effect in alleviating any of the symptoms, and on inspection after death, either no vestige of disease could be discovered in the brain, or at most, there was but a slight turgescence of the blood-vessels.

I trust that I have honestly made the case strong enough against the universal applicability of blood-letting in the treatment of Apoplexy; I trust that I have done enough, and that right fairly to prove that the sound and learned medical practitioner is often imperatively called upon to avoid blood-letting in many apoplectic attacks; but, notwithstanding all this, I am fully convinced that blood-letting is safe and useful in some cases; even COPEMAN, the great opponent of blood-letting in Apoplexy, says that in his opinion, the only cases in which bleeding is proper, are those which occur in plethoric habits, and where in addition to the symptoms of what is generally understood by a full habit, there is *evident distension or fulness of the superficial vessels of the head and neck*, and that it is rarely necessary to carry the bleeding beyond the point of relieving entirely the external visible fulness of the vessels. COPLAND admits the safety and benefit of blood-letting where there is slowness and fulness of the pulse, stertorous or strong breathing, and a tumid, flushed or livid countenance. RAU says, bleeding may be necessary in those rare cases of true plethora where the brain and nervous system is overwhelmed by the excess of blood, and in violent congestions of noble organs, such as the brain or lungs, where there is imminent danger of Apoplexy in the former, and of suffocation in the latter. In these cases the bleeding simply averts the present danger, but does not cure the disease : this has to be accomplished by appropiate medicines, and if this be not attended to, every drop of blood may be taken away without relieving the patient; beyond a certain moderate point, we weaken the body by abstraction of blood, without lessening the quantity circulating in the brain. [PETERS.]

7. COCCULUS.

(*a*.) Dr. BLACK says that this remedy somewhat resembles Nux-vomica in its action; it is most indicated when the patient has not entirely lost consciousness, although it is more homœopathic to stupor than Nux; the best indications for its use are the presence of: Violent pains, especially in the forehead; severe headache with much vertigo, nausea and vomiting; numbness, sometimes of the hands, sometimes of the feet; or transient fits; and paralysis of one side.—Brit. Jour. Hom., vol. 5, p. 56.

(*b*.) It is used, perhaps, more frequently, to prevent Apoplexy, and against apoplectic-vertigo, than in the fit itself, although it may prove useful in many cases of gastric-, nervous-, and convulsive- or epileptic-Apoplexy. NOACK and TRINKS recommend it in Nervo-apoplectic conditions with hemiplegia; in congestion of the brain and Apoplexy, even after profuse blood-letting; when there is great nausea with a tendency to faint; dizziness with inclination to vomit; attacks of dizziness with feeling of intoxication, dulness of the head, nausea, pressing and beating in the temples, alternate falling asleep of the feet and hands, difficulty in speaking, thinking or reading; severe headache with nausea and vomiting; headache with feeling of emptiness and hollowness of the head, increased by eating and drinking; when there is vertigo, with nausea and falling down without consciousness; vertigo, as from intoxication, and stupid feeling in the head, as if he had a plank before it; vertigo, when raising himself in bed, as if everything turned around, with inclination to vomit, obliging him to lie down again; headache with inclination to vomit, as if he had been taking an emetic; stupid feeling in the head, with cold sweat on the forehead and hands. Attacks of paralytic weakness. Apoplexy of the left side; *epileptic- or convulsive-Apoplexy*, in which the patient first feels as if intoxicated, then becomes quite still, and stares for a long time at one spot, without hearing or answering any questions, then falls down unconscious, writhing and muttering unintelligible words, with involuntary emission of urine, spasms of the limbs, convulsive clenching of the fingers, paroxysmal choking in the throat, the mouth being open as if he would vomit, the hands being cold, the face covered with cold sweat, the eyes glassy and protruded; after the attack he is partly unconscious and bewildered. PEREIRA says it is homœopathic to nausea, vomiting, staggering, trembling and convulsions; 3 or 4 grains of it have proved homœopathic to nausea and fainting, although it is frequently added to malt liquors for the purpose of increasing their intoxicating powers. TAYLOR says it is homœopathic to vomiting and intoxication. ATTOMYR regards Cocculus as indispensable in some of the consecutive affections of Apoplexy, especially against the weakness and irritability of the stomach, weakness and dizziness of the head, and the paralysis. He regards it, however, as more homœopathic to epilepsy than to Apoplexy. Others regard it as most homœopathic to asthenic Apoplexy, when the face is pale and sallow, but puffy and bloated, the pulse feeble and easily compressed, the respiration heavy and laborious; especially when these symptoms have been ushered in by headache, giddiness, loss of memory, illusions of hearing, inarticulate speech, and inclination to somnolency.—PETERS.]

CASE 35.—A maiden, aged 18, slender, and not yet menstruated, fell suddenly to the ground.

Symptoms.—Her face was red, and glowing hot; her eyes closed, eyeballs in constant rotation, and her pupils much dilated; breathing short and noiseless, scarcely to be heard for hours together; pulse full, hard and frequent; entire unconsciousness.

Treatment.—Bleeding was followed by groaning respiration, restless and anxious moving of the left arm and leg; the right side was entirely insensible to severe pricking with needles. She then received Cocculus, 12th dilution, and in the course of one hour she moved herself, turned over upon her side, her breathing became more quiet, but stronger and more equal, and she opened her eyes, although still without consciousness, or ability to speak. Consciousness returned at the end of four hours, but perfect paralysis of the right side remained; at the end of twelve hours feeling and power of motion began to return in the paralyzed parts. Recovery in two days more.—Annals, vol. 4, p. 47. Dr. TIETZ.

CASE 36.—Mr. L. had suffered for a long time with vertigo, which returned daily at 11 A.M. Whenever he looked up, he had a tendency to fall to the left side; when he stooped it seemed as if he would fall backwards, so that he was obliged to hold on to something quickly. He often had stitches of pain in the top of the head, and pains in the back and sacrum.

Treatment.—Two doses of Cocculus caused some improvement, but Causticum 30, effected a cure.—Archiv, vol. 17, part 1, p. 6. Dr. B. of D.

CASE 37.—A youth, aged 17, had suffered with attacks of dizziness recurring every fourteen days, and lasting for several days.

Symptoms.—Vertigo while sitting, when rising from bed, or from a chair, also while standing, but most frequently after dinner, and attended with a feeling of intoxication, and stupidity, with nausea, pressing and throbbing in both temples, and alternate falling asleep, first of the feet, then of the hands.

During the attacks he could scarcely speak; afterwards he had difficulty in reading and thinking.

Treatment.—Nine doses of Cocculus 15, one dose every six days, cured him entirely.—Gen. Hom. Jour., vol. 8, p. 70. Dr. ELWERT.

Dose. The 12th and 15th dilutions have been used successfully. In other cases the same doses as recommended for Nux may be given.—PETERS.

8. CONIUM-MACULATUM.*

GENERAL REMARKS.—According to ATTOMYR, the principal homœopathic remedies against Apoplexy are: Belladonna, CONIUM, Hydrocyanic acid, Hyosciamus, Opium, and Plumbum.

According to CHRISTISON, Conium acts as specifically in causing paralysis of *motion*, as Aconite does in producing paralysis of *sensation*. It is homœopathic to palsy, first of the voluntary muscles, next of the chest, finally of the diaphragm, causing asphyxia from paralysis, without insensibility, and with slight occasional twitches only of the limbs.

In several soldiers, it proved homœopathic to such drowsiness that they seemed to drop asleep while conversing; but they soon became giddy with headache; in one case there was such a state of insensibility, that the patient could only be roused for a few moments, his face was bloated, pulse only 30, and extremities cold.

It is also homœopathic to great congestion of the head, with an unusually fluid state of the blood.

Conium also differs very widely from Bellad., Stramon., and other narcotic remedies, in not producing violent orgasm, commotion, and active congestion of the blood; POHLMANN found after taking one-third of a grain of Conium, that his pulse fell from 70 to 59, with slight dizziness, and a remarkable sensation of heaviness in the arms and legs, but especially in the left arm. VOGT thinks that it checks the arterialization of the blood, and renders it much more venous. ABLES also thinks that it acts sedatively on the arterial system. SOBERN-

HEIM asserts that it diminishes the frequency of the pulse, and relaxes the muscular, and vascular fibres.

It exerts a similar depressing action on the brain; it is not only much more apt to be homœopathic to paralysis and coma, than to delirium and convulsions, but it causes a most intense passive stagnation, and venous congestion of the blood about the head, and brain. In this respect it acts almost antagonistically to Ferrum; (see page 154); and in like manner as this latter remedy is, perhaps, the most homœopathic to true *arterial* congestive plethora and Apoplexy, so is Conium the most homœopathic remedy to true, simple, and uncomplicated *venous* plethora and Apoplexy.

Its action upon the functions of the brain are also decidedly depressing; it is homœopathic to weakness of the intellectual faculties, loss of memory, inclination to shun society, yet with fear of being alone, dread of thieves, and liability to be easily frightened; to want of mental energy, unfitness for exertion, confusion of ideas, as if from drowsiness, slow conception of ideas, ready forgetfulness, hypochondriacal indifference, dejection of mind, &c., all pointing to a torpid and sub-paralytic state of the brain, which may easily be followed by Apoplexy.

It is also homœopathic to apoplectic attacks, connected with, or dependent upon derangement of the liver; according to VOGT it is homœopathic to excessive distension of the vessels of the vena-porta system, with great enlargement of the liver, and profuse effusion of bile. PETERS).

(*b.*) According to ATTOMYR, Conium is indicated when the following

Premonitions of Apoplexy occur:

Vertigo, in which everything seems to turn around in a circle; dizziness when rising up from stooping, with feeling as if the head would split; dizziness, which is more severe while lying down, and then attended with the feeling as if the bed turned around; dizziness on going up stairs, he was obliged to hold fast to something, and for a few moments did not know where he was. Dulness of all the senses. Confusion and heaviness of the head; persistent stupefaction of the head, with constant inclination to lie down. Dimness of sight. Roaring in the left ear with hardness of hearing, aggravated while eating. Roaring in the ears, as if from a wind-storm, increased from after dinner until bed-time, aggravated by mental exertion, but particularly by lying down in bed; it was also noticed at night when he awoke.

Bleeding from the nose, gritting of the teeth, difficulty of speaking, waterbrash, nausea and inclination to vomit.

Dead feeling of the left hand, especially when clenching the fist; numbness of the fingers, falling asleep of the legs while sitting; numbness and coldness of the fingers and toes. Trembling of all the limbs, and incessant trembling. Great lassitude, relaxation of body and mind, nervous debility, fainting fits. Sleepiness during the day, so that he can scarcely keep his eyes open while reading; drowsiness, even while walking in the open air; sleepiness in the afternoon, so that, in spite of all his exertions to the contrary, he was obliged to lie down and sleep. Sleep disturbed by unpleasant dreams.

Conium is indicated in *attacks* of Apoplexy when the patient lies without consciousness, in a deep sleep, and breathes with extraordinary difficulty and exertion, (see Apoplexy of the Medulla-oblongata, page 168); when the breathing is slow and difficult; when the pulse is unequal in force and quickness, large and slow pulsations being followed at irregular intervals by several small and quick pulse-beats; slow, weak pulse; pulse small, hard and slow, only 30 beats per minute. Protrusion of the eyes, dilated pupils, followed by contraction of the pupils.

Paleness of the face; blueness, or bluish and swollen state of the face; blueness of the face, as if crowded with venous blood, as in strangled persons. Constipation, involuntary discharge of fæces while asleep. Suppression of urine, ischuria, frequent urination, with inability to retain the urine. Paralysis and coldness of the extremities. ATTOMYR.

From the powerful action which Conium exerts upon swellings and exudations, it is very probable that it will also aid powerfully in the absorption of apoplectic clots; and from its depressant action on the vascular system, it may prove antipathic to the inflammatory irritation which is so apt to set in around the clot. PETERS.

Dose. No cases of Apoplexy have as yet been reported, as cured by Conium. NOACK advises 1 or 2 drops of the pure tincture per dose, or of the 1st or 2d dilution. Those who prefer them, may use the globules, either dry upon the tongue, or in solution. PETERS.

9. CROTALUS.

CASE 38.—A man was suddenly attacked with Apoplexy.

Symptoms.—Headache, oppression of the chest, and burning fever with quick pulse; inability to speak; deep slumber, from which he could not be roused; muttering to himself.

Treatment.—Crotalus 30 effected a speedy cure. Genl. Hom. Jour., vol. 39, p. 280. Dr. WEBER.

10. CUPRUM- AND PLUMBUM-ACETICUM.

GENERAL REMARKS.—BEER, of Vienna, in 5 cases, found Copper to be homœopathic to very severe headache, slight delirium, convulsive movements of the legs, great exhaustion, and somnolence, which in 3 cases amounted to coma. From CHRISTISON'S remarks we also learn that it is often homœopathic to violent headache and other affections of the brain, in which symptoms of narcotism appear first, and are followed by irritation.

It is also peculiarly homœopathic to Apoplexy which arises from disorder or disease of the liver; to the brain-affections which are so common in bilious persons, and in those who have acute or chronic jaundice, although we will soon see that Phosphor. also deserves attention.

From DANA'S American edition of TANQUEREL'S work on *Lead Diseases*, we learn that Lead is decidedly homœopathic to some varieties of coma and partial Apoplexy. It is so when the patient suddenly falls into a comatose state in the midst of an appearance of good health, or during the course of severe colic. In the highest degree of this variety of disease, the patient is immovable, the limbs gathered upon the body, the eyes closed or half closed, and snoring may be heard like that from one in a sound sleep; from time to time the patient utters heavy groans, but if spoken to he cannot be roused from the comatose state in which he is plunged; still at times, if he be pinched sharply, he may open his eyes, look around, and then fall again into his lethargic sleep without replying to any question. Involuntary automatic movements of the head, trunk, and limbs take place from time to time; the pupils may be dilated or contracted, and light either has no effect upon them or else causes them to slowly contract; sensibility and motion are lessened, but not abolished; the jaws are firmly clenched; and from time to time there may be an abrupt motion of the lips accompanied with a strong expiration, a movement common in Apoplexy, and often called "smoking the pipe."

Lead is also homœopathic to a sub-delirious form of coma; the patient after having been plunged into a sleep, more or less profound, seems to awake suddenly, opens his eyes, nearly always mutters the same unintelligible words, or distinctly pronounces them without any meaning; he may turn, and turn again in his bed, rise and take the most fanciful postures, and then finally fall back into his first sleep. If he be briskly aroused from his lethargic state, he at first opens his eyes a little, then closes them immediately, or if he opens them completely they look fixed and haggard, and if he then be questioned with much earnestness he will sometimes look fixedly at the person without speaking, or else he replies in a stammering, very laughable and sing-song manner; there is a constant tendency to repeat the same, or similar sounding words.

Sometimes when the patients are awakened from their stupor, their harsh jargon often expresses discontent, and they turn with ill humor away from their interlocutor; sometimes when they are awakened, they articulate the first words of a reply, and mutter the rest as they fall again into their stupor. In some cases they can give a rational reply if it does not require more than one word, such as yes or no. All the organs of the senses are blunted.

Lead is also homœopathic when these two varieties of simple coma and sub-delirious coma occur in alternation, or appear and disappear without any particular order of occurrence. Lead is peculiarly indicated when the above states set in without premonitory symptoms, and almost instantaneously; but it is very rare that the comatose variety occurs alone, without being preceded or followed by delirium or convulsions.

Lead-Atrophy of the Brain.

In 21 cases Lead proved homœopathic to a flattening and shrinking of the convolutions of the brain, with increase or diminution of the firmness or cohesion of the medullary substance, and of the size of the brain. In 19 cases, to yellowness of the substance of the brain; in 32 other cases there was serous infiltration, more or less slight; congestion of the membranes of the brain, more or less great; and diminution of the consistence (softening) of the white cerebral substance, without any change of color.—Tanquerel says, that the shrinking and flattening of the cerebral convolutions deserve serious examination, because they have been noticed by numerous and skilful observers, and consequently are worthy of the highest credence—in some of these cases there was also an increase of the volume and consistency of the brain, in fact, an hypertrophy; but in other cases there was also a flattening of the cerebral convolutions, with diminution of the size of the brain, in short there was either an atrophy, or at least a shrinking, or condensation of the cerebral mass. In other cases there is only a turgescence of the cerebral tissue.

It will be seen that if homœopathy be true, Lead must prove a most important remedy in some of the most serious chronic affections of the brain; in acute swelling of the brain, in hypertrophy, in white or yellow softening, in atrophy and induration of the brain.

Rokitansky in particular has laid great stress upon the more or less frequent occurrence of premature atrophy of the brain in Apoplexy, associated or not with manifest premature senility of the whole organism—he thinks it a very important condition in itself, but it also becomes still more so from its immediate and subsequent consequences. These consequences are:

(*a.*) Congestion of the brain, or *Hyperæmia ex vacuo*, giving rise to those transient or protracted attacks which simulate Apoplexy, and are so frequent in old age.

(*b.*) *Actual Apoplexy*, with hæmorrhage, is one of the most common consequences of atrophy of the brain, and the congestion to which it gives rise.

(*c.*) *Œdema of the brain* is a very common occurrence in the atrophied brains of the aged and imbecile—it may be chronic or acute.

Atrophy when it involves the whole brain and has reached a certain degree, terminates fatally either by paralyzing the brain, or through some of the consequences described above. (See page 165.) PETERS.

SCHMID found Cuprum-acet. exceedingly useful in nervous Apoplexy marked by loss of consciousness, twitchings of the face, distortion of the mouth, partial paralysis and distortion of the tongue, paralysis of the tongue, immobility of one or the other limb.—Hygea, vol. 12, p. 127.

Dose. NOACK advises 1 grain doses of the 1st, 2d, or 3d trituration; or 3 or 4 grains of the 100th, 150th, or 200th, in a tumbler of water, a tablespoonful to be given every quarter, half, one or two hours. PETERS.

10. FERRUM.

See pages 18 and 19.

11. IPECAC.

CASE 39.—In an attack of nervous and serous Apoplexy, attended with dizziness, paralysis of the lips, inability to speak, flow of spittle out of the mouth, and paralysis of the limbs, much good was accomplished with Ipecac.: but Cocculus was necessary to perfect the cure. (See case 17.) Dr. RUMMEL.

12. GLONOINE.*

This extraordinary remedy promises to be useful against headaches, congestion of the brain, and congestive apoplectic attacks. It is particularly indicated, according to HERING, against throbbing headache, aggravated by shaking the head, and attended with great quickness of the pulse, which may range as high as 120 per minute, and even more; it is more homœopathic to these symptoms than any known remedy.

It is also indicated against: "sensations of swelling about the face and neck; uncertainty of step; dizziness from moving the head; heaviness of the head, especially over the eyes, and extending to the ears; dull headache, with warm sweat on the forehead. Headache ascending from below upwards, especially on the *top* of the head; from within outwards, especially in the temples, with feeling as if the brain were swelling, or getting too large; fulness in the head, especially on the top, with throbbing and heat. *Congestion to*, *and heat* of the head. *Throbbing* in the forehead, *temples* and vertex, extending back into the nape, increased by every step, and by every motion of the head. A bruised and sore feeling in the head. The pain, heat and fulness of the head are peculiarly apt to ascend from below upwards, i.e., to commence in the chest, nape of the neck, or occiput, and then pass up into the upper part of the head. Shaking of the head aggravates the pain very much. The headache is attended with quick pulse, redness of the face, and perspiration of the forehead, with redness of the eyes, heat in the eyeballs and lids, soreness and aching of the globe. HERING.

There may be sparks, spots, and dimness before the eyes; fulness and noises, with sense of stoppage of the ears; pain and stiffness of the jaws; nausea and vomiting; increased flow of clear, spastic urine; (an unfavorable sign in Apoplexy, according to SCHŒNLEIN); suppression of menses, with congestion to the head and chest, or with headache and fainting fits.

Also oppression of the chest, sobbing, violent palpitation of the heart, pain and stiffness of the nape of the neck (from congestion of the brain); pain, throbbing and fulness in the nape; pain, heat and shivering down the whole of the back; heaviness, weakness, and numbness of the arms, with pain and trembling; fainting fits; throbbing, crawling, thrilling, and curious feeling of warmth through the whole body, moving from above downwards; twitchings of the fingers; yawning, with congestion to the head; sleepiness; feeling of warmth, especially in the face, and ascending from the pit of the stomach to the head; perspiration, especially on the face.

HERING also advises it against the effect of mental-concussions or shocks, fright, or mechanical injuries of the head; in congestions of the head, Apoplexy, headaches, and sun-stroke.

CASE 40.*—Dr. ZUMBROCK, subject to frequent attacks of headache, almost always after taking cold, and always on damp days; they generally lasted a whole day, or longer; always commenced in the occiput, and spread from there over the whole head; were increased by shaking the head, but relieved by gentle walking, especially in the open air. During the attacks his face became red, he could not see distinctly, and he had black specks before the eyes.

Treatment.—Aconite and Bellad. did not relieve, but Glonoine 1-300 relieved him quickly and permanently for months.—HERING upon Glonoine, p. 52.

CASE 41.*—A patient, with frightful arthritic pains in the head, and vomiting, followed by a fainting fit, was very quickly relieved by Glonoine, but not cured—in several other cases it only produced transient relief. Dr. GEIST.

CASE 42.*—Flushes of heat and congestion of blood to the head, in a lady predisposed to Apoplexy, were quickly relieved by Glonoine. Dr. OKIE.

CASE 43.*—In two cases of throbbing headache in the forehead, and between both temples, with violent palpitation of the heart, and throbbing of the carotids, speedy relief was induced by Glonoine 2. Dr. DURHAM.

CASE 44.*—A young man, from working in a garden, in the hot sun, was taken with nausea, violent headache, which soon became throbbing, and attended with fever; his face had a yellowish red color, his eyes were fixed, dull and glassy, pupils contracted, pulse quick and small, he could scarcely speak, and had frequent retching to vomit.

Treatment.—This case, and several similar ones, were quickly cured by Glonoine. Dr. CAMPOS, of Norfolk.

CASE 45.*—A delicate woman had headache upon the vertex and in the temples, which, without being throbbing, increased and diminished in intensity, and some of the exacerbations were so severe that she almost wished to die; her pulse was small, weak, and not quick.

Treatment.—Relieved quickly by Glonoine 12. Dr. HERING.

CASE 46.*—Rev. WAAGE had severe symptoms from an over-dose of several hundred globules, but remained free from an accustomed sick-headache from Nov. to May, *i.e.*, for six months.

Symptoms.—The attacks occurred at every opportunity; commenced suddenly with the illusion, as if the focus of the left eye were changed; he then saw everything half-light, half-dark, and felt as if he must die; in half an hour inclination to vomit set in, he was obliged to sit down, and then it seemed as if a cloud rose up and melted away, when his sight would be restored, but the most violent headache would arise and persist until he vomited. This headache was always on the left side. Dr. HERING thought the attacks would ultimately lead to Apoplexy, if not cured.

Treatment.—Every variety of homœopathic treatment had been tried without benefit until Glonoine was given. Dr. HERING.

CASE 47.*—An aged nurse, suffering with chronic disease of the heart, was frequently attacked with violent headaches, lasting all day, especially in damp, foggy weather. The pain was tearing, ascended from the occiput up to the vertex, where it became throbbing; motion and stooping increased it; lying down relieved it; she also had a sense of fulness, as if from rush of blood to the nape of the neck and head.

Treatment.—Relieved in one hour by Glonoine 12; this

high potency did not relieve other attacks, and Platina had to be resorted to. Dr. RAVE.

CASE 48.*—Congestion of blood to the head in a pregnant female, attended with paleness of the face, loss of the senses, and falling down unconscious, with cold sweats.

Treatment.—This and other cases were relieved by Glonoine 6, or 12, or 30. Dr. HERING.

CASE 49.*—Many cases of headache just before menstruation, or during the monthly period, or just after it has ceased, or when it does not appear, especially when there is fulness of the head, with or without redness of the face and eyes, with throbbing pains, or the most violent throbbing and rending ones, may be relieved almost instantaneously by Glonoine 6, 12, or 30. Dr. HERING.

CASE 50.*—A plethoric girl, ever since she began to menstruate, became subject to attacks of congestion to the head, alternating with rush of blood towards the heart; her face was pale at times, red at others, and such attacks sometimes occurred five or six times a day; she was apt to fall down insensible.

Treatment.—Glonoine, repeated every two hours, cured this case, and also another in which there were alternations of congestion to the head and heart, with loss of consciousness, spasms, and frothing at the mouth. Dr. OKIE.

Dose. In these cases, and those already reported in my book on Headaches, (p. 115,) the 1st dilution was used in one case; the 2d in one; the 3d in three instances; the 6th in four cases; the 9th in two; the 12th in six; and the 30th in two cases. It is probable, from the experience of WAAGE, if larger doses had been used in some of the cases, the result would have been far better. PETERS.

13. HYOSCIAMUS.

GENERAL REMARKS.—Dr. Schneller experienced from 1⅓ grains of the extract: confusion of the senses, weakness of sight, some difficulty of speaking, and a by no means disagreeable state, like that of slight intoxication. From 2 grains:

confusion in the forehead, afterwards of sight and hearing, followed by restless sleep. From 3½ to 4 grains: dull frontal headache, followed in seven hours by cloudiness and weakness of sight, and slowness of the pulse. From 4¼ to 4¾ grains: confusion of the head, frontal headache on the left side, dimness of vision, frequent inclination to yawn, and sleepiness. From 11¼ grains: giddiness, reticulated vision, frontal headache on the right side, and sleepiness.

Choquet, in the persons of two soldiers, found it homœopathic to giddiness, stupidity, speechlessness, with dull and haggard look, dilatation of the pupils, and such great insensibility of the eyes to light, that the lids did not wink when the cornea was touched; their pulses were small and intermitting; breathing difficult, jaws locked, and mouth distorted by risus sardonicus.

Christison asserts that it is homœopathic to loss of speech, dilatation of the pupils, coma and delirium, generally of the unmanageable, but sometimes of the furious kind. Also to that singular union of delirium and coma which has been termed *Typhomania*. Wibner found it homœopathic to profound coma, but when the prostration and somnolency went off, extravagant delirium set in, and the patient became quite unmanageable. Christison also says that it is homœopathic when delirium precedes coma, and when the coma passes off, the delirium is apt to return for some time. Loss of speech is regarded as one of its most common effects. Vogt admits that it is homœopathic to vertigo, heaviness of the head, sleepiness, confusion of the head and headache, and when the senses commence to deceive one, so that taste and smell are diminished, noises are heard in the ears, and illusions of vision, such as flimmering before the eyes and double vision, occur. In one case it caused impotence which lasted for eight months.

According to Attomyr, Hyosciamus is indicated against the premonitions of Apoplexy, when there is vertigo with dimness of sight, and staggering to and fro like a drunken person; when the memory is weak, spirits depressed, with redness of the face and dilated pupils ; when the nose is apt to bleed, the speech difficult and inarticulate, with sense of crawling and falling asleep in the hands and limbs; great debility, disinclination to move or work, inclination to faint; great drowsiness, with gritting of the teeth.

It is homœopathic in attacks of Apoplexy with snoring respiration; against those profound and long-continued slumbers which are apt to end in Apoplexy; when epileptic attacks occur in alternation with apoplectic conditions. When the patient falls suddenly to the ground with entire loss of consciousness; when the breathing is quick and rattling, interrupted by snoring and choking.

When the eyes are fixed and inclined to squint; or are open and roll from side to side; or are protruded forwards, and move convulsively; the pupils being widely dilated. When the patient's face looks as if he were drunk, or is distorted, bluish, or earth-colored, and the jaw is dropped. Or when the color of the face varies from being pale and cold, to a bluish, or red and swollen state, or to a brownish red color.

When there is inability to speak or swallow, the throat being contracted or paralyzed, so that the patient is obliged to spit out the things which he has taken into his mouth.

Also when there is looseness of the bowels, with urging to urinate, retention of urine, or paralysis of the bladder.

Hyosciamus acts more like Opium than any other remedy, except that it is more apt to cause nervous irritations of various muscles, marked by twitching of the eyes and face, and jerkings of the limbs. It is homœopathic in those cases in which Opium seems indicated, yet the pupils are much dilated. It acts more powerfully on the vascular system than Conium, yet not so much as Bellad. and Stramon. PETERS.

CASE 51.—An unmarried lady, aged 59, fell into a comatose state, with frequent snoring, from which she could only be roused imperfectly for a few moments by hard shaking, and loud speaking; still she could answer no questions, neither could she swallow; her excretions were passed involuntarily. Her face was red, the veins of the body were distended, her pulse quick and full; this condition of things had already lasted for several days; and there was much numbness of the hands.

Treatment and result.—A few drops of Hyosciam. 3 were put in a wineglassful of water, and a teaspoonful given several times a day, with such good effect that she was almost well in ten days. Bellad. perfected the cure.

In the course of the following year the same patient was suddenly attacked with bloating of the face, staggering-dizziness, distortion of the mouth, twitching of several muscles of the face, with entire inability to speak, although she was perfectly conscious.

Treatment.—She was perfectly restored in six days, by means of Laurocerasus 3, given as above directed for Hyosc. Dr. Elwert.

Drs. Ozanne and Ladelci have used Hyosc. with benefit, as an intercurrent remedy in several cases of Apoplexy.

Dose. Same as recommended for Conium.

14. HYDROCYANIC-ACID.*

General Remarks.—Black says it is indicated in Apoplexy, when the patient is quite insensible, the pupils immovable, the breathing stertorous and slow, the pulse feeble and only 30, the features spasmodically contracted, eyes fixed and staring, and turned up, the chest heaving convulsively and hurriedly.

Attomyr thinks it homœopathic when there is dizziness, with inclination to sleep, and the head seems to turn round and round. When the eyes are half opened and fixed; pupils dilated and immovable; when the face is sunken, dingy, and gray; breathing difficult and rattling, or slow and almost imperceptible; the pulse small, contracted, and infrequent, or neither quick nor slow, but irregular as regards the force of the beats.

Dose. Noack advises 1 or 2 drop doses of the 1st, 2d, or 3d dilution, repeated every half, one, two, or four hours, in acute and severe cases. Peters.

15. IGNATIA.*

General Remarks.—The action of this remedy is very similar to that of Nux, and like it, it is best suited to Apoplexy when attended with convulsions.

CASE 52.*—A man, aged 38, had had an attack of Apoplexy, which weakened his memory of names, but left him tolerably able to attend to his business. But he was again seized with a violent attack; he was copiously bled, but his face and lips still continued livid and swollen; his teeth were clenched; frothy and bloody saliva exuded from his mouth; his breathing was stertorous, and he had general convulsions. He was bled again without relief, and matters seemed growing worse and worse, the patient remaining quite insensible. Dr. Gachapin then, in despair, proposed to his colleague the trial of a homœopathic remedy, the indication for which seemed precise, but as this was his first trial of homœopathy, he admitted that he could not predict the result. His colleague consented, and 1 drop tinct. Ignatia, was given in a spoonful of water; this dose was soon repeated, as the patient could not swallow all of the first. In five minutes, the convulsions were violently increased, but they soon began to abate, and gradually ceased. In half an hour consciouness began to be restored, and he soon recovered.—Brit. Jour. Hom., vol. 5, p. 51.

16. NUX-VOMICA.

General Remarks.—[Dr. Black suggests that Nux may prove homœopathic to the paralytic cases of Apoplexy, in which there is often but little loss of consciousness; it is, however, far more homœopathic to Apoplexy which follows epileptic or other convulsive attacks. According to Wood and Bache it acts specifically and principally upon the nerves of motion; its operation is evinced at first by a feeling of weight and weakness, with tremblings in the limbs, and some rigidity on attempting motion. It also sometimes produces pain in the head, vertigo, *contracted* pupil, and dimness of vision, while sensations analogous to those attending imperfect palsy, such as formication and tingling, are apt to be experienced on the surface. If the remedy be pushed a little farther, there will be a tendency to permanent involuntary muscular contractions, as in lock-jaw, but at the same time frequent starts or spasms occur, as from electric shocks; finally, severe and long-continued spasms arise.

To FOUQUIER belongs the credit of first applying it in the cure of paralytic affections; WOOD and BACHE say that his success was such as to induce him to communicate to the public the result of his experience. Other physicians have since employed it with variable success, but the experience in its favor so much predominates, that it may now be considered a standard remedy in palsy. It is a singular fact attested by numerous witnesses, that its action is directed more especially to the paralytic part, exciting contraction in this, before it exerts any perceptible influence upon other parts. It has been found more successful in general palsy and paraplegia, than in hemiplegia, and has frequently effected cures in palsy of the bladder, incontinence of urine from paralysis of the sphincter, amaurosis, and other cases of partial palsy. WOOD and BACHE also say, that upon the same principle it has been found useful in obstinate constipation from deficient contractility of the bowels; but how do they explain its curing obstinate spasmodic asthma and chorea, which they assert it does?

It may prevent Apoplexy in debilitated persons with scanty urine, and constipated bowels, for PEREIRA says, it usually promotes the appetite, assists the digestive process, increases the secretion of urine, and renders the excretion of this fluid more frequent, while in some cases it acts slightly on the bowels.

PEREIRA also says, it is homœopathic when the patient has a feeling of weight and weakness in the limbs, with increased sensibility to light, sound, touch, and variations of temperature, with depression of spirits and anxiety. Also when the limbs tremble and a slight rigidity or stiffness is felt; finally, when the patient experiences some difficulty in keeping the erect posture, and frequently staggers in walking.

It may also prove homœopathic to Apoplexy of the cerebellum (see page 169), as TROUSSEAU and PIDOUX say it is apt to affect the muscles of the penis, rendering the frequent diurnal and nocturnal erections quite inconvenient, even in those who, for some time before, had lost somewhat of their virility. PEREIRA alludes to two cases of paralysis in which Nux caused almost constant nocturnal erection, while females experience more energetic venereal desires, as proved by confidential communications on this point, which cannot be doubted.

Nux-Softening of the Brain.

According to CHRISTISON both it and Strychnine are homœopathic to softening of the brain and spinal cord, congestion of the brain and its membranes, and effusions of serum and blood. In one case the vessels of the brain were gorged, the membranes of the spinal cord highly injected, and four patches of extravasated blood were found between the spinal arachnoid and the external membrane; fluid blood flowed in abundance from the spinal cavity, where the veins were gorged; the pia mater was injected, and the spinal column *softened* at its upper part, and here and there almost pulpy. There was also congestion and softening of the brain. In another case ORFILA and OLLIVIER found it homœopathic to much serous effusion on the surface of the cerebellum, and *softening* of the whole cortical substance of the brain, but especially of the *cerebellum*. BLUMHARDT, too, found it homœopathic to *softening of the cerebellum*, and congestion of the cerebral vessels, together with *softening* of the spinal cord, and general gorging of the spinal veins. CHRISTISON says, this is some confirmation of an opinion advanced not long ago by FLOURENS that Nux acts particularly on the cerebellum. THOMSON found it homœopathic to much congestion of the whole membranes and substance of the brain and cerebellum, and even some extravasation of blood within the cavity of the arachnoid, over the upper surface of the brain (See Meningeal Apoplexy, page 171). WATT found it homœopathic to *softening* of the substance of the brain, and lumbar part of the spinal cord.

CASE 53.—A man, aged 63, much addicted to the use of coffee, fell suddenly to the ground.

Symptoms.—He lay snoring, in an unconscious condition; the spittle ran out of his mouth; when loudly spoken to, he opened his eyes, muttered to himself, and then fell again into slumber; his eyes were dim, and the corners filled with purulent matter; the organs of deglutition, and his legs, were entirely paralyzed; his jaw hung down on the right side; he had no fever, but his pulse was full and slow; he grasped towards his head, with his right hand; he had a large, protruding inguinal hernia.

Treatment and result.—Nux-vom. 30 was given him to smell, and five drops were added to an injection; in the course of four hours his consciousness commenced to return, and he attempted to speak. Nux 30 was given internally, and in the course of the following night his rupture was reduced spontaneously; the next morning his speech could be understood, and he could swallow without difficulty, but complained of heaviness of his head, and dizziness. After taking several doses of Arnica 9, he was entirely restored in eight days.—Archiv, vol. 8, part 2, p. 81. Dr. SCHÜLER.

CASE 54.—Lady S., aged 55 years, was attacked with Apoplexy.

Symptoms.—She lay on her back, with rattling respiration; her eyes were fixed, dim, and did not move even when the cornea was touched; the pupils were dilated; thick white mucus collected in the mouth, and her whole body was cold, and without feeling.

Treatment and result.—One drop of Nux 1 was given in water, and repeated in a quarter of an hour; in ten minutes a tetanic spasm set in, and lasted for two hours, the previously relaxed limbs becoming stiff and rigid; when this subsided she lay quietly, her breathing became regular, a gentle perspiration broke out over the whole body, and although she was unconscious and unable to swallow, still she seemed sensible to touch. One drop of Opium 6 was given, and in one hour she opened and moved her eyes, made signs that she recognized her friends, then fell asleep, and perspired profusely, after which she began to speak. In three days more, she was entirely restored, although very weak.—Gen. Hom. Journ. vol. 24, p. 216. Dr. SCHOLZ.

CASE 55.—A man, aged 49, of medium size, but apoplectic build, had often suffered with rush of blood to the head. He was attacked with confusion of the head, dizziness, and trembling of the limbs.

Treatment.—Aconit. and Nux in repeated doses cured him entirely (see cases 2 and 10).—Hygea, vol. 8, p. 34. Dr. KÄSEMANN.

CASE 56.*—A stout, healthy woman, aged about 50, had been remarkably well until the morning of the same day, when she began to complain of pain in the head and giddiness; her head and face were hot, mouth drawn to one side, the left arm numb, pulse full and strong, but natural in frequency; she complained of dull pain, with fulness in the head, and great drowsiness.

Treatment.—Nux-vom. 3, one drop per dose, to be repeated every quarter of an hour for two or three times, and then every two or three hours, as soon as improvement was observed; by the next day all the above symptoms had disappeared, but she still had a disagreeable dull sensation in the head and slight numbness of the left arm. The Nux was continued every six hours, and by the evening she was quite well, and remained so for at least two months.—Brit. Journ. Hom., vol. 5, p. 49. Dr. BLACK.

CASE 57.*—A lady aged 51, short-necked, very stout,

face generally flushed and eyes suffused, was suddenly seized with Apoplexy, sank down heavily and became insensible, while stooping over a sick friend. In twenty minutes she recovered her consciousness, but could not open her eyes; her face was flushed, pulse imperceptible, limbs and bowels cold; she had numbness of the tongue, with stammering on attempting to speak.

Treatment.—Hot bottles were applied to her feet, and one drop of tinct. Nux was put in six table-spoonfuls of water, and one teaspoonful given every half hour for two hours, and then every three hours. She became warm in the course of an hour, and then gradually and steadily improved until she was quite well.—Brit. Journ. Hom., vol. 5, p. 52. Dr. KER.

CASE 58.*—Mrs. B. was suddenly seized with Apoplexy; she had been under homœopathic treatment for some weeks, for numbness of the right hand and arm, and tingling sensation in the ends of the fingers; the fingers were occasionally œdematous; numbness of the right leg; weakness of the whole right side; a painful and indescribable feeling of apprehension; occasional difficulty in pronouncing words; stammers, and says what she did not intend to say; confusion of ideas; sensation in the top of the head as if electrical sparks were being emitted; pain, occasionally in the left temple; dizziness at times, but rarely; the right hand apt to be colder than the left; pulse 70, and weak. She was of a full habit of body, with a short, thick neck, red face and suffused eye; she passed much urine, which deposited a white sediment; bowels were regular; she was troubled with piles, which bled profusely sometimes, and then gave relief to most of her symptoms; her menses were ceasing gradually, and change of life was taking place. She never had any appetite for breakfast, and had nausea immediately afterwards; her appetite was generally not good, tongue coated with a whitish fur, and fulness in the pit of the stomach; she was also apt to have a pricking sensation over the face.

Treatment.— For these symptoms she had taken Nux,

Opium, Bellad., Puls., and tinct. Sulph., with benefit, when the sudden death of a friend excited her greatly, and brought back most of the above symptoms, in addition to violent palpitation of the heart and intense headache, and finally, after making some exertion in a stooping posture, she fell down heavily in a comatose state.

Symptoms.—Her face was swollen, eyes turned up, and breathing stertorous; she remained half an hour in a state of insensibility, and then began to recover consciousness, but there was icy coldness of the extremities, and of the whole surface of the body; her pulse was scarcely perceptible; she had much headache, with sensation of pricking on the top of the head; she could not swallow, spoke with great difficulty and very indistinctly; her eyes were shut, and could not be opened; the stertorous breathing changed to slow, full respiration.

Treatment.—Hot bottles were applied to the abdomen and to the limbs. One drop of tinct. Nux-vom. was mixed in a tumbler half full of water, and one teaspoonful given every half hour. The next day, the skin was warm, pulse stronger, and headache slight, but she had acute pain in the pit of the stomach occasionally; she could open and shut her eyes, and had somewhat recovered the use of her faculties, although there was still a great tendency to mistake objects, and call things by wrong names. Nux was given every four hours. On the following day she was very much better, with the exception of her headache; the pain was acute, and darted from one temple to another, and there was a tendency to faintness. Bellad. 3 was given, without much relief for a day or two; but it was continued, and, in eight days more, she was well enough to go to church.—Brit. Jour. Hom., vol. 7, p. 169. Dr. KER.

CASE 59.*—A carman, aged 50, very steady and temperate in his habits, was seized, whilst loading his cart, with dizziness and staggering, which caused him to hold by a post to prevent falling. He recovered himself a little, and attempted to drive, but had not proceeded many steps before he fell two or three times upon his hands, and when he got up, could not stand without support. He became confused in his sight, and could scarcely distinguish the road. He had now a general aching in the head, with a sensation of swimming and lightness, as soon as he moved; his forehead was hot, his pulse slow and throbbing; no thirst, tongue moist and clean, and bowels regular.

Treatment.—Nux-vom. 6, every four hours. The next day he was so much better as to be able to walk out, as he only had a slight headache, with a little dizziness at times, and occasional singing in the right ear; his appetite was better. Continued the Nux, and in three days he was much better still, although he yet had a little dizziness when he stooped, or walked fast. China 3, two doses at intervals of six hours, then Sulph. 12, also two doses at the same intervals of time; he was so much relieved in two days more, that he could stoop without inconvenience, was cheerful and active. Took Conium 6 twice a day, for a momentary return of swimming of the head, recurring once or twice a day.—Hom. in Acute Diseases, p. 175. Dr. YELDHAM.

CASE 60.*—Mrs. M., aged 50, tolerably stout, and generally healthy, had felt heavy in the head for the last fortnight; finally she was seized with a heavy dizziness, as if she had received a blow on the head; this passed off, and she felt pretty well for a time, when she again felt as if struck violently on the right side of the head, and lost all consciousness, without falling from her seat, but her head fell to one side, and her breathing became stertorous. This condition lasted for some hours, when she gradually revived, but found that she had lost the use of the right arm, leg and foot. Her head felt like a dead weight, and there was pain at the top of it; she vomited as soon as she came to, although she had eaten nothing indigestible.

Treatment.—Nux 3, every four hours; by the next day she was much improved, her head felt nearly well, but was somewhat heavy at the back part; the use of the leg and arm had returned to a great extent. She continued Nux, and on the following day there was still further improvement; she had almost recovered the entire use of her limbs, but had had a slight threatening of a relapse, in a feeling of faintness, and numbness in the tongue, and deep-seated pain in the head. Lachesis 12, three times a day, perfected the cure.—Hom. in Acute Diseases, p. 178. Dr. YELDHAM.

CASE 61.*—A man, aged 70, of herculean stature, robust of his age, stout, plethoric, and accustomed to stimulants, was seized with severe pain in the head, followed in a short time by paralysis of the right side of the face, numbness and partial loss of power of the right arm. His head was heavy and confused, but he was able to sit up, and speak rationally and collectedly, but his articulation was considerably impaired; his mouth was completely drawn to one side, but the paralysis did not extend to the tongue; he complained of a sense of fulness and thickness about the throat; his head was hot, his pulse firm and regular, and a little quick.

Treatment.—Nux-vomica 6, every four hours; on the next day his head was much relieved; it was not so heavy and confused, and also cooler to the touch. He repeated the Nux every six hours, and then only once a day for eight or ten days; the muscles of the face, arm, and hand gradually recovered their tone, and at the end of fourteen days there was scarcely any trace of the attack remaining.—Hom. in Acute Diseases, p. 179. Dr. YELDHAM.

CASE 62.—A lady, aged 27, eight months pregnant, and of a phlegmatic temperament, had suffered for several weeks with dizziness, both while at rest and when moving about; she was often in danger of falling, especially after dinner; she had aching pains in the forehead, intermingled with sharp stitches, especially early in the morning, while in bed; burning in the stomach after every meal, and frequently recurring flashes of heat.

Treatment.—She was entirely cured by 4 doses of Nux 18, six globules each. In her next pregnancy, a similar dizziness and headache were relieved by Nux 18.—DIEZ, p. 176.

CASE 63.—Mrs. L., aged 54, who had not menstruated for seven years, was suddenly attacked, ten days ago, with dizziness, which was so much increased by stooping, and looking upwards, that she was obliged to hold on to something to prevent her falling; she also had slight signs of blind piles. She had been bled by another physician in order to prevent Apoplexy.

Treatment.—After taking Nux 12, she was entirely relieved of her vertigo, on the following day.—DIEZ, p. 177.

CASE 64.—A powerful man, aged 40, without any peculiar predisposition to Apoplexy, had suffered with dizziness for four years; he also had had itching of the skin for ten years, ever since an attack of itch.

Symptoms.—The dizziness was preceded by a tense headache, with heat in the forehead, both disappearing when he was quiet; then the vertigo set in suddenly like an electric shock, so that his senses seemed to leave him, although he did not fall down; attacks of dizziness even occurred during the night, and waked him up from his sleep; he generally awoke early. His digestion was good, except that he was occasionally troubled with heart-burn. Although naturally of an equal temper, if he became irritable, passionate, or anxious, vertigo would set in, preceded by yawning.

Treatment.—Nux-vom. was given, one dose every three days, and soon removed everything, except slight traces of vertigo. Then six doses of Sulphur, at intervals of eight days, cured him entirely, and he remained well for years.—Hygea, vol. 3, p. 12. Dr. GRIESSELICH.

CASE 65.—A patient, aged 55, had been obliged to keep his bed for sixteen weeks.

Symptoms.—He is scarcely ever able to get or sit up; even the slightest change in the position of his head, such as occurs in eating, brought on such a turning and falling vertigo, with dimness of vision and nausea, or even retching and vomiting, that he was obliged to desist. When he was obliged to rise, he could not walk without assistance, from fear of falling. He had heaviness and aching in the head, loss of appetite, and constipation, with violent hiccough.

Treatment.—After taking Nux 3, two drops per dose, every night and morning, he was soon relieved of vertigo, nausea, and vomiting.—Gen. Hom. Jour., vol. 34, p. 88. Dr. ELWERT.

CASE 66.—A man, aged 36, of delicate constitution, remained dizzy, after an attack of nervous fever; he staggered while walking, and often came near falling; he also had a permanent pain in the left side of his chest, increased by coughing and breathing.

Treatment.—Bryon. 3 relieved his side, but the dizziness did not leave him until after he had taken Nux 3.—Dr. DIEZ, p. 177.

According to RÜCKERT, the clinical indications for the use of Nux, in the above cases of dizziness, are: The sudden occurrence of vertigo, coming on like an electric shock, with loss of consciousness, but without falling; attacks of dizziness while asleep at night, so that he seems to waver or stagger in his sleep; inability to sit or stand up; every motion of the head, even in eating, brings on a turning-, staggering-vertigo, with dimness of vision and nausea; dizziness when stooping, or looking upwards, with danger of falling.

Dose. The pure Tincture was used in four cases; the 1st dilution in one case; the 3d dilution in five cases; the 6th in two cases; the 12th in one case; the 18th in two cases; the 30th in one case. The doses were repeated every quarter, or half hour, in urgent cases; every two, four, or six hours in less severe attacks. NOACK advises one drop doses of the 1st or 2d dilution, repeated every one, two, or three hours.—PETERS.

17. OPIUM.

GENERAL REMARKS.—The indications for the use of Opium in Apoplexy are so well known, that it will be unnecessary to dwell long upon them; still, as SCHMID truly says, it deserves the first place in the attention of the physician who treats disease according to the law "*similia similibus curantur.*" It is most indicated when the face is of a mahogany red color, the pupils very much *contracted*, the sleep profound, the limbs motionless, but not absolutely paralyzed, the pulse full and slow, skin hot and perspiring, the urine retained or suppressed, and the bowels obstinately costive (see pages 159 and 160). *Nux-vomica* is most homœopathic, when the face is pale or livid, the pupils much *contracted*, and the limbs powerfully convulsed, or rigidly contracted. *Belladonna*, when the face is much flushed and bloated, the pupils excessively *dilated*, the limbs either motionless, or but slightly convulsed. *Hyosciamus*, when the face is pale or flushed, pupils dilated, and twitchings of the eyeballs, muscles of the face, and risus sardonicus, are present. *Aconite*, when the face is pale or livid, the pupils much *contracted*, pulse very feeble, and much numbness and tingling are present.—PETERS.

(*b.*) ATTOMYR's indications for the use of Opium are the presence of dull stupefaction, with dimness of the eyes, and extreme weakness; or great activity of mind, and inclination for earnest and important labors.

Unusual redness of the face, with swelling of the lips; very red face, with wild, protruding and very red eyes; open and turned-up eyes; paralysis of the eyelids. Spasms of the facial muscles, convulsive trembling of the face, lips, and tongue. Distortion of the mouth.

Oppressed, difficult, and irregular breathing. Respiration at times loud and snoring, then heavy, and then again very weak. Panting, loud and difficult breathing; single, slow respirations, followed by absence of breathing for several moments; long and sobbing respiration; short and snoring respiration, with absence of breathing for half a minute; loud, difficult and rattling respiration. Snoring in sleep.

Pulse weak, suppressed, small and slow; pulse at first full and slow, then weak; slow pulse and breathing; pulse large and slow, with slow, heavy, and deep breathing.

Numbness and insensibility of the limbs, coldness of the body, paralysis of the arm and limbs.

Heavy, stupid sleep; unrefreshing sleep, with profuse perspiration; dreamy and restless sleep, with frightful or pleasant dreams.—ATTOMYR.

CASE 67.—A man, aged 50, addicted to the use of spirituous liquors, oppressed with much care and sorrow, had suffered for a long time with sleeplessness, anxious dreams, and congestions of blood.

Symptoms.—The attack was preceded by vertigo, dulness and heaviness of the head, dulness of the senses, difficulty of hearing, noises in the ears, indistinct speech, staggering walk, fixed staring before him, and sleeplessness, followed by asthmatic oppression of the chest, spasmodic jerkings of the limbs, loss of consciousness, and an apoplectic condition.

Treatment.—He was bled, and had ice applied to his head; consciousness returned in a few hours, attended with the following condition: Excessive excitement; he laughed much, spoke much unconnected and confused stuff; he did not know those around him, and kept grasping constantly towards his head; his face and eyes were red, and his pupils dilated. Tinct. Opium, in 1 drop doses, at suitable intervals, removed all the preceding and subsequent symptoms, and even prevented a return of the attacks.—Gen. Hom. Jour. vol. 5, p. 305. Dr. KNORRE.

CASE 68.—A man, aged 75, with inclination to Apoplexy, the premonitory symptoms of which had often been removed by *Bellad.*, suffered with the following symptoms: Indifference to everything; he spoke little, stared fixedly before him; could not readily recollect himself; the right corner of his mouth was drawn up more than the left; his pulse was full, soft, and bounding.

Treatment.—Bellad. 1, two drops per dose, every three hours, did not relieve him at all; then Opium 2d dilution, one drop every two or four hours, removed the apathy, mental confusion, and distortion of the mouth so completely, that, by the fourth day, the patient could be regarded as cured. —Gen. Hom. Jour., vol. 21, p. 233. Dr. FRANK.

18. PHOSPHOR.

GENERAL REMARKS.—This remedy may be useful in some of those cases of Apoplexy occurring in debilitated subjects, in which Ammonia is generally relied upon. It is a powerful, diffusible stimulant; exciting the nervous, vascular and secreting organs. It creates an agreeable warmth in the body, increases the frequency and fulness of the pulse, augments the heat of the skin, heightens the mental activity and muscular powers, and operates as a powerful sudorific and diuretic.—PEREIRA. It is homœopathic to Apoplexy of the cerebellum, and that which arises from great excitement of the sexual organs (see page 169). It is also homœopathic to Bilious Apoplexy (see page 183). DIERBACH recommends it in the last stages of Typhus and Apoplexy, when the exhaustion of the body has reached its extremest degree, and speedy death is to be feared; when the pulse is small, sunken and soft; the limbs cold; hiccough has set in, with difficult swallowing, coma, rattling respiration, cold, clammy sweats, and even when the death-struggle seems to have set in.—PETERS.

CASE 69.—A maiden, aged 21, with short and muscular frame, fell down suddenly in the yard, on a cold, misty morning, and seemed dead.

Symptoms.—Loss of consciousness; the powers of life seemed quite extinct; she was motionless, pulseless and breathless; her face was red, but the rest of her body cold; neither speaking, shaking, or rubbing her, produced any sign of consciousness, but she seemed to feel deep pricks with a needle in the soles of the feet.

Treatment.—She was restored by the use of Phosphor 60. Dr. SCHMID.

CASE 70.—A woman, aged 75, who had been reduced by previous blood-letting and hæmorrhage, was attacked with Nervous Apoplexy, and seemed in a hopeless condition.

Treatment.—She received Phosphor 1st dilution, 3 drops per dose; signs of life returned in a quarter of an hour, and then she took only 1 drop per dose, every hour. At a later period, she took 1 drop of the 6th and 12th dilution, every night and morning. In 10 days she was able to leave her bed.—Gen. Hom. Jour., vol. 1, p. 67. Dr. STURM.

CASE 71.*—A man, aged 35, of full habit, healthy, but anxious about business, arose in the morning not quite well; he was dizzy and staggered, but went down town, where he became stupid and heavy, lost his way, and wandered about; a friend brought him home; he was cold, and when put to bed soon became stupid and unconscious; his face was flushed.

Treatment.—He took Bellad. 3; reaction with fever soon set in, and Aconite was given; but he remained unconscious, his breathing became stertorous and snoring, and he could not be roused. Then Opium, 2 drops of the tincture, was put in a tumbler half full of water, and a teaspoonful given per dose; improvement soon commenced; he could be roused, and was able to put out his tongue. The next day he was comparatively well.—Minutes of Pathologico-Therapeutic Society. Drs. BALL and KINSLEY.

CASE 72.*—A lady in the habit of taking heavy suppers, with wine, went to bed not very unwell, but her husband was awaked at night by her noisy breathing and snoring; her face was flushed, and she could not be roused.

Treatment.—Tinct. Opium, 1 drop per dose, every half hour; she could be roused at the end of six or eight hours, and recovered with paralysis of one eyelid and arm, which lasted for two or three months. Is now well.—Ibid. Dr. BALL.

CASE 73.*—A child who had been sick for three or four days, finally became stupid, and could not be roused. It recovered entirely under the use of Opium.—Ibid. Dr. BALL.

CASE 74.*—A man, subject to attacks of dizziness, fell down insensible, and remained unconscious for twenty hours;

then he slept heavily, but could be roused; his skin was hot, and pulse 65.

Treatment.—He recovered under the use of Opium, aided by Aconite and Arnica.—Ibid. Dr. STEWART.

CASE 75.*—An old woman, addicted to the use of liquor, was found lying speechless and powerless upon the floor; her mouth was drawn to one side; the right arm and leg were paralyzed.

Treatment.—She was bled, and remained for twenty-four days in a very precarious state, but finally recovered entirely under the use of Opium 3, Bellad. 2, and Hyosc. 3.—Brit. Jour. of Hom., vol. 5, p. 65.

CASE 76.*—A man, aged 41, not very robust, had felt queer and confused in the head, for a week; purgatives did not relieve him; he staggered and reeled like a drunken man, appeared to have lost nearly all command over his movements; the left arm hung powerless by his side, and the left leg was scarcely more obedient to his will. He could not sit up without being held; his head dropped down, he spoke thickly and indistinctly, breathed spasmodically, and was very sleepy.

Treatment.—Opium 3 was given every two hours. The next day he felt better, could walk more steadily, and raise his left arm; his head was still light. Under the use of Nux 6, and Bryonia 6, for indigestion and cough, he recovered perfectly in about ten days.—Dr. YELDHAM.

APPENDIX.

ON THE NATURE AND TREATMENT

OF

SOFTENING OF THE BRAIN AND PALSY.

Softening of the Brain is so closely related to, and so frequently connected with Apoplexy, that it would be almost inexcusable to pass it over entirely here. Rochoux, and others, even maintain that the texture of the brain is almost invariably softened prior to the occurrence of apoplectic effusions, which they suppose are occasioned by the imperfect support afforded under these circumstances to the blood-vessels of the brain. Although exceptions to this rule are by no means few, Rowland admits that, in many cases of Apoplexy suddenly fatal, the brain is not only found softened, but also bearing the marks of previous disease.

Again, one of the most remarkable varieties of the disease is the *Apoplectic Softening*, so called from the suddenness and severity of the attack; comatose seizures are common to all its forms, but sometimes the case assumes all the peculiarities of Sanguineous Apoplexy; although precursory symptoms of some kind generally precede these attacks, such as headache, failure of intelligence, inaptitude of expression, pains and weakness of the limbs, or other marks of disturbance of the brain; but these warnings are generally extremely indistinct, when the comatose attack occurs.—Rowland.

The relation of this disease to Apoplexy is also manifested in the manner of death; in seventy fatal cases, the death was comatose in as many as forty, either from a sudden apoplectic seizure, or by stupor gradually increasing to coma; in six of these cases the death was sudden; the patients being taken off unexpectedly while in their usual health, or were found dead, no danger having been immediately apprehended. It is sometimes exceedingly difficult to distinguish the coma of Apoplectic-softening from that of Hæmorrhagic-apoplexy, and ROWLAND even thinks that many of the premonitory symptoms, usually enumerated among the precursors of true Apoplexy, are referable, in reality, to Softening of the Brain. Thus, in seventeen cases out of twenty, of *Hæmorrhagic-apoplexy*, in which a clot of blood was found in the brain after death, the attacks were sudden and entirely without warning; in the remaining three cases of Apoplexy, the precursory signs were headache, vomiting, vertigo, loss of recollection, drowsiness, and, in one instance, convulsions;—while, on the other hand, in twenty cases of *Softening of the Brain*, the comatose seizure was preceded by premonitory signs in all but two cases. In sixteen cases out of eighteen, headache was a prominent symptom before the attack; it generally came on severely, either a few hours, or sometimes several days, before the appearance of more decided symptoms; there was more or less loss of motion prior to the comatose attack in twelve cases; the Palsy was ingravescent in five cases, gradually increasing from a slight feebleness of the limb, to more or less complete paralysis. In thirteen of the cases of Softening, the intellectual faculties were disordered in some degree very early in the disease; in seven cases, some symptoms connected with speech or articulation were observed before the sudden or apoplectic seizure.—ROWLAND.

Hence we may draw the conclusion that, in the majority of cases in which the attacks are quite sudden, or without evident warning, the probability is great, that the case is one of Sanguineous- or Hæmorrhagic-apoplexy; while, when there are many precursory symptoms, the probability is equally great that Softening is present. Headache and giddiness, however, are common to both affections at their commencement; but in Softening, the subsequent course is more characteristic. The dulness of comprehension, vacancy of expression, forgetfulness, especially in regard to language, and hemiplegic threatenings leading to an apoplectic seizure, are finally sufficient to indicate the presence of Softening.

The apoplectic paroxysm is precisely alike in both diseases; but in the one case, the frequent transitory character of the coma, its sudden termination and frequent repetition, resembling, in this respect, the epileptic paroxysm, are characteristic of Softening. The presence of contraction of the palsied limbs is also a very reliable sign of Softening; but increase of sensibility of the paralyzed part is not, for they commonly become painful when a clot exists, either from the irritation of the clot, or from the occurrence of inflammatory Softening about it, or from an irritation probably depending upon a curative process going on in the brain.—ROWLAND.

Apoplectic-softening corresponds to one variety of red-softening in which the blood is either stagnated in the minute vessels of the softened part, or else infiltrated into it, or both combined. In recent cases the softening has a deep- or dusky-red tint, which passes into a dark brown. There are no exudation corpuscles, coagulable lymph, or pus globules to be detected by the microscope; venous congestion, hyperæmia, and extravasation of blood, are the principal appearances besides the Softening.

Treatment.—Nux and Opium are the most important remedies.

Of course all cases of Softening of the brain are not apoplectic in their nature; some are acute, others inflammatory, or ataxic, or chronic, or latent. There are as many pathological varieties, viz., red, white, yellow, and dark softening; also softening from œdema, and fatty degeneration of parts of the brain.

INFLAMMATORY SOFTENING.

According to ROWLAND, the symptoms of this variety are not always as clearly defined as might be expected, for the disease is usually confined to a small portion of the brain. The attack does not often commence with a distinct chill, or the other phenomena that mark the onset of inflammation in vital organs; in some cases, however, there are acceleration of the pulse, heat of skin and scalp, and other signs of fever, especially when the disease occupies the surface of the brain. The first circumstance to excite attention is usually headache, which is not always severe, but it is excessively harassing; the pain seems to dart through the brain, and to proceed from the centre of the organ, occupying now one spot, now another, but having no fixed seat; it is always *paroxysmal*, and sometimes intermittent. Accompanying the headache there may be confusion of thought, and a settled apprehension that the mind will be destroyed; at night, restlessness, excitement, and delirium come on, and sometimes a convulsive paroxysm. These cases are apt to be attended with nausea and vomiting.

Shortly afterwards, signs present themselves that foreshadow the coming danger; unusual sensations are felt in one or both limbs of the same side; tinglings, prickings (*pins and needles*), or numbness, with some degree of weakness, alarm the patient with threatenings of palsy. At this period the headache has probably fixed itself in one region, which in many cases is on the side opposite to that of the limbs whose functions are impaired.

The second stage of the disorder now begins; the delirium and restless excitement, the feeling of apprehension or terror, give way to stupor, or indifference; the headache and vomiting cease, and the patient lies in a state of mental and bodily torpor; the memory fails, there is great difficulty in comprehending questions, and in recollecting words suitable for a reply; the face is dull and heavy, the pupils contracted, or sometimes dilated, and insensible to light; the paralysis of one side becomes more confirmed; the pulse is slow; the skin at one time flushed, at another covered with a clammy sweat; the tongue is reddish and inclined to dryness; the appetite bad, and bowels constipated.

The further progress of the disease varies in different patients. Many have an attack of coma or somnolence from which it is impossible to arouse them; several such seizures may occur within a short period of time; or with the senses apparently intact, and the intelligence in some degree remaining, the power of utterance is suspended, and not a syllable can be formed upon the lips, (Hyosc.) The palsied limbs are variously affected; they are often extremely painful (Acon.); sometimes they are moved convulsively (Bell., Stramon., Op.); at others kept in a state of tonic spasm, by the action of the flexor muscles, the limbs remaining permanently contracted, (Nux, Plumbum, Ignat.) This peculiar contraction of the muscles is regarded as characteristic of softening of the brain. —ROWLAND.

In other cases, the patient sinks gradually into coma (Opium); emaciation proceeds rapidly (Iodine); the pulse is quick, and sometimes intermitting (Glonoine); the tongue is parched and encrusted in the centre (Opium, Plumbum, Glonoine, or Alumina); the teeth and gums are covered with sordes; the eyelids are glued together; bronchial râles are heard in the chest; the patient becomes stupid, cannot swallow, passes his evacuations involuntarily (Hyosc.); and finally sinks into the most profound insensibility (Hyosc. and Opium).

Inflammatory Softening of the brain corresponds with one variety of Red-softening, viz., that in which plastic exudation, and a large proportion of coagulable lymph, are mixed up with blood globules. The prevailing color of the affected part of the brain is a pale red, the substance of the brain being uniformly permeated with an inflammatory exudation; but ruptures of small vessels, and bleeding into the softened part, often occur, causing dark red patches, from blood which has been extravasated at various times; streaks or stripes of a yellow and green color may also be met with, from the coagulation of the fibrin of the exudation; and finally, we may also find white spots, from an occasional piece of brain which has escaped disease. All these other shades are planted upon, or mixed with the more extensive paler reddening arising from

21

the infiltration of the cerebral tissue with the fluid part of the inflammatory exudation.—ROKITANSKY.

ATAXIC, CHRONIC, AND LATENT SOFTENING.

The ataxic form is characterized by extreme depression of the vital powers, either in consequence of previous disease, or from original weakness of constitution. The chronic form approaches gradually, and almost imperceptibly; it is most common in aged persons, and before the patient makes any complaint, the danger may be perceptible to others in his altered manner and failing intellect; the headache is seldom very severe or distressing, neither is the nausea or vomiting; but the faculties become clouded, the memory fails, the speech is slow, hesitating, and incongruous; familiar names cannot be uttered, nor familiar objects recognized. These premonitory symptoms may last for months; then follow more marked symptoms, such as difficulty of speaking, numbness, formication or pricking of the limbs, and especially of the fingers, partial loss of power and motion, as shown for instance in one leg dragging in walking, and in the inability to grasp objects firmly. *Contraction of the limbs* in these chronic cases is much more frequent than entire palsy, whereas the reverse holds good in acute Softening; still it may be absent in about one-fourth of the cases. Pains in the limbs and joints usually accompany these contractions, and they are generally much aggravated by motion, but not increased by pressure. There is commonly a partial, but scarcely ever a perfect loss of sensation in the paralyzed and flexed limbs. The face becomes partially distorted, and the features are devoid of expression; the memory is gradually lost, the ideas become confused, and all reasoning power disappears. The paralysis gradually extends; the power of retaining the contents of the bladder and rectum disappears; the limbs waste away, and yet the force with which they are flexed is almost incredible; and thus the patient sinks, utterly unconscious of his own pitiable condition. In some cases the flexure ceases, and the limbs relax shortly before death.—DAY.

Such are the ordinary symptoms of *chronic* Softening; it may go on for years; while 11 cases of *acute* Softening terminated fatally in two days, 26 other cases before the fifth day, 43 cases before the ninth day, 7 cases between the ninth and twentieth days, and 9 more cases between the twentieth and thirtieth days.—DAY.

In these cases, the pathological appearances may be either Red-softening, from chronic venous congestion and capillary hæmorrhage; or White-softening; yellow patches on the convolutions; or Yellow-softening, with more or less fatty degeneration. These different varieties of course call for quite different treatment.

According to ROKITANSKY, *Yellow-softening* is founded upon a chemico-pathological process. The yellow color is owing to the presence of a thin, yellow, acid fluid, containing a number of broken, extremely varicose, primary tubes, with their contents of swollen blood globules, very transparent fat globules of various sizes, and some yellow amorphous pigment. FREMY considers the brain to consist of Cerebric acid, either free, or combined with Soda and Phosphate of lime; of Oleophosphoric acid, both free and in combination with Soda; of Olein and Margarin; of small quantities of Oleic and Margaric acids; of Cholesterine, water, and of a substance resembling white of an egg, but composed of 7 parts of albumen, 5 parts of fatty matter, and 80 parts of water. The Oleophosphoric acid, which is usually yellow, is very variable in its composition and combination, and readily separates into Phosphoric acid and Olein from very slight causes. ROKITANSKY thinks that obstruction of the blood-vessels near the softened part, from deposit of atheroma, or impermeability of them from pressure, and the consequent impeding and interruption of the circulation in one portion of the brain, may cause a lower state of vitality there, somewhat similar to that which occurs in senile gangrene, and thus allow of the liberation of an acid or acids, viz., the phosphoric, and one or more of the fatty acids, which then play a more important part in the farther process of Yellow-softening. This conjecture is somewhat supported by the very decided acid reaction of the fluid contained in the softened spot.

Another important phenomenon in Yellow-softening is the remarkable degree of swelling of the brain which Yellow-softening produces; softened spots, of the size of half a cubic inch, or of a nut, give rise to quite a disproportionate turgescence. From these facts it may readily be conjectured that the symptoms of Yellow-softening are severe and acute. ROKITANSKY says, that it appears to be always, and often rapidly fatal, still idiopathic Yellow-softening may last a longer time; but the secondary variety, that which forms around apoplectic clots or inflamed patches of the brain, often runs a rapid course. It corresponds more nearly to the so-called acute ataxic variety than any other.

Treatment.—Arsenicum, Secale, and Phosphor are homœopathic to that stage which resembles senile gangrene. If the presence of atheroma can be conjectured by the presence of peculiar hardness and inelasticity of the superficial arteries, then the remedies pointed out for Atheroma (see page 174,) will be brought in play. If the Softening be brought about by a violent tonic, tetanic spasm, or constriction of the blood-vessels, similar to the violent contraction of the muscles which is so characteristic a sign of Softening of the brain, then Nux, Ignatia, Angustura, or Conium, and Opium, may be useful. The excessive swelling of the softened part, and consequent pressure upon the healthy part of the brain, together with presence of an intensely acid fluid in the diseased part, may call for Kali-hydroidicum, Baryta, Kali-carb., or Phosphor.

White-softening of the brain.—According to ROKITANSKY, this consists in a loosening and subsequent maceration of the substance of the brain by an interstitial effusion of serum. Like œdema in general, it sometimes takes place without any inflammation; at other times it is unquestionably so far inflammatory, that a certain quantity of coagulable lymph, capable of assuming an elementary organization, is poured out with the serum. Examples of it are furnished in the more or less acute forms of œdema which occur in the neighborhood of patches of inflammation, and more especially in the œdema which accompanies acute meningitic hydrocephalus, and destroy the tissue around the ventricles of the brain. In such cases of Softening, the characteristic products of inflammation may generally be discovered with the microscope in the diffluent portion of the brain.

This disease apparently approaches in its character the acute inflammatory, erysipelatous, or œdematous inflammation, similar to that which is so specifically caused by Arsenicum, Cantharides, Rhus, Euphorbium, Marsh Marigold, and other remedies.

TREATMENT OF SOFTENING OF THE BRAIN, AND PALSY.

As there is but little experience in the homœopathic school in the treatment of this disease, even in its more common form, and much less in all its varieties and complications, it will be well for us to ascertain what has been accomplished by other physicians; in how far their experience agrees with the rules of the homœopathic school; and how much remains for us and others to point out, *ab novo*, either theoretically or practically.

Arsenicum.—According to ROWLAND, this exerts a well-known beneficial influence in some nervous affections. For several years he has been in the habit of prescribing the *Liquor Arsenicalis* in palsy, and other conditions depending upon Softening of the brain. It is, he says, best suited to the chronic form, or, at least, to that in which all activity and excitement have ceased, and where the vital energy is deficient. In such cases, this remedy is frequently of much benefit, and appears to give renewed strength and firmness to the nervous system. It even seems to possess a curative power in this complaint; in several instances, I (ROWLAND) have observed permanent improvement follow its administration, and in two patients the cure was almost complete. According to Homœopathy, Arsenicum should prove curative against that variety of *white* Softening which arises from inflammatory œdema. Christison admits it to be homœopathic to "gorging of the vessels of the brain, effusion of serum into the ventricles, inflammation of the brain, and even extravasation of blood"; *i. e.*, both to the œdematous or white variety of Softening, and to the apoplectic, hæmorrhagic, or red Softening. Turgescence of the vessels, *i. e.*, congestive or red Softening, has been mentioned in several published cases; and Christison himself has met with it, and in one case found "gorging of the vessels of the brain, inflammatory adhesion of the dura mater to the membranes beneath, and *effusion of eight ounces of serum into the lateral ventricles.* In another case, Christison admits it homœopathic to the apoplectic variety, as the patient became apoplectic, and a recent clot of blood was found in the right anterior lobe.

We have also seen that *Palsy, and Contraction of the limbs*, are among the most common symptoms of Softening of the brain, yet Christison says that *Arsenicum* is homœopathic to Palsy, and Rowland, we have seen, asserts that it cures paralysis.

Christison says a common nervous affection to which Arsenicum is homœopathic is partial Palsy; paralysis in the form of incomplete paraplegia is very indicative of Arsenic, and incomplete paralysis of one or more of the extremities, resembling Lead-palsy, is often one of the last symptoms which continues. Dehaen relates a distinct example in which *Ars.* proved homœopathic to Palsy; cramps, tenderness and weakness of the feet, legs, and arms, increased gradually until the whole extremities became at length almost completely palsied; the power of motion returned first in the hands, and then in the arms. Christison says than an excellent account of a set of similar cases has been given by Dr. Murray of Aberdeen; in four cases, *Arsen.* proved homœopathic to great muscular debility; in two cases, to true partial Palsy; in one case, the power of the *left* arm was lost altogether, and six months after, he was unable to bend the arm at the elbow-joint; in another case, it was homœopathic to great general debility, long-continued numbness, and pains in the legs.

In another case, *Ars.* was homœopathic to a dysenteric attack, followed by feebleness of the limbs, almost amounting to Palsy, attended with irritative fever, diarrhœa, and faintness, followed by great *stiffness*, numbness, and loss of power in the joints of the hands and feet. Another case, somewhat similar to the preceding, was observed by Mr. Lachese, of Angas, in which Arsenicum proved homœopathic to convulsions, followed by almost complete Palsy of the limbs. Christison also says, a well-marked case of the same nature was noticed by Professor Bernt; the paralytic affection consisted of loss of sensation, and of the power of motion in the hands, and of loss of motion in the feet, with *contraction* of the knee-joints. Dr. Falconer is also quoted as having frequently witnessed the homœopathicity of Arsenicum to local Palsy, and alludes to one case in which the hands only were paralyzed; also to two others, in which the Palsy spread gradually from the fingers upwards, until the whole arms were affected. On the whole, then, Christison admits, Arsenic is quite homœopathic to local Palsy, even to the most obstinate and intractable cases, as in the person of a cook, who had had perfect Palsy of the limbs for the greater part of a long life. Occasionally, Christison also asserts, it is homœopathic when the limbs are *rigidly bent, and cannot be extended.* It was homœopathic in another case, in which the limbs were *contracted* as well as palsied.

Nux-vomica.—The undoubted and even extraordinary homœopathicity of this drug to Softening of the brain has already been sufficiently alluded to on page 263.

Ferrum is recommended by Rowland, owing to the frequent alliance of Softening of the brain with anæmia, or fatty degeneration of the brain or other organs, in order to improve the condition of the blood by making it richer in fibrin and red particles; it certainly will not increase the quantity of fibrin, although it will aid in the production of the red coloring of the blood. In two cases of recent hemiplegia, in old and debilitated patients, the symptoms gradually improved, ROWLAND says, under the use of Iron, until voluntary motion was restored. Several old paralytic patients, with mental infirmity, also improved in some degree, but the medicine subsequently lost its power; in some it was afterwards injurious, while others could not bear Iron in any form or dose. Some of these latter cases might have been benefited by Plumbum.

Plumbum.—The homœopathicity of this remedy has also been sufficiently dwelt upon, on page 252. As its action is almost diametrically opposite to that of Ferrum, it might be used with advantage in those cases which are aggravated by Ferrum without subsequent improvement.

Iodide of Baryta is recommended by NOACK, and Agaricus deserves particular attention in the first stages of the disorder (see page 140). The effects of Agaricus there detailed are wonderfully similar to those of an adynamic condition of the brain, which may easily lead to Softening.

Opium.—Singularly enough, although ROWLAND is an allopathist, he says, that there are circumstances which not only warrant the administration of Opium, but considerable relief is derived from it; it even seems most appropriate to the cases where the brain is extensively disorganized, and sometimes stupor or coma may be warded off by a small dose of morphine, or a few grains of Dover's powder.

Symptomatic treatment.—According to ROWLAND, the most frequent affection of the intelligence in Softening of the brain, is feebleness of the intellectual faculties, slowness of apprehension, or imbecility; to these, Baryta and Conium are the most homœopathic remedies. Wild or noisy excitement, or delirium, is rarely observed, except in the first stage of acute Softening, especially of the convolutions; and even this is only transient, soon giving way to the torpor of the brain, which more properly belongs to the disease; in fact, the continuance of high delirious excitement would even warrant a pretty confident opinion that the structure of the brain is still sound—Bellad. and Stramonium will be most indicated. Attacks of lethargy, somnolency, and coma form a most important and characteristic feature of Softening of the brain; it is very peculiar that these attacks are generally transient and frequently repeated; in chronic Softening, paroxysms of insensibility or coma may return at intervals for months or years, and it is remarkable that the intelligence in these patients undergoes less permanent injury than in that form in which the disease is not marked by such accessions of stupor; after the patient has been for some time previously in a state nearly approaching to imbecility, or somnolency, an attack of coma will frequently remove a great portion of the oppression, and be followed by a sense of relief and greater firmness in the exercise of the intellect, and in fact, at times the mind will become sufficiently buoyant to permit the patient to attend to his usual avocations. Another circumstance peculiar to Softening of the brain, is the abrupt manner in which consciousness is restored; at one hour the patient will be suffering under the symptoms of deep apoplexy, and at the next he may be found with his memory and judgment in a great measure regained, and even sitting up and conversing cheerfully.—ROWLAND. These attacks are not always owing to congestion of the brain, to spasm, or to the sudden supervention of acute disease; for in many instances the death-like pallor, the thready pulse, the suddenness and frequency of the attacks, and their rapid termination, rather point to sudden exhaustion, debility, or adynamia of the brain. Opium, Hyosc., and Agaricus are the most important homœopathic remedies.

Sometimes that species of imbecility which is manifested chiefly in the manner and actions, and on that account called by the French *delirè d'action*, accompanies Softening of the brain; the patients are occupied continually with some employment, often without motive, almost without consciousness, and are generally very restless and irritable; they dress and undress frequently, busy themselves in unmeaning preparations, and continually repeat the same act; finally, they become completely demented, the mind is hopelessly clouded, the expression vacant and idiotic, and the limbs become paralytic. Agaricus, Hyosciamus, Spigelia, Bellad., and Stramonium are much indicated, although Arsenicum is sometimes indispensably necessary, or *Plumbum*.

When the speech is very much affected, Hyosc. is the best remedy.

In the paralysis, Arsenicum, Nux, Plumbum, Secale, Staphysagria, and Acidum oxalicum deserve attention. It should be recollected, however, that Palsy from softening of the nervous centres sometimes subsides without treatment, especially when the attack has been sudden; it is hard to understand why a condition occasioned by a permanent lesion should be capable of spontaneous removal, but so it is.

When the lower limbs are paralyzed, I wish to call attention to Secale, and Acidum oxalicum. Secale acts so specifically upon the lower portion of the spinal marrow, and experience with it has been so frequent and beneficial, that its name need merely be mentioned to awaken that attention which it deserves. But the specific action of Acidum oxalicum is not so well known; in one case, Christison says it proved homœopathic to great lassitude and weakness of the limbs, and numbness and weakness in the back, so severe that the patient could scarcely walk up stairs; in another case, the first thing complained of was acute pain in the back, gradually extending down the thighs, occasioning great torture ere long; in a third case, the patient complained more of the pain shooting down from the loins to the limbs than of any other symptom. It is also homœopathic to general numbness approaching to Palsy; to headache, extreme feebleness of the pulse, and a sense of numbness, tingling, or pricking, especially in the back and thighs. In another case, it proved homœopathic to " a feeling as if the hands were dead, to loss of consciousness for eight hours, then to lividity, coldness, and almost complete loss of power of motion in the legs: the patient recovered in fifteen days."

The treatment of the stiffness, rigidity, and contraction of he limbs, so common in Softening of the brain, has already been alluded to (see Nux).

Convulsions and convulsive tremblings require Nux, Ignat., or Mercurius.

The perversions of sensation, such as delusive feelings of heat and cold, or tingling or pricking sensations are most homœopathically treated by Aconit. rad. The same remedy will relieve the excessive sensitiveness of the skin and muscles of the paralyzed side, even when it is so great that the least touch causes exquisite suffering, although Agaricus should not be forgotten.

The headache is best treated by Glonoine.

Blindness of one or both eyes, or indistinctness of vision, or flashes of light, or black specks before the eyes, may be met by Bellad., Plumbum, Pulsatilla, or Phosphor; contraction of the pupils, if persistent, finds its homœopathic remedy in Opium or Nux; its antipathic antagonist in Bellad., Hyosc., or Stramonium.

When there is deafness or noises in the ear, *China* is indicated.

In the distressing nausea and vomiting which sometimes attend the acute form of the disease, Cuprum aceticum, or Zincum, may be thought of, in addition to the usual remedies.

When the respiration and pulse are slow, Opium, Plumbum, Aconite, and Digitalis should be thought of.

GENERAL REVIEW

OF THE

TREATMENT OF APOPLEXY, ETC.

---

1. ACONITUM NAPELLUS.

It may be used antipathically in full doses, when the face is flushed, skin hot, pulse full, strong and quick, pupils dilated, with severe pains, and great sensitiveness of the skin and nerves. Or, it may be used homœopathically in small doses, when the face is pale and sunken, skin cool, pulse weak and slow, pupils contracted, and much numbness and tingling are present.

2. ABSORBENTS.

A very important part of the treatment of hæmorrhagic Apoplexy, is that which has for its object, the safe and rapid absorption of the clot. Of course this should not be attempted too soon, or renewal of the bleeding might occur. Nitrate of Potash and the alkaline carbonates possess the power of dissolving fibrin and prevent its coagulation. Arnica, Baryta, Conium and Phosphor, also seem to possess the power of hastening absorption of the clot; while Nux-vomica, if used too freely, is apt to induce white Softening of the brain around the coagulum.

3. AGARICUS MUSCARIUS

Is homœopathic to enfeebled states of the brain, when the patient is giddy, weak, apt to tremble, and troubled with loss memory, and dimness of vision; when the patient's memory fails him, and he loses his way, does not recognize his friends, and is inclined to sleep. It may also prove homœopathic to Softening of the brain, and true hæmorrhagic Apoplexy. It is homœopathic to bilious Apoplexy, with jaundice and enlargement of the liver; also to those cases which are preceded by unusual wakefulness, and excitement or irritation of the brain, especially when there is much twitching of the face and limbs, with dilatation of the pupils and glistening of the eyes.

4. ARNICA MONTANA

In traumatic Apoplexy, or that which occurs after blows and falls upon the head. In hæmorrhagic Apoplexy, to check the bleeding and promote the absorption of the clot; in serous Apoplexy, to aid the absorption of the watery fluid; in Apoplexy followed by paralysis, especially in the earlier stages, before more active remedies, such as Nux-vom., are admissible.

5. BARYTA

In torpid and chronic cases, to promote the absorption of the clot. Against tendency to Apoplexy from excitement of the sexual organs; in Apoplexy of the cerebellum, with much pain in the back of the head. In the Apoplexies of delicate, and old people.

6. BELLADONNA.

It may be given homœopathically in small doses, when the face is flushed and bloated, the carotids beating violently, eyes red, pupils widely dilated, pulse full, hard and strong, and slight convulsions are present. RÜCKERT says it has effected cures in aged patients, from 60 to 70 or 80 years old, of powerful, heavy and plethoric constitutions, i. e., in those with the true apoplectic habit; especially when there was unconsciousness, *swollen and red*, or else pale face; protruding and reddened eyes, with *dilatation* of the pupils; loss of sight, smell, and speech; presence of muttering and and stammering; *distortion* of the mouth; twitchings of the face; involuntary flow of spittle and fluids from the mouth; protrusion and swelling of the tongue; pulsation of the carotids; *difficulty* or inability to *swallow;* involuntary urination; grasping at the genitals; groaning and snoring; *obstructed respiration;* paralysis of the limbs, either of the right or left side; *fulness*, tension, quickening, or retardation of the pulse; coma, or *sopor*. The most characteristic and important indications are printed in *italics*.—PETERS.

It may be used antipathically in full doses, in anæmic and atrophic states of the brain, when the face is pale, pupils contracted, head dizzy and weak (from insufficient supply of blood,) pulse slow and small, and urine scanty.

7. BLOOD-LETTING.

According to WATSON, this is required when the patient is plethoric, the pulse full, hard or thrilling, or else oppressed, large and slow; and if there are obvious external signs of great congestion to the head, such as great throbbing of the carotid and temporal arteries, turgid state of the veins of the face and scalp, great turgor or flushing of the face, or else a bloated and livid appearance of the same. If the patient's skin be pale and cold, his pulse feeble and flickering, bleeding will probably insure his death. RAU, who was second to none but HAHNEMANN in Homœopathy, also admits the propriety of occasional blood-letting.

7. COCCULUS

Is most homœopathic to gastric Apoplexy, when there is emptiness and hollowness of the head, dizziness, with great nausea and tendency to faint, falling asleep of the feet and hands, difficulty in speaking and thinking, &c.

9. CONIUM

Is most homœopathic to Apoplexy from pure and uncomplicated venous congestion, and congestive Apoplexy, when the face is bloated, purple or livid, the skin rather cool, pulse slow and feeble, pupils contracted, and the breathing extraordinarily difficult and oppressed. It will also aid in the absorption of the clot in hæmorrhagic Apoplexy, by arousing the activity of both the venous and lymphatic systems; and is decidedly homœopathic to the debility and paralysis which precedes, or follows Apoplexy.

CUPRUM

Is allied in its action to Nux, Plumbum, Cocculus, Ignatia;

it is homœopathic to Apoplexy when preceded by, or attended with convulsions, viz., in spasmodic and nervous Apoplexy; also in bilious Apoplexy. It may prove antipathic when the complexion of the patient is unusually white and clear; when there is a deficiency of bile, not only in the liver and bowels, but also in the whole system; and when paralysis is a predominant symptom.

FERRUM

Is apparently, although not absolutely allied in some of its actions, to Bellad., Glonoine, Opium and Phosphor; but it is more homœopathic to true arterial plethora and Apoplexy, than any of these remedies, except Glonoine and Phosphor. It is somewhat antagonistic in its action to that of Conium, Hydrocyanic Acid, and Plumbum. It is homœopathic to violent arterial congestion to the head, with powerful beating of the heart and arteries, great redness and heat of the face, heat of skin, severe head-ache, heat and fulness of the head, and dizziness, from rush of blood to the head. It is also homœopathic, both symptomatologically and pathologically, to hæmorrhagic Apoplexy, especially when there has been a feeling as if the brain had received a sudden shock, or had been rent asunder, soon followed by faintness and sense of sinking, owing to rupture of a blood-vessel and pouring out of blood in, or upon the brain.

It is antipathic to the Apoplexies of anæmic and debilitated persons; when the skin and lips are bloodless, the body thin and feeble, the extremities cold, the mind weak and the pulse feeble.

IPECAC

Is most suitable in gastric and nervous Apoplexy, especially when there is much nausea, and great asthmatic difficulty of breathing.

GLONOINE

Is most homœopathic to sudden and violent congestive Apoplexies. It may prove the most antipathic remedy to anæmia and atrophy of the brain, when the patient is in imminent danger of dying from an enfeebled and bloodless condition, especially when sudden and alarming syncope sets in from great depression of the heart, arteries and brain; it may act almost as promptly as transfusion of blood.

HYOSCIAMUS

Is most homœopathic when there is a high state of nervous excitement, with more or less delirium and twitching of the muscles.

HYDROCYANIC ACID

Is most homœopathic to Apoplexy attended with extreme exhaustion and prostration.

IGNATIA

Is indicated under almost the same circumstances as those which require Nux.

NUX-VOMICA

Is most homœopathic in convulsive Apoplexy, when the limbs are in a state of permanent and rigid contraction, especially if the face be pale or livid, and the pupils *contracted.* It is allied in its action to some of the effects of Arnica, Cocculus, Cuprum, and Ignatia; it is somewhat antagonistic to Belladonna, but especially to Opium, Conium, Plumbum, and Hydrocyanic Acid.

OPIUM.

According to Rückert, it is most indicated when there is congestion to, with violent roaring in the head; loss of consciousness; or excitement with laughing, and confused, erroneous talking; restlessness; redness of the face and eyes; contracted pupils; grasping at the head; drawing of the tongue to one side; difficulty of speaking and swallowing; groaning and anxious respiration; coldness and paralysis of the limbs; softness, fulness, or weakness of the pulse; and coma.

PHOSPHOR

Is homœopathic to the most active and sthenic cases of Apoplexy, with much arterial, congestive and febrile excitement. It is antipathic to the Apoplexies of debilitated persons, when the exhaustion has almost reached its extreme degree, the pulse being small, sunken, rapid and soft, the limbs cold; when hiccough has set in, with rattling respiration, and cold and clammy sweat.

STYPTICS.

Among the remedies treated of in this book, which may be used as styptics, Plumbum-Aceticum, Opium, and Ferrum deserve particular attention; Arnica and Ipecac. may also come in play.

TABULAR REVIEW.

BY RÜCKERT.

	Acon.	Arn.	Baryta.	Bell.	Coccul.	Cuprum.	Ipec.	Hyosc.	Nux.	Opium.
Chewing and gritting of the teeth,	..	..	..	Bell.	..	..	..	..	..	..
Coma, (deep sleep),	..	..	Bar.	BELL.	Cocc.	Cupr.	..	..	..	..
Consciousness, loss of,	Acon.	Arn.	..	BELL.	Cocc.	..	..	..	Nux.	Op.
" undisturbed.	..	..	..	Bell.	..	..	..	..	..	..
Difficulty of speaking,	..	Arn	..	BELL.	..	Cupr.	Ipec.	..	Nux.	..
" swallowing,	..	..	..	Bell.	..	..	..	Hyosc.	Nux.	Op.
Distortion of the mouth,	..	..	..	BELL.	..	Cupr.	..	..	..	Op.
Eyes, dim and fixed,	..	..	..	..	..	..	..	..	Nux.	Op.
" congested with blood,	..	..	..	Bell.	..	..	..	..	..	..
" squinting,	..	..	..	Bell.	..	..	..	..	..	..
" rolling of,	..	..	..	..	Cocc.	..	..	..	..	..
Face, corpse-like and pale,	Acon.	..	..	Bell.	..	..	..	..	..	..
" red and swollen,	..	Arn.	..	BELL.	Cocc.	..	..	Hyosc.	..	Op.
Forgetfulness,	..	Arn.	Bar.	..	..	..	..	..	..	..
Groaning and gurgling in sleep,	..	..	..	BELL.	..	..	..	..	..	..
Head, heat of,	Acon.	..	..	..	..	..	..	..	..	..
" grasping at,	..	..	..	..	..	..	..	..	Nux.	Op.
" roaring in, and in ears,	..	..	..	Bell.	..	..	..	..	..	Op.
Heart-beats, slow and trembling,	Acon.	..	..	..	..	..	..	..	..	..
Jaw, dropped,	..	Arn.	..	Bell	..	..	..	..	Nux.	..
" locked, with spasms of face,	..	..	..	..	..	Cupr.	..	..	..	..
Limbs, cold and stiff,	Acon	..	..	Bell.	..	..	..	..	Nux.	..
Lying as if dead,	..	Arn.	..	..	..	..	..	..	..	Op.
Mucus, thick in and about mouth,	..	..	..	..	..	..	..	..	Nux.	..
Muttering and mumbling,	..	..	..	Bell.	..	..	..	..	Nux.	..
Paralysis of sensation on right side,	Acon.	..	..	Bell.	..	..	..	..	..	..
Paralysis of bladder,	..	..	..	..	..	..	..	Hyosc.	Nux	..
" of the limbs,	..	Arn.	..	..	..	Cupr.	Ipec.	..	Nux.	..
" of the left side,	..	Arn.	..	BELL.	..	..	..	..	..	Op.
" of the right side,	..	..	..	Bell.	Cocc.	..	..	..	..	..
Pulsation of the carotids,	Acon	..	..	Bell.	..	..	..	..	..	..
Pulse, full,	Acon	Arn.	..	Bell.	Cocc.	..	..	Hyosc.	Nux.	Op.
" hard,	Acon.	..	..	..	Cocc.	..	..	..	..	..
" intermitting,	..	Arn.	..	..	..	..	..	..	..	..
" not intermitting,	Aeon.	..	..	..	..	..	..	..	..	..
" not to be felt,	Acon.	..	..	..	..	..	..	..	..	Phos.
" quick,	..	..	..	..	..	..	..	Hyosc.	..	..
" slow,	..	..	..	Bell.	..	..	..	..	Nux.	..
" tense,	..	..	..	Bell.	..	..	..	..	..	..
" weak,	..	..	..	..	..	..	..	..	..	..
Pupils contracted,	ACON.	..	Baryt.	..	..	..	..	..	Nux.	..
" insensible and dilated,	Acon	..	Baryt.	BELL.	Cocc.	..	..	..	Nux.	Op.
Respiration, infrequent,	Acon.	..	..	Bell.	..	..	..	..	..	..
" rattling,	Acon.	..	..	Bell.	..	..	..	..	..	..
" deep,	..	..	..	Bell.	Cocc.	..	..	..	..	..
" scarcely perceptible,	..	..	..	..	Cocc.	..	..	..	..	Phos.
Skin, warm,	Acon.	..	..	..	..	..	..	..	..	..
Salivation,	..	..	..	Bell.	..	..	Ipec.	..	Nux.	..
Tongue, paralyzed, and drawn to one side,	..	..	..	..	..	Cupr.	..	..	..	Op.

A

TREATISE

ON

NERVOUS DERANGEMENTS

AND

MENTAL DISORDERS.

ON THE

NATURE AND CAUSES

OF

MENTAL DERANGEMENT.

Mental derangement is made to include all derangements of the intellectual and moral functions. The primitive type of all the forms of derangement is supposed to consist in an excess or perversion of some one of the natural passions or emotions of the mind. Among the insane we find the same ideas, the same errors, the same passions, the same misfortunes which elsewhere prevail. The insane world is the same as the sane world, but its distinctive characters are more noticeable, its features more marked, its colors more vivid, its effects more striking, because the insane man displays himself in all his nakedness; dissimulating not his thoughts, nor concealing his defects; lending not to his passions seductive charms; nor to his vices deceitful appearances. If we reflect upon what passes through the mind of even the most sensible and virtuous person for a single day, what incoherence shall we notice in his ideas and determinations from the time that he awakes in the morning, until he retires to rest at night; and how many foolish, wicked and offensive impulses. His sensations, ideas and determinations, have some connection among themselves, only when he arrests his attention, and then only does he reason and exert mental control. The insane no longer enjoy the faculty of fixing and directing their attention, and this privation is the primitive cause of all their errors. All reasoning and mental control presupposes an effort, and we are not naturally reasoning, and self-denying beings; that is to say, our ideas are not instinctively and naturally conformed to objects, our comparisons correct, our reasonings just, and our actions proper, except by a succession of efforts of the attention, and a ready submission to the results of the consequent reflections. In the insane, the impressions are so vivid, fugitive and numerous, and the ideas so abundant, that they cannot fix their attention sufficiently and justly upon each thought, object, or idea; while with the monomaniac, the attention is so concentrated, and the ideas so few, that it cannot turn itself aside upon surrounding objects and accessory ideas. Hence a vicious, or imperfect mental and moral training is a powerful predisposing cause of derangement. There may be error in two opposite directions. The brain may be prematurely stimulated to exertion by the ambition of the child, or the parent; or the evil passions may be allowed to develop themselves unchecked, through a weak and injudicious indulgence. In the former case, especially if the patient be of a naturally highly nervous or enthusiastic temperament, the brain is often brought into a state of excitement and irritation, which requires but a slight additional excitement to become decidedly morbid; in the latter, the character is left unprovided with the due safeguards against the temptations, annoyances, disappointments, and necessary struggles of life, and the mind sometimes breaks down under the first serious conflict. Mental and moral training is essentially necessary to those who have naturally any strong passion in excess, such as ambition, pride, love of applause. The one-sided, enthusiastic, conceited, or careless person, will also be very apt to neglect the proper care of his or her body, natural functions, diet, rest, &c., and hence, various bodily derangements will soon be ready to add their quota to natural predisposition, or acquired tendency to mental derangement.

In accordance with these views, the profession or business of men has great influence over the number of the insane. The proportion is vastly greater among classes whose brains are kept in a perpetual turmoil, either of passion, or of intellect, than among those who pursue a tranquil course of moderate industry and enjoyment. It has also been observed that the number of insane is greater in a community, in proportion to the political and religious freedom of the population; that is, to the opportunity they enjoy of working out their own purposes, whether in relation to this world, or the next, in the manner most agreeable to themselves. Excitement, powerful effort, and want of mental balance and control are always greatest in such communities. Perhaps there is no country in the world, in which the insane are proportionally more numerous than in America.

Excessive mental excitement, whether intellectual or emotional, is probably the most common cause of insanity. Every excess pre-supposes a want of judgment and mental control, and consequently, forms the first great step towards derangement. Excessive study; perplexing metaphysical or religious investigations; over-indulgence of the imagination; struggles for power, influence, or wealth; religious or political excitement; violent anger; excess of revenge, jealousy, or hatred; the agitations and perplexities which arise from the entanglements of engrossing business speculations, household cares, domestic unhappiness, and especially the remorse from vicious, or criminal indulgence. Early mental training is especially necessary to ward off the bad effects of fear, disappointment, grief, despair, reverses of business, loss of friends, triumph of enemies, abuse of confidence, betrayed affections, public disgrace, general destitution, bodily pain and disease. The mental emotions and imagination should be controlled, and the reasoning faculty and judgment developed, in order to prevent insanity; for in the insane, the *reasoning faculty* is always deranged, although not abolished; the patient can often follow out trains of ratiocination with considerable correctness, and sometimes, even with much ingenuity; but he is apt to change abruptly from one course of thought to another, before the first is completed; each idea that presents itself, however irrelative, becomes the starting point of a new succession of thought, which is in its turn, soon interrupted; and his intellectual action is thus broken up into disjointed fragments, which are fitted to no useful purpose; he often, besides, mistakes some slight semblance, some mere shadow of association, a similarity of sound in a word, for example, for a legitimate link in a chain of reasoning, and thus, even when starting from correct premises, is led into the most egregrious errors. The *judgment* is perhaps more perverted than any other faculty. It is the quality of mind which is most rarely perfect in health, and which, therefore, may be expected to be most defective in mental unsoundness. The maniac cannot duly appreciate his relations to the world around him, cannot shape his course in accordance with the various interests, opinions and feelings of others, and is therefore constantly encountering difficulties and vexations. The *imagination* in mania, is often greatly excited, fruitful in its suggestion, not unfrequently brilliant in its illusive picturing, but always deranged; the pictures which it forms, like the workings of the insane reason, are without due relation of parts, mere jumbled assemblages of the grotesque, the ludicrous, the wild, the fearful; shifting too, like dreamy phantasms, to which it is probable they bear no slight resemblance. Early control of *temper*, is all important to those predisposed to insanity, for in general, the maniac is more irascible than in health, surrenders himself more readily to every impulse, is often suspicious, revengeful, and malicious. Excesses of pride, ambition, and vanity, are frequently witnessed. Steadiness of the affections and feelings, should be cultivated, for among the most common results of the disease, is an alteration of the natural affections; the dislike of the insane for their former nearest and most intimate friends, is almost proverbial; while the feelings are exceedingly unstable; the patient passes rapidly from one state to another; the mental chords vibrate in quick succession with the whole gamut of the passions.

It is unnecessary to follow out this idea farther here; it is as important, however, to pay equally great attention to physical and hygienic training; derangements of the stomach and liver dispose to the melancholic forms of madness, and especially to hypochondriasis; nothing is more common than to see a depression of spirits approaching to mental derangement, consequent upon dyspepsia, functional disease of the liver, derangement or constipation of the bowels, and the superaddition of delusion or hallucination, converts the affection into insanity. Such affections occasionally clear off like mists before the sun, under the use of proper regimen, exercise, diet, relaxation from care and business, judicious anti-bilious or laxative, or other means; avoidance of alcohol, tobacco, strong tea, or coffee, &c., &c.

Of 1000 cases of Insanity collected by Barlow:

110 arose from drunkenness;
73 " " excessive ambition;
73 " " excessive bodily or mental labor;

69 arose from misfortunes;
54 " " chagrin;
47 " " disappointed love;
29 " " religious enthusiasm;
26 " " political events;
12 " " ill usage;
9 " " crimes, remorse, or despair;
78 " " epilepsy;
71 were born idiots;
69 arose from old age;
39 " " accidents and injuries;
17 " " poisonous effluvia;
100 " " consequences of disease;
115 " " unknown causes.

Of 704 cases in males, 346, or one-half, were deranged from *moral* causes; and only 156, or one-fourth, from *physical* causes.

Of 1094 cases in females, 489 arose from *moral* causes, and 282 from *physical* causes.

The principal *moral* causes in these 346 cases in *males* were:

Reverse of fortune in 86 cases;
Anxiety . . . " 69 "
Religion . . . " 45 "
Love . . . . " 18 "

Principal *moral* causes in 489 insane *females*, were:

Anxiety . . . in 79 cases;
Religion . . . " 69 "
Loss of relatives " 62 "
Love . . . . " 57 "
Fright . . . . " 50 "
Reverse of fortune " 49 "

The principal physical cause in 156 insane males, was: Inemperance in 80 cases.

In females, puerperal disease in 117 cases out of 282.

In 490 cases of INSANITY from *moral* causes, ESQUIREL found

136 cases caused by domestic troubles;
71 " " " disappointed affection;
91 " " " misery and reverses of fortune;
46 " " " fright;

45 cases caused by	political events;
9 " " "	fanatacism;
32 " " "	jealousy;
16 " " "	anger;
17 " " "	wounded self-love;
13 " " "	excessive study;
2 " " "	misanthropy;
12 " " "	disappointed ambition.

In 730 cases from *physical* causes:

255 were caused by	hereditary tendency;
70 " " "	apoplexy;
64 " " "	progress of age;
16 " " "	convulsions of mother during pregnancy;
13 " " "	epilepsy;
16 " " "	sun-stroke;
16 " " "	falls and blows upon the head;
25 " " "	fevers;
38 " " "	critical period of life;
74 " " "	menstrual disorder;
73 " " "	puerperal disorder;
9 " " "	syphilis;
32 " " "	mercury;
28 " " "	intestinal worms.

In 482 cases of MELANCHOLY:

110 cases arose from	hereditary predisposition;
60 " " "	domestic trouble;
48 " " "	reverses of fortune;
42 " " "	disappointed affection;
40 " " "	change of life;
35 " " "	puerperal state;
30 " " "	libertinism;
25 " " "	suppressisn of menses;
19 " " "	abuse of liquor;
19 " " "	fright;
18 " " "	anger;
12 " " "	wounded self-love;
10 " " "	falls upon the head;

8 cases arose from jealousy;
6 " " " masturbation.

In 299 cases of MANIA from moral causes:
91 cases arose from domestic trials;
71 " " " disappointed affection;
43 " " " fright;
25 " " " reverse of fortune;
22 " " " wounded self-love;
19 " " " want;
17 " " " jealousy and anger;
10 " " " excessive study.

Of this long array of the causes of insanity the effects of many cannot altogether be warded off, and the unfortunate sufferer must bear up as well as his religious and moral training will enable him to do. Although, drunkenness, excessive ambition, excessive bodily and mental labor, religious enthusiasm, crimes, excessive anxiety, fanaticism, jealousy, anger, misanthropy, libertinism, fear, &c., &c., can be and should be controlled; still misfortunes, chagrin, disappointed love, ill-usage, disease, reverse of fortune, loss of relatives, domestic troubles, misery, wounded self-love, with or without hereditary tendency, will fall heavily on all, and too heavily on some. Religion and moral training must soften their influence, or the result will be disastrous. Dr. RAY thinks that defective or perverted education is one of the most productive causes of insanity. The gross neglect, he observes, of the moral powers, those which guide the passions and determine the notions, is the crowning defect of the education of our times, ruinous in its consequences to the health, both of body and mind. At home, children should be taught to acquire the power of governing passion and resisting the impulses of the lower appetites, of discerning the nicer shades of right and wrong, of sacrificing self to the call of benevolence and duty, and amid trial and change, steadily keeping in view the great purposes of life. How many of this generation complete their childhood scarcely feeling the dominion of any will but their own, and obeying no higher law than the caprice of the moment. The legitimate result in the education of our times is, that finally the ordinary virtues of life are degraded to a very low rank. Patient and persevering industry, with its slow and moderate rewards, honest frugality, and a temperance that restrains every excess, frequent and faithful self-examination, clear and well-digested views of duty, become distasteful to the mind, which can breathe only an atmosphere of excitement, craving stimulus that rapidly consumes its energies, and destroys that elasticity which enables it to arise frcm every pressure with new vigor and increased power of endurance.

A very large class of the insane, however are formed by bright and sensitive spirits, fully alive to every emotion of pain or pleasure; over-conscientious and honorable; too anxious to perform every duty, and comply with every exaction upon them; if to this be added natural weakness of body, and some ill health, with frequent and sudden trials and misfortunes, then reason often gives way under them.

Of 28,548 cases collected from all sources and treated *allopathically*, 10,757 were cured, and 2955 died, leaving 17,781 in a more or less hopeless state of mental derangement. In March, 1844, of 984 cases in the Hanwell Asylum, only 30 were regarded as curable. Of 11,976 cases accumulated in the British Asylums in 1851 and 52, only 953 were cured, 1183 died, and 9840 were left uncured. At the York Retreat the average proportion of recoveries during the forty-four years it had been in operation, in 1846, amounted to nearly forty-seven per cent. The general average of relapses, is from ten to seventeen to thirty per cent; and second attacks may occur four, five, eight, fourteen, or even nineteen years after the first.

The liability to relapse after a recovery from a first attack is scarcely less than fifty per cent, or one in every two cases discharged as recovered; five out of ten recover, and five die sooner or later during an attack; of the five who recover, not more than two remain well during the rest of their lives; the other three sustain subsequent attacks, during which at least two of them die. The interval of mental health may last from ten to twenty years, during which the individual may enjoy all the comforts cf social life. Of 1300 recoveries, 206 were known to have relapsed; of 51 other recoveries, 11 relapsed in less than one year. Of 320 other recoveries, 47 were visited with a second attack of insanity; 7 with a third attack, 1 with a fourth and 1 with a fifth. The relapses therefore amounted to about seventeen per cent on the recoveries. Still, cases of mental improvement, caused by attacks of insanity have been recorded by several writers. Dr. CHANDLER says, he has known a few persons who recovered to become better citizens than they were before. Their minds and feelings acquired strength and soundness by the disease, and by undergoing the process of cure, as some musical instruments are said to be improved by being broken and repaired again. Of 244 cases by NEUMANN only 131, or fifty-three and a half per cent recovered from the first attack; of these 131 recoveries, only 45, or eighteen per cent remained permanently free from mental disorder; while 86 had one or more subsequent attacks, and only 20 of the 86 were sane at the time of death. Hence of 244 cases, only 65 were sane at the time of death, or twenty-six and a half per cent. In females sixty-seven per cent relapse; in males sixty-five per cent. Of insane under twenty years of age, fifty-five per cent recover; between twenty and thirty years, fifty-two per cent; between forty and sixty years, forty-six per cent; between sixty and eighty, only twenty-eight per cent.

Of curable cases, those of one month's duration, eighty-three per cent recover; of from one to three months, seventy-eight per cent recover; those of from three to six months' duration, fifty-nine per cent; six to twelve months, thirty-five per cent; twelve to eighteen months, eighteen per cent; eighteen to twenty-four months, only ten per cent; and those of two or more years' duration only four per cent are restored.

Again, according to JARVIS, of 57,794 cases in males, 23,677 recovered; of 53,946 cases in females, 23,704 were cured; leaving 64,359 of both sexes more or less hopelessly insane. Although the females recovered in an excess of nine per cent over the males, still they are rather more subject to relapses.

Of 112,143 cases, 20,458 died, and the mortality increases in proportion to age; in those insane from twenty to thirty years of age, the mortality is from three and a half to five per cent; from thirty to forty years, three to seven per cent; forty to fifty years, three and a half to nine and a half per-cent; fifty to sixty years, four and a half to six and a half per cent; sixty to seventy, six to seven per cent; seventy to eighty, eight and a half to twelve per cent; eighty to ninety, twenty-one to thirty per cent.

Mean mortality in all ages, four and a half to seven and a half per cent. In the English Asylums the mortality varied from 5.30 to 11.27 per cent. The cures, from 22.48 to 59.0 per cent.

PINEL says, recoveries generally take place within five or six months; at York Asylum fifty per cent of the recoveries occur within three months; ESQUIROL in 2005 cases had 604 recover in the first year, 497 in the second, 86 in the third, and only 41 in the seven following years, leaving 777 hopelessly insane.

Of all the circumstances which affect the comparison of the recoveries and mortality of the insane, when treated in asylums, the stage or duration is the most important; the probability of recovery, in cases brought under care within three months of first attack, is as four to one. In cases not admitted until more than twelve months after the attack, the probability is less than one to four. On the other hand, the mortality is greater in recent than in chronic cases, viz., seven per cent in the former, and only four and a half per cent in the latter.

The probability of recovery is greater, from four to twenty per cent, in women than men; and the excess of mortality in males varies from thirty-four to seventy-two per cent.

Of 112 cases of recovery in New-York State Asylum, 36 had been insane only one month, or under; 44, between two or three months; 18, from four to seven months; 9, from seven to twelve months; and 3 over twelve months. Ten of these 112 cases were cured in two months and under; 6 in three months; 54, in from four to seven months; 27, in from seven to twelve months; 13, in from one to two years; 2, in two years.

Of 1355 cases not insane over one year, no less 1089 recovered, leaving only 266 more or less hopelessly insane. GALT, in the Eastern Asylum of Virginia of 14 recent cases, cured 12, which success he regards as unexampled; he used Opium in enormous doses, from six to twelve grains, or from two to three grains of Morphine, three times a day; he also had Opium smoked in pipes mixed with tobacco. MOREL gave Opium to the extent of nine grains in twenty-four hours, without satisfactory results; so that very large doses seem to be required.

The early and proper treatment of insanity is all important; it is said that scarcely a single case recovers when left to run its course either unchecked, or only partially checked by irregular treatment. In every case, the first thing necessary is to subject the patient to some control, more or less strict, according to circumstances; control is one of the most important remedial means; it is a great mistake to suppose that the insane can be reasoned out of their delusions, or that remonstrance will prevent their absurd conduct; argument and remonstrance are generally prejudicial, unless the patient be under control, and so far recovered that he may be regarded as somewhat convalescent.

The great question is whether this control shall be at home, by means of medicine, or in asylums. WOOD is in favor of an early removal to an asylum, because insane persons are very apt to contract aversion for their nearest friends and relatives, and are consequently liable to perpetual irritation from their presence. Instead of being soothed by their kind offices and affectionate attentions, they are often excited into paroxysms of rage. Besides the patient often requires control; he has lost his own self-control, and some opposition to his will is absolutely essential. But such opposition and control from persons from whom he has before experienced nothing but kindness, and perhaps submission, become sources of perpetual vexation, and sustain an excitement highly calculated to aggravate and fix his disorder, &c., &c.

On the other hand, WILLIAMS says, in an incipient case of *mania*, it is far better to treat it at the patient's house; this is infinitely preferable to removal. The patient can be placed under control, and the degree of restraint which may be necessary can be properly adapted by having one or more attendants. It is always in early cases that so much may be done; and more persons recover during the first six weeks after being attacked, than in the aggregate of all other subsequent periods. If this be true in acute attacks, in those cases which come on more slowly, removal to an asylum must not be delayed too long; the patient may get somewhat better, but will almost certainly relapse soon after he again begins to mingle in the world. After the first two or three months of insanity, the longer an efficient course of treatment is postponed, the less is the chance of success.

The seat of insanity is probably in the cineritious, or grey portion of the brain; in a few cases the irritation may be inflammatory in its nature, but in the very largest portion it is merely nervous. Very few cases commence with delirium, fever, furred tongue, thirst, heat of skin, and loss of appetite; in the larger portion the temperature of the skin is not raised, although there may be some heat of the head, similar to that caused by a fit of passion, or any irritation; of 222 cases seen by JACOBI, only 22 or 23 had fever, and some of these were hectic, or fever from other causes than the mania. It may be asserted without fear of contradiction that no pathologist could in nine-tenths of all the cases of mental derangement which prove fatal, take upon himself to say from an examination of the brain, whether the person during life had been of sound mind or not. BURNETT thought insanity a blood disease depending upon a derangement, or mal-assimilation of those particular materials of the blood, Carbon and Phosphorus, which constitute the bulk of the elementary tissue of the brain and nervous system—insanity in some cases is immediately caused by the deterioration of the fatty matter of the blood, by which the Carbon and Phosphor are unable to combine in healthy proportions and make sound nerves and brain. In proof of this BENCE JONES found an increase of phosphates excreted during a paroxysms of mania; and another remarkable feature in the urine of the insane is the excess of Ammonia, in the form of Carbonate, Urate, Hydro-chlorate, or the Ammonio-magnesian phosphate.

My own opinion is that the irritation in the brains of many deranged persons is very similar to that which occurs in scrofulous ophthalmia and spinal irritation. In both these diseases the redness, congestion or inflammation of the eye or spinal marrow is very slight, although the irritation is very great. It is very true that the diseased changes, which pathologists may generally expect to find on examining the heads of lunatics in a great majority dissections will be:

1st, Infiltration of the pia-mater with serum,

2d, Congestion of the brain and its membranes,

3d, Effusion into the ventricles.

In 67 cases, 53 had the third; 53, the first; and 38 the second; 30 also had the arachnoid thickened and opaque; in 26 the color of the brain was altered; 15 had effusion of blood in the skull; 62 had the organs of the chest disordered; 30, those of the abdomen.

That insanity is often connected with a tuberculous or scrofulous diathesis is evident from the fact that of 1540 cases of death in insane persons, no less than 200 died with consumption, or about twelve per cent; cases of marasmus not included. HITCHMAN says that there is much reason to suppose, that in the insane, the organs of the chest are more frequently diseased than those of the abdomen. Consumption is common, but in a masked form; sometimes tubercles form and even tubercular excavations take place, without manifesting any of those distressing symptoms of cough, expectoration and restlessness, so common in the sane.

In 145 cases examined by Dr. HITCHMAN the dura-mater was adherent to the skull in about one-third of the cases, especially in those long insane, and advanced in years.

In 115 cases the arachnoid was more or less opaque and thickened, and contained a considerable quantity of serous fluid. These conditions are almost invariable accompaniments in chronic cases of insanity; in 22 cases out of 27. In recent cases the arachnoid does not adhere as closely to the pia-mater, nor is there so much thickness, opacity, or serous effusion; thus in 165 recent cases the arachnoid was thickened and opaque in 62 instances only.

In 118 cases the pia-mater was venously congested and infiltrated with sub-arachnoidean fluid. In chronic cases the pia-mater is almost invariably found thickened and altered; it becomes much thickened, can be removed from the brain in large pieces without laceration; is sometimes dark from the congested state of its blood-vessels; frequently œdematous, and bathed in a muddy fluid, resembling diluted jelly. The pia-mater is even more frequently affected in chronic lunacy than the arachnoid itself. The choroid plexuses were simultaneously congested, and contain cysts, and sand.

Pachionean glands were much enlarged in twenty, mostly old patients.

The convolutions of the brain were sunken, atrophied or soft in 72 cases out 119, and all these had either been insane for a long time, or were in a state of extreme imbecility or dementia. Seen through the thickened pia-mater, the convolutions have a brownish hue owing to the presence of large quantities of serum.

In advanced dementia, the surface of the convolutions when cut, sometimes was dark in hue.

In acute mania, the grey substance of the convolutions is apt to have a pink or roseate color.

In 64 cases in which the patients had long been insane or imbecile, the grey substance was pale or blanched.

The white part of the brain was softened in 19 cases ; greatly congested in 12.

There are quite a variety of forms of mental derangement.

1st, MANIA, or *general delirium*, including

a) mental derangement without fury ;

b) mania, with fury.

2d, MONOMANIA, or delirium limited to one, or a few objects, with a predominance of one passion.

a) *Monomania of pride*, the subjects of which imagine that they are possessed of great riches or power ; that they are generals, princes, deities, &c.

b) *Gay monomania ;* according to Esquirel, true monomaniacs are always gay and expansive, affording a striking contrast to hypochondriacs.

Haschisch and Aurum are perhaps the most homœopathic remedies against gay monomania (see Appendix).

c) *Sad monomania*, or the melancholy of the ancients, lypemania of Esquirol ; these patients are deranged on one or a few subjects, with a predominance of sadness, or depression ; are apt to fear that they are dishonored, condemned to death, imprisoned, &c. ; some are under the influence of a continuous or irresistible fear.

d) ***Religious monomania***, including Demonomaniacs, Theomaniacs, Ascetics, &c.

The insanity of masturbators is sometimes thought by their friends to be caused by religious anxiety, because the first evidence of it noticed, was an extraordinary anxiety about their salvation, an inordinate fear of future punishment; or abandoning all occupation but that of reading or holding a bible, as if reading; or praying, or mumbling incoherent sentences in an attitude of prayer at improper times and places, &c.

Another class, frequently placed under the head of religious anxiety, are religious monomaniacs whose insanity is undoubtedly referable to dyspepsia, habitual indigestion and constipation. BRIGHAM.

e) *Erotomania.* This is very different from nymphomania and satyriasis; it bears the same relation to these, what the ardent affections of the heart, when chaste and honorable are, in comparison with frightful libertinism; actions the most obscene, shameful and humiliating characterise the latter, while the erotomaniac neither desires, or dreams even, of the favors to which he might aspire from the object of his insane tenderness. In erotomania the eyes are lively and animated, the look passionate, the discourse tender, and the actions expansive: but the subjects of it never pass the limits of propriety.

In two cases of Dementia and two of Mania, caused by masturbation, the Muriate tinct. of Iron in large doses was found to be the best anaphrodisiac which SMITH could employ; appearing to be the real agent in the cures which followed its use. Nymphomania in one case was cured by Bromide of Potash in fifteen grain doses, three times a day. In the treatment of masturbation BRIGHAM preferred Conium, Camphor and Belladonna, and thinks that he has indubitable evidence of its power. WOOD thinks that in excitement of the venereal propensity, Dulcamara, very freely employed, is perhaps the most efficient remedy—Muriate of Baryta also deserves attention.

f) *Kleptomania*, or monomania for stealing.

g) *Pyromania*, or mania for incendiarism.

h) *Suicidal* and Homicidal monomania.

In suicidal insanity, the Meconite, and Hydrochlorate of Morphia often act like a charm, if uninterruptedly and perseveringly given, until the nervous system is completely under its influence. FORBES WINSLOW has witnessed the most distressing attacks of this form of insanity radically cured by this treatment when every other has failed. He has also seen the suicidal impulse removed after the administration of a few doses of Belladonna.

3d, HALLUCINATIONS.

a) Hallucinations of sight; seeing of phantoms, imaginary or absent persons, of forms, or colors.

b) Hallucinations of hearing; these are the most frequent of all; are found in at least two-thirds of all hallucinated persons; consist in noises in the head and ears; hearing of sounds, voices, cries, &c.

c) Illusions of touch; these are common.

d) Illusions of taste and smell, are rare.

e) Illusions about one's internal organs, in which the patient imagines various extraordinary conditions of his internal organs, that he has snakes or reptiles within him; or is filled with sulphurous vapors which will suffocate him, &c.

LEURET's treatment of Hallucinations consists in the frequent use of the douche, taking care while the patient is in the bath to speak on all the subjects connected with his insanity, and making him give rational replies; he was not contented so long as there was or appeared to be a mental reservation in his words; he obliged the patient to admit that he was mad or deranged; the douche was repeated daily and the same system of questioning, &c., continued until the patient fully understood that he was in the wrong, and was anxious to recover his health and reason.

4th, DEMENTIA, or general feebleness of the mental faculties.

5th, IDIOCY.

6th, PUERPERAL MANIA, or mental derangement of lying-in-women.

a) MENTAL DERANGEMENT soon after confinement.

b) do. do. during or after protracted nursing.

7th, DELIRIUM TREMENS.

8th, MENTAL DERANGEMENT from poisoning with narcotics, Opium, Stramonium, Haschisch, &c., &c.

9th, GENERAL PARALYSIS of the insane.

In eight cases, the structure of the brain was firm and tough; so tough in one case that the brain could be lifted without breaking it.

BLOODLETTING.

WOOD says, to bleed and otherwise deplete copiously for insanity alone, even in its early stages, is he is convinced, a highly injurious practice. Without having the least influence over the delusions of the patient, it lowers the grade of his vital force, and renders him less able to support the more or less wearing influence of the mental disease on the bodily health. It is even thought by some to dispose to a more rapid decline of mania or monomania into dementia; and to diminish the chances of a subsequent cure, or at least to protract the duration of the disease. Dr. Kirkbride, the intelligent superintendent of the Pennsylvania Hospital for the Insane, informed Dr. Wood, that depletion is in his estimation the great error in the primary treatment of insanity. It is not uncommon to mistake some frequency of the pulse and heat of head, which may be the mere results of the functional disturbance of the brain, for indications of active febrile excitement, and the violent maniacal paroxysms as proofs of cerebral inflammation. There can be no greater errors than these. The pulse is often much accelerated by the want of sleep and the various agitations of the patient, without fever or inflammation, and indeed may in many instances *be most happily composed by Opium and other cerebral-stimulants.* The maniacal paroxysms, though frequently attended with signs of general and febrile excitement, are a purely nervous affection, occur as well in debilitated as in elevated states of the system, and may be quite compatible with a stimulating or supporting treatment; instead of being relieved they are in some instances decidedly aggravated by the loss of blood.

In his remarks on bleeding in insanity, Dr. Patterson, of the Indiana Hospital for the Insane, uses the following language: Raving mania can be much more permanently controlled by the use of the warm bath, cold applications to the head, warm foot-baths, mild cathartics, and in some cases by nauseants. Bleeding quiets the patient temporarily, but the excitement returns with greater fury, and the system is less able to bear it than before. So far as I have observed the practice, bleeding does not accomplish the desired object, but the contrary; for it impoverishes the blood, reduces the strength of the patient, and thereby renders the nervous system more excitable.

Dr. Hanbury Smith, of the Ohio Asylum, says that during the year 1851, the idea of depletion was entertained in no one case by any of the medical officers; and those who had lost blood previously to their admission proved exceedingly difficult to restore, sank into hopeless dementia, or died. It may be considered as a settled thing that at the present time depletion is exceedingly hazardous, and commonly contra-indicated in insanity; the liberal use of stimulants proves eminently curative; immediately after the action of a cathartic, sometimes previously to, or during that action, he gives his patient from four to six ounces of wine, or an equivalent portion of brandy, together with the most nourishing and easily digested food. Maniacal excitement commonly ceases very quickly under the above treatment.

Bell's disease or typhomania is a peculiar form of mental derangement becoming quite common, particularly in large cities, and one in which the unpractised physician is almost certain to pursue a deleterious course of treatment; the patients almost invariably die after general bloodletting; a fatal result can only be avoided by active stimulation.

In 913 or perhaps 1806 cases, Dr. Kirkbride did not practise venesection for *insanity* in a single instance; he may have done it for apoplexy, or congestion of the brain, but never for mania, melancholia, or any of the maladies generally included under the name of insanity.

Dr. Rush is the great authority in favor of bloodletting, but in his time, in the early part of the present century, the system of treatment at the Bethlehem Hospital for the Insane, consisted of bleeding, purging and vomiting in the spring months. A certain day was appointed on which the patients were bled; another when they were purged; another when they were vomited. They were all bled in May, and again in June, the precise time depending on the weather. This was the best treatment in Rush's time; for the physicians of the Bethlehem Hospital, were among the most eminent in London.

The physicians of probably 19/20ths of the institutions for the insane, not only in America and Great Britain, but in France, Prussia, and Austria condemn the practice of general bleeding in insanity, unless it be in rare and exceptional cases.

In puerperal mania Smith says, bloodletting is preëminently contra-indicated; in this matter all authorities agree; Churchill, Pritchard, Esquirol, Haslam, Gooch, and Burrows are equally opposed to it; even where local inflammation is discovered, other means should be used.

In the treatment of acute mania with violence, raving and consequent exhaustion, Dr. Brigham employed seclusion, hot baths, with cold applications to the head and free evacuation of the bowels. In no case did he find local or general bleedings admissible; but on the contrary nutritious diet and brandy-punch are generally required.

Dr. BENEDICT, of the New-York State Asylum, says, he cannot too strongly urge his medical brethren to abstain from bloodletting in insanity; his plan of treating very acute insanity is directly opposed to depletion. Not one ounce of blood was drawn from 825 patients, 54 of whom were deranged less than one month. He resorts to stimulation in many cases with great freedom, and has seen the best evidences of its propriety.

Dr. CURWIN, of the Pennsylvania State Asylum, says, that he must call attention to an error which is very extensively prevalent, and which consists in the almost invariable resort to bloodletting in all cases of insanity. All hospital experience proves that the loss of blood in any form of insanity, is almost uniformly attended with unpleasant effects, prolonging the period of cure, and in many cases placing the patient hopelessly beyond the reach of any benefit to be derived from subsequent treatment. Insanity is essentially a nervous disorder, and must be treated as such.

PURGATIVES.

WOODWARD says: if bleeding is injurious, active purging is still more so. In torpid states of the bowels he preferred the Tinct., or Pulv. Guaiac; has been most successful with it in dyspepsia and distress after eating; it invigorates the stomach, acts on the skin and bowels, and in females is an emmenagogue; the powder is the most useful, if the principal object is to act upon the bowels.

FORBES WINSLOW says in the early stage of insanity, and throughout its whole course, the bowels are often in an obstinately constipated condition. The concentration of nervous energy in the brain appears to interfere with that supply which should proceed to other structures. There is no class of agents which act so certainly and effectually in relieving the mind when under the influence of depressing emotions, as cathartics. The bowels are often found gorged with fecal matters, and immediate relief follows full action on the bowels. I have seen several cases of great despondency, obstinacy and invincible taciturnity attended with, and caused by excessive costiveness, cured at once by a single dose of purgative medicine.

NARCOTICS.

Of these OPIUM is the most important. In acute mania, if there is much excitement, many physicians have great confidence in GRAVE'S combination of Opium and Tartar-emetic, and in the proportions originally proposed by him. Afterwards if the head be not very hot, full and repeated doses of Opium are given; also in cases marked by extreme irritability, restlessness and want of sleep, with moist, flabby and tremulous tongue, natural or dilated pupils, frequent, irregular and weak pulse, cold and relaxed skin; then commonly with wine, and always with excellent effect. See GALT'S Opium treatment, page 52. WOOD says, independently of the advantageous influence excited by narcotics in quieting irritation, controlling excessive nervous excitement, and producing sleep, they probably operate in another mode in the cure of insanity. When kept steadily under their influence, the brain is rendered in some measure insensible to those morbid impressions which have a constant tendency to disturb it. Though the patient may not be restored to reason, yet the irregular mental movements are much repressed, the proverbially cheering influence of the drug restrains the tumult of the feelings, and a condition of the brain is induced, in which a continued presentation of rational objects of reflection, and sources of a healthful interest, may gradually accustom the organ to a sound mode of action; while the morbid trains of reflection, and the perversions of the passions are gradually obliterated from want of renewal. After the removal, therefore, of physical derangement, no medicine is so efficient as Opium in favoring a return to a healthy state of function. It must be given in such quantities as to produce and maintain a decided impression, and must consequently be increased with its continued use. After the brain has been restored to a perfectly healthful state of action, the Opium should be gradually diminished, and the patient should not be considered well until the medicine can be entirely dispensed with. WOOD has known patients in the most violent state of maniacal excitement, after being put asleep by Opium, to awake in the morning quite composed and rational. In some cases Opium will aggravate the cerebral disorder; when this passes off the patient will be found in a better state than before the aggravation; new quantities will be followed by fresh exacerbation, and these in their turn by still more decided improvement. It is an unpleasant way of treating the patient, but a cure will follow quite as certainly, as if none but the most pleasant results had followed. WILLIAMS says, physicians have been much divided in opinion respecting the propriety of exhibiting narcotics when there is furious delirium, it having been frequently noticed that even when sleep has followed very large doses, yet the patient has awoke with aggravated symptoms; and hence although the sleep may for some hours have appeared tolerably easy and natural, yet from the subsequently increased frenzy on waking, it has been thought unadvisable to continue the narcotic. Other physicians would immediately repeat the dose and still larger ones if required. WILLIAMS thinks that the stimulating powers of the *Hydrochlorate of Morphia* are so slight as to be scarcely perceptible, the sedative effect being immediately induced.

1) Against an atrophied, or softened condition of the nervous matter, FORBES WINSLOW thinks more can be done towards a cure than is generally supposed. He has in several instances seen brain disease exhibiting all the legitimate features of ramollissement, yield to the persevering use of Iron, Phosphor, Zinc and Strychnia, combined with generous living. In general paralysis from inflammatory softening of the brain, BOYD gave the Liquor Hydrargyri bichloridi, to eight males; two improved, and one who had been confined to his bed for several weeks and in a very helpless state, became able to sit up in a chair and feed himself. Another who was of very dirty habits, became cleanly, and gained in weight 21 lbs. in six months; two cases gradually became worse, and four remained stationary. See also my Treatise on Apoplexy and Softening of the Brain, p. p. 149 to 155.

2) In some chronic forms of insanity, in dementia and persistent monomania connected, as it was supposed with morbid

thickening of the dura-mater, and with interstitial infiltration of that membrane, as well as exudations on its surface, FORBES WINSLOW has seen marked benefit from the persevering use of a strong ointment of Iodide of potassium combined with Strichnine rubbed over the scalp.

In other cases apparently quite beyond the reach of improvement or cure, where the mental symptoms were supposed to be associated with effusions of serum in or about the brain, he has applied Iodine externally, and given small doses of Iod., Merc., and Digitalis internally, with considerable benefit.

FOOD, TONICS AND STIMULANTS.

It has been unquestionably proved, by long and well tried experience that a good and liberal scale of diet is necessary for the insane. A scale of diet above that which the person would take if well and surrounded by the comforts of home, is certainly required by those confined in an asylum. We will find that when the diet is deficient that the mortality is invariably higher and the amount of cures less. All authorities agree upon this point, in chronic insanity.

3) Cases sometimes present themselves where the patient determinately refuses to take either food or medicine. The refusal of food may be connected with the determination to destroy life, or it may be associated with delusive impressions. Upon examination we often find, in these cases, great gastric derangement, obstinate constipation, considerable tenderness of the pit of the stomach, bilious disorder, foul tongue and offensive breath, with other symptoms of a morbid condition of the digestive organs. In some of these cases the determination to refuse nourishment arises from a positive loathing of food; or from a delusion of taste, everything appearing to the patient, bitter, disgusting or poisonous; or the unhappy patient imagines that he is commanded either by good or evil spirits not to eat.

Such cases can be speedily cured by removing the visceral derangement, if there be any, or by specific remedies, if the digestive organs be sound.—FORBES WINSLOW.

MELANCHOLY.

The principal remedies against this form of mental derangement, are: 1st; Arsenicum, Aurum, Bellad., Calcarea, Causticum, Graphite, Ignatia, Lachesis, Natrum-mur., Pulsatilla, Rhus-tox., Sulphur and Veratrum. 2d; Cocculus, Hellebore, Hyosciamus, Lycopod., Mercur., Nux, Phosphor., Platina, Sepia and Stramonium. 3d; Aconite, Anacard., Carb.-anim., Crocus, Digit., Nitric and Phos.-acid., Ruta, and Staphysagria.

Aurum is indicated when the patient is sad and feeble, with desire for solitude; when he fears to have lost the love and consideration of others, with profound chagrin and weeping; great desire for death, with religious pre-occupation, with tears and prayers; great anxiety in the region of the heart, with great weakness and exhaustion, so that one feels as if dying; scrupulous inquietude; timidity; all attended with derangement of the liver.

Calcarea. When there is dejection and sadness; restlessness, with commotion of the blood; great disposition to fear and apprehension; fear of misfortuue or of losing one's reason; despair about one's health; want of interest and will; disgust for work.

Natrum Muriaticum. When there are frequent accessions of melancholy, with abundance of sombre thoughts, and recalling of unpleasant events long since passed; want of self-confidence, with great inclination to weep; the least trifle, solitude for a short time, the slightest look from others will produce tears; even the thought of unpleasant occurrences brings on a flood of tears. Inclination to remain absorbed in thoughts for hours; frequent attacks of complete unhappiness and despair; sudden paroxysms of anxiety as if one had committed a crime. Graphite and Causticum are indicated under almost similar circumstances.

Veratrum. When the melancholic patient has nausea and frequent chills; is taciturn or obstinate, or sits in a corner absorbed in thought. Verat., Hellebore and Cocculus are particularly suitable in melancholy when attended with marked derangement of the stomach, bowels or liver.

Phosphorus, Platina and Sepia are often useful in extreme cases of nervousness and melancholy in females, with marked derangement of the urinary and sexual organs, suppression of the menses, &c.

HYPOCHONDRIA.

The principal remedies against this disorder are: Calcarea, Sulphur, Conium, Ignatia, Petroleum, Staphysagria, Gratiola, Sabadilla and Zincum.

SABADILLA is the principal remedy, when the patient has illusions about the state of his internal organs, that his stomach is ulcerated, abdomen disorganised, scrotum swollen, &c., &c.

ZINC is regarded by RADEMACHER, as one of the most powerful and specific brain-remedies. He says that it may be styled a *Metallic Opium.* It will allay the most violent neuralgic pains, headache, toothache, earache, ischias, &c. It is useful against obstinate sleeplessness, and will cause sleep in deranged and delirious persons; but its use must be continued after sleep has been produced, and the patient must be waked up regularly to take his medicine, or else he will finally awake just as much deranged and delirious as ever.

Singularly, he also states that Zinc may be used in the soporose states, which so frequently attend brain-affections, and which are closely allied to delirium, or at least are frequently followed by it. Under its use the patient will finally awake himself, still one will notice when the patient is aroused hourly to take his medicine, that his mental powers are gradually returning to a natural state, and finally he will awake spontaneously; still the remedy must be used some little time afterwards.

RELIGIOUS MELANCHOLY.

The principal remedies are: Bellad., Hyosc., Opium, Platina and Sulphur.

MISANTHROPY.

The most useful remedies are: Muriate of Ammonia, Aurum, Cicuta, Ledum, Manganese, Nitric-acid, Stannum and Sulphur.

MURIATE OF AMMONIA is useful against melancholy, connected with marked disorder of some or many of the mucous membranes, derangement or enlargement of the liver, enlargement of the womb and ovaries; also when the patient has a well-marked mucous fever, the tongue being coated with tough, white mucus, with great inclination to perspiration, so that the sweat breaks out from the slightest exertion, the urine being strong and ammoniacal, and some diarrhœa is present, with discharge of tough, glassy mucus from the bowels; in some cases, the attending fever has a seven-day type.

CICUTA, Aethusa and Bovista are supposed to be useful against melancholy and other cerebral affections, arising from suppression of eruptions; also against spinal irritation from the same cause.

LEDUM is useful against brain-affections, attended with violent headache, restlessness, oppression of respiration, cough, sleeplessness, pains in the limbs, increased flow of urine, itching, eruptions or pustules upon the skin, contractions of the limbs, gouty and rheumatic pains, &c.

STANNUM is homœopathic to extreme nervousness, such as is sometimes seen in persons who have become exhausted by loss of blood, excesses, or a long-lasting sickness, attended with considerable loss of flesh; misanthropy and invincible repugnance to conversation.

SUICIDAL MONOMANIA.

The principal remedies are: Arsenicum, Aurum, Belladonna, Drosera, Hyosciamus, Antim.-crud., Alumina, Spigelia and Staphysagria.

Belladonna and Morphine have been recommended by Forbes Winslow. (See p. xv.)

NOSTALGIA.

The principal remedies are: Capsicum, Mercurius, and Phosphoric-acid.

MANIA.

The principal remedies are supposed to be, 1st, Bellad., Canthar., Hyosc., Stramon., and Veratrum.

2d, Agaricus, Arsen., Cannabis., Crocus., Cuprum., Kali., Lycopod., Lach., Merc., Phosph., and Secale.

3d, Aconite, Anacard,, Camph., Conium, Moschus, Natrum, Nitric.-acid., Nux-v., Plat., Plumbum, and Tart.-emet.

The first set of these remedies is most useful in *Acute Mania.* In this disorder the following symptoms generally appear immediately before the full development of the disease. Every natural thought and feeling is exaggerated. At first this is scarcely noticeable; but, after a short time, the exaltation becomes more and more manifest; soon we observe former objects of quiet and unobtrusive affection are treated with the most persuasive and endearing fondness, and at the same time, those that may have once incurred the displeasure of the patient, are spoken of with a bitterness and angry vindictiveness totally inconsistent with the previous character of the individual. The patient is evidently becoming more and more a creature of impulse, and cannot fix his attention upon the ordinary employments of the day, but is wandering with strides increasing in rapidity from one thing to another. As the excitement increases, the wildness and often redness of the eye, begin to attract attention, and finally actual raving ensues.—PERKINS.

The same author says: "If a strong, plethoric and physically healthy man becomes the subject of acute mania, if the head is hot, eyes injected, face flushed, pulse full and strong, and at the same time, if the patient is violent and noisy, the physician would naturally be tempted to a trial of general blood-letting. Let him on no account yield to his inclination, for there is hardly any form of insanity in which blood-letting is admissible. In every case in which it has been employed within the writer's knowledge, it has proved highly injurious."

Most of the other remedies are suitable in *Chronic Mania.* Anæmia is a common accompaniment of this disease, and a state of the system decidedly below par, is too often met with. In these cases, the only efficient allopathic remedies are tonics and sedatives. Conium and Iron are used with great success, Morphine may be used with marked good results.

ANTAGONISTIC STATES OF THE MIND.

Anacardium may be used when the patient seems to have two opposite wills, one of which excites him to do that which the other would like to prevent. Is inclined to laugh when he ought to be serious, and does not incline to laugh, even when tempted by ludicrous things.

Sepia when he imagines things, which he does not want to imagine; uses wrong expressions, which he knows are wrong; proposes to himself things which are contrary to his intentions; is in contradiction with himself, and altogether in a disagreeable mood; has paroxysms of laughter and weeping in alternation, without either resulting from a corresponding frame of mind.

Phosphorus when the patient laughs against his own inclination, being very sad.

Capsicum and *Staphysagria* when he is merry, but nevertheless inclines to get angry and be quarrelsome.

ANTIPATHIES.

Conium may be given when the patient is inclined to dislike every one who passes him, would like to lay hold of them, and abuse them.

Cicuta when he abhors all mankind, hates their follies, and seeks solitude.

Aurum when many persons are offensive to him.

Ammon.-mur. when there are involuntary antipathies to certain persons.

Calcarea when there is an aversion to most men.

APATHY.

Antimonium-crud. may be given when the patient is completely apathetic, does not leave her bed, does not speak, desires neither to eat or drink, but eats readily what is offered and feels hungry.

Argentum-nitricum, when there is apathy with great debility and tremulous weakness.

GAY MANIA.

The principal remedies are: 1st, Aurum, Bellad., Crocus., Lycopod., Platina, Opium, Stramon., and Verat.

2d, Aconite, Anacard., Cuprum, Hyosc., Lachesis, Natrum-m., Nux-mosch., Phos., and Phosphoric-acid.

Belladonna is suitable when there is a merry craziness, with laughing and singing; when the patient tries to compose songs, and sings merry, but utterly senseless tunes, or whistles occasionally, but refuses either to eat or drink; or sings or hums different airs, or smiles a long while to himself, or is disposed to sing or whistle, with frequent bursts of laughter, or is wild and wantonly merry, with inclination to quarrel without cause; or when the patients tear off their clothes, run out into the street, partially or wholly naked, gesticulating in a strange manner, dancing, laughing, uttering and demanding foolish things.

Cicuta-virosa, when the patient becomes heated while asleep, wakes up, jumps out of bed, dances, laughs, does all sorts of foolish things, claps her hands, &c.

Cuprum when he sings merry songs.

Hyosciamus when the patient dances, laughs in an absurd manner, makes ridiculous gesticulations like a clown, or performs funny tricks like a monkey.

Opium, when the patient's mirth and bliss increase until he becomes irrational.

Stramonium, when one seems as if in an ecstacy, and beside himself; when he seems filled with pleasant fancies, expresses his wishes by signs, and runs about for some days, exceedingly busy with his phantasies, and quite cheerful; or when he dances, gesticulates, laughs and sings; or has paroxysms of constant talking, or breaks out into loud laughter, or violent rage.

MANIA WITH FURY.

Cuprum is indicated against mania attended with full, quick pulse, red and inflamed eyes, wild looks, incoherent speech, and rage, every paroxysm terminating in perspiration.

Opium against furious mania with distortion of the features, swelling of the head and face, protruded and congested eyes, bluish redness and swelling of the lips, paroxysms of rage, with rolling on the floor, and threats against his own relatives, whom he does not seem to recognize.

Hyosciamus, when the patient is alternately ludicrous, solemn, or furious; dresses himself in a priest's gown over his shirt, puts on fur boots, wants to go to church in this guise, in order to preach, or officiate at mass, and furiously attacks all those who attempt to prevent him.

RELIGIOUS MANIA.

Lachesis, when the patient supposes himself doomed to eternal punishment.

Stramonium, when the patient kneels down, stretches out his hands, with pious looks, but starts up from the least opposition, with wild cries and violent gestures.

Aurum, when the patient imagines that she is irretrievably lost, with depression of spirits, followed by shouts and screams.

Baryta, when he has all sorts of sad notions about his future destiny, and deems himself utterly lost.

Crocus is also suitable against religious melancholy.

SUICIDAL MANIA.

Arsenicum, when there is great indifference to life, with inclination towards suicide.

Aurum. Excessive desire for death, with melancholy; notion that he was not intended for this world, with anxiety amounting to a desire to commit suicide, attended with derangement and cramps in the stomach and bowels.

Belladonna. Distaste for life, with desire for death, wishes some one to kill him, attempts to jump out of the window; anxiety and desire for death, alternating with paroxysms of fury.

Carbo-vegetabilis. Despair with weeping, every thing seems clothed in the darkest colors, inclination to suicide, with irrascibility, desire for death, because he thinks that he is most unfortunate.

Nux-vomica. Inclination to commit suicide, with palpitation of the heart, and great anxiety; desire for death, because his great agony of mind allows him no repose; inclination to commit suicide, because his present pains and misfortunes seem insupportable to him.

Sepia. Discouragement with absolute despair, attended with moroseness; distaste for life in an extreme degree, because he thinks that he cannot endure his pitiable condition, and that he will be irretrievably lost in this world if he continues to live.

Alumina. Whenever he sees blood or a knife, he is seized with a crowd of terrible ideas, attended with an inclination to kill himself, although he has a horror of suicide.

China, is indicated when there is a distaste for life, with melancholy, anxiety and feverish heat which drives him to his bed, attended with inclination to suicide, although he dreads to carry it into execution.

Mercurius, when there is disgust for life, from want of courage to meet its trials and mortifications; or desire for death, from an insupportable indifference for every person and thing, even those which are most loved.

Nitric-acid, when there is disgust for life, with discontent; desire for death, although one is afraid to die.

Phosphorus, when there is disgust for life, because the whole world seems gloomy and terrible; tears alone bring relief, and they are followed by the most extreme apathy.

Platina, when there is a distaste for life, as if one was not suited to the world as it is, attended with great agony about the heart, fear of dying, and depression of spirits; disgust for the whole world, with inclination to weep.

Staphysagria. Desire for death, from an insupportable hypochondriacal indifference to everything; disgust for life, from anxiety and disquieting thoughts.

Sulphur. Disgust for life, from discouragement and sadness, and from the feeling of being exceedingly unhappy.

Of 74 cases of mental alienation treated homœopathically, by Dr. Wittfeld, in his private Asylum at Meurs, near Hamburg, 9 were hopelessly incurable, and had been dismissed as such from other institutions; they were only admitted to be taken care of; 2 were dismissed within the first fortnight, on account of irregularities on the part of the patient's friends; 4 were laboring under incurable organic diseases, such as softening of the brain and tabes dorsalis; they died respectively in 3, 8, 10 and 21 days, so that no opportunity occurred of healing their mental affections. Deducting these 15 cases, there were 59 cases submitted to homœopathic treatment; of these 29 were dismissed cured; 19 more or less improved, and 11 uncured and unimproved.

Of the 29 cured, only 1 had a relapse after 2 years; the remaining 28 continued perfectly well.

Of these 29, 4 were cured within 4 months; 6 within 6 months; 10 within 12 months, and 9 within 2 years.

The average length of treatment for all was $14\frac{11}{29}$ months; for those cured within 12 months, the average length of treatment was $6\frac{10}{26}$ months; for those cured within 2 years, $23\frac{2}{8}$ months.

It thus appears that nearly one half of all the cases were cured, and not $\frac{1}{5}$ of the whole number were dismissed without improvement. Dr. WITTFELD says such success, cannot be shown by any other Asylum; but it will be seen by reference to pages viii, ix and x, that the dominant school seems to cure quite as many, if not more, although relapses seem to be much more frequent under allopathic than homœopathic treatment.

Among the 29 cured homœopathically, 13 were affected with furious mania; 9 with imbecility or melancholy; and 7 with hallucinations or monomania.

The disease upon admission had lasted, in one case which was cured, above 9 years; in 2, above 4 years; in 5 above 2 years; in 8 above 1 year; in 10 above 6 months; and in 3 above 4 months.

The medicines chiefly used by Dr. WITTFELD were Bellad., Cicuta, Digitalis, Phosphor. and Stramonium, for *Furious mania;* Arnica, Ambra, Selenium and Sepia, for *Imbecility;* Ignatia and Hyosc., for the consequences of *Grief* and *Unfortunate Love;* Secale, Nux-vom., Arsenicum, Staphysagria and Conium in many different kinds of derangement. Teucrium and Viola-odorata, were also frequently used; Hellebore and Veratrum very seldom.

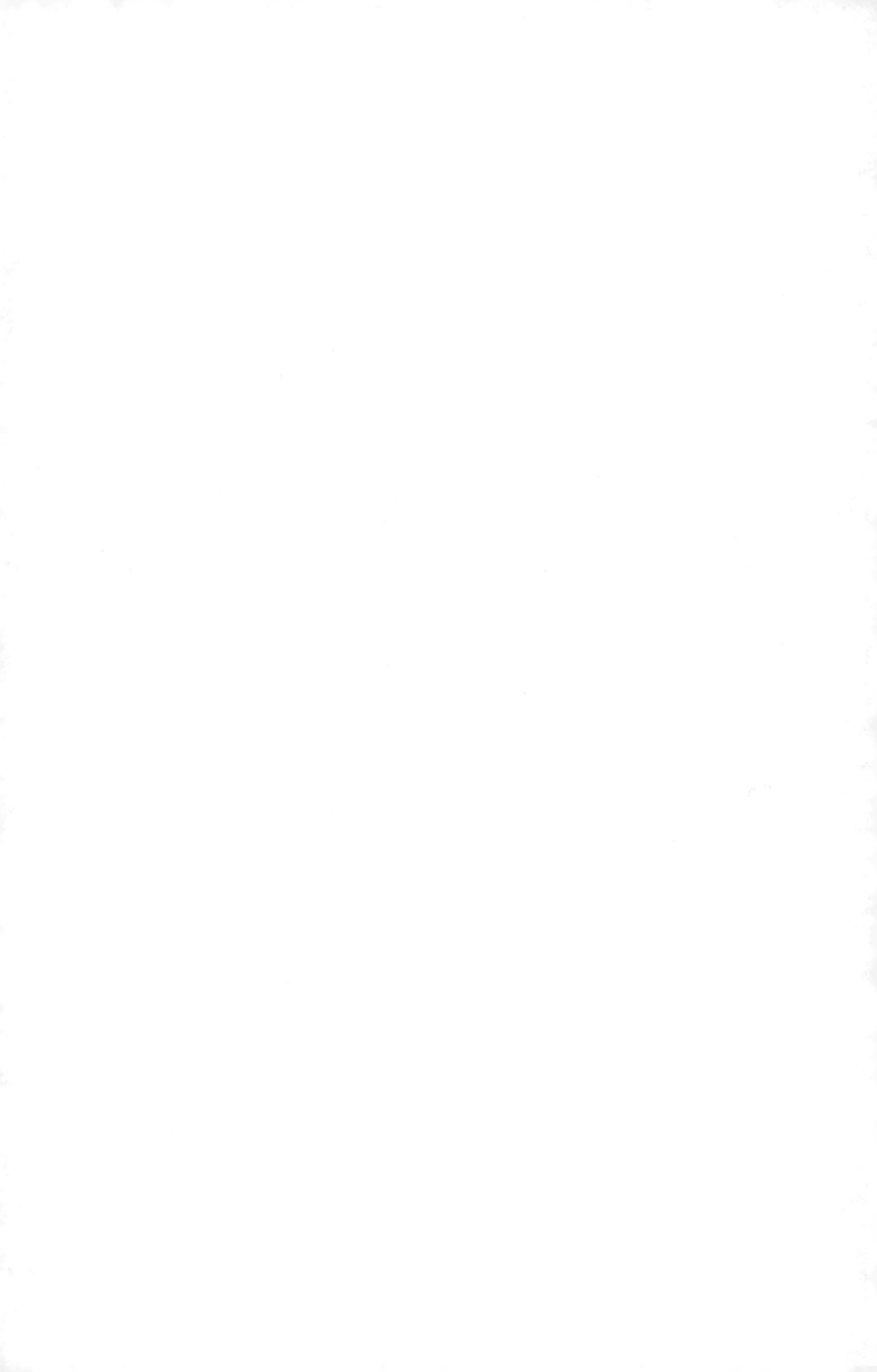

NERVOUS DISEASES

AND

MENTAL DERANGEMENT.

CHAPTER I.

CASES IN WHICH A SINGLE REMEDY PROVED DECIDEDLY USEFUL—ARRANGED ALPHABETICALLY ACCORDING TO THE REMEDIES.

1. ACONITE.

GENERAL REMARKS.—Aconite is particularly indicated where there is excessive irritability either in the bodily or mental sphere, and this hyperæsthesia is a frequent attendant in certain forms of mental derangement. It is also suitable in that form of mania in which the vascular system is principally involved, and which increases to phrenzy, evidently occasioned by a hyperæmic and inflammatory state of the brain and its membranes, with a decided tendency to dropsical effusions. Febrile and acute mental affections may be relieved by Aconite. In the action of Aconite paroxysms of anxiety often predominate, and it has been found useful in various forms of mental depression.

Hygea, Vol. 23, part. 4, p. 259.—GRIESSELICH.

Besides the more well known effects of Aconite it is particularly apt to produce the most singular sensations of bodily deformity, similar to those which occur in a limb when it is asleep. Sensations of thickness, swelling, or distortion or displacement of the features, limbs, &c., &c. arise under its use, while the intellect is less comparatively unclouded, and seem so real that the experimenter is obliged to examine himself in a glass or appeal to his friends for re-assurance of being in his sound and undeformed state. Hence it may prove curative in some of those forms of hypochondria and illusion in which the patient imagines that various wonderful transformations have taken place in some one or the other of his internal or external organs.

There is but little old school experience with Aconite in Insanity; J. M. Cox, in 1816, said that it had been extolled by some, but it was too uncertain, and apt to constipate. Milligan, in 1841, says that Pinel admits that bleeding is now rarely employed by him; he sees many patients cured without bleeding, and many remain incurable after being bled. When there is much excitement and increased action of the heart and arteries, it will be found that Aconite in fractional doses will procure a state of calmness more rapidly than detraction of blood. PETERS.

CASE 1.—A young woman, aged 20, fancied that she would die during her second confinement, and in spite of a favorable issue of her delivery, expected a speedy death, especially as she had violent congestion of blood to, and excessive oppression of the chest, to the point of suffocation, with intermission of the pulse.

Acon. 30. removed all ideas of death in the course of two hours and restored her equanimity.

Archiv, Vol. 7, part. 2, p. 42.—GROSS.

[The whole affair was probably hysterical.—PETERS.]

CASE 2.—A joyous young woman, æt. 20, became depressed during her first pregnancy, and believed firmly that she would die in her confinement.

A profuse flooding followed the otherwise regular delivery of the child and placenta, and the patient now expected a speedy death. Her body was covered with a cold viscid sweat, she took leave of her relatives, raved about her approaching dissolution, lay perfectly quiet, but her countenance expressed great internal agony about the heart, while she occasionally cried that nothing would help her, and that she must certainly die. Paroxysms of agony set in, she lost her consciousness, and convulsions of the arms occurred. After Acon. 24, she fell into a slumber, and awaked with renewed cheerfulness.

Archiv, Vol. 9, part. 1, p. 114.—BETHMAN. See also Case 95.

[This second case seems very like the first.—PETERS.]

REVIEW. Anxiety and fear were present in all three cases, especially of approaching death in cases 1 and 2 (see Materia Med. Pur. Sympt. 537—40.), occurring in puerperal women with congestive or even inflammatory conditions.

Dose.—$\overline{24}$ and $\overline{30}$ with speedy relief.

Fear indicates an affection of the organ of *Caution*, and Aconite may be supposed to act upon that part of the brain occupied by it.

2. ANACARDIUM.

General Remarks.—*a*) It is indicated in mental affections, with decided loss of memory, sluggish flow of thought, apathy and anæsthesia, &c. In general, Anacardium promises much in hypochondria and melancholy.

Hygea, Vol. 23, p. 265.—Griesselich.

b) It causes a hypochondriacal and gloomy condition, loss of courage, fear of approaching death, misantrophy; anxiety, want of moral tone, a wicked, godless, inhuman and hard-hearted state of mind. Also a state in which one seems to have two wills, one of which restrains one from do that to which the other impels. Sensation as if the spirit were separated from the body.

Hahnemann, Chron. Diseases, Vol. 2, p. 156.

c) Anacardium is generally regarded as a spicy aromatic stimulant, which primarily exerts an exciting effect upon the brain, inducing unusual excitement of the imagination, with great flow of fresh ideas, which one must follow, the whole gradually passing over into entire absence of thought and utter stupidity. It has also been said to cause great acuteness of the memory, with vivid recollection of the slightest and long forgotten things; great activity of mind, with inclination towards astute investigations, followed by aching pains in the forehead, temples, and occiput, by a bruised feeling in the brain, and by stomach-ache.

It also causes weakness of digestion, flatulence, profound hypochondriacal humor and derangement of the liver, marked aching pain in the hepatic region, light colored a-bilious stools, &c.; hence it may be found as useful in some of the dyspeptic and hypochondriacal disorders of literary men, as Nux has been decreed to be.

Besides simple excitement of the intellect, imagination and memory, Anacardium may cause a pleasant and joyous excitement, followed by laughing at serious things, and gravity about laughable occurrences, &c.—Stapf asserts that it causes quite opposite effects, viz, both increase of mental activity and torpor.

—Franz experienced very decided increase of memory and mental activity within one hour after taking it.—Hahnemann experienced both exaltation and depression, but does not tell us which occurred first.—Ruckert has dwelt almost entirely upon the depressing effects of Anacardium.—Peters.

CASE 3.—A man, æt. 30, tall thin, of a consumptive constitution, and suffering with chronic pectoral and abdominal affections, suppressed an itch-like eruption with lead water, after which he fell into a state of mental derangement.

Symptoms.—He believed that he was composed of two persons, and that several men slept in his bed. When he drank any thing he supposed that it did not get into his body and nourish him, because his stomach was torn in two, or that some one was concealed in his body, who swallowed every thing away from him.

Ipec., Verat. and Bellad. helped him but little, while *Anacard.* 6 cured him quickly.

New Archiv, Vol. 3, part. 1, p. 23.—Wahle.

CASE 4.—A widow, æt. 64, after undeserved mortification fell with a state of mental confusion, in which she talked constantly in stupid and irrational manner. She was cured in fourteen days by Anacard. $\frac{}{30}$.

Allg. Hom. Zeit. Vol. 13, p. 23.—Lobethal.

CASE 5.—A maiden, æt. 22, of a sensitive disposition, and somewhat over-educated for her station, and disposed to religious enthusiasm, was taken sick suddenly after violent mental emotion and separation from her lover. In the beginning she was violent, and was treated allopathically from Jan. to April 21; latterly a melancholic condition had been developed. Hyosciamus was useless, while Anacardium given on the 25th, restored the patient so rapidly that she could be regarded as cured by the 30th April.

Pract. Beiträge, Vol. 4, part. 1, p. 15.—Schindler.

Review.—From the above few observations, Anacardium would seem most suitable, when the patient is melancholic and shy, suspicious and troubled with illusions about his own body.

Doses.—6th, 24th, and 30th, the last in repeated doses.

According to Phrenology, *Anacard.* seems indicated against mental delusions which lead to fixed ideas, hence, in disorders of the organ of *causality*, also in want of proportion in the activity of the organ of benevolence, compared with those of *combativeness* and *destructiveness*.

3. ARSENICUM.

GENERAL REMARKS.—*a*) Paroxysms of anxiety, which drive one out of bed at night.—Fear of death.—HAHNEMANN. Chronic Diseases, Vol. 5, p. 497.

b) Arsenic is especially indicated in periodical recurrences of melancholy, when there are night-aggravations, paroxysms of agony about the heart, with intermitting pulse and rapid failure of the strength.

Hygea, Vol. 23, p. 9.—GRIESSELICH.

Although OTTO says that Arsenicum causes melancholy, this does not deter COX from asserting that when there is great debility and relaxation the continued use of Arsen. might contribute to recruit the system and restore reason; nor HALLORAN from saying, "where chronic insanity has decidedly assumed the periodical type, and also notwithstanding the intervals, together with the paroxysms, has obtained the most desirable balance, without terminating in health, recovery may be greatly promoted by the cautious introduction of Arsenicum—he will not undertake to say that such instances have been numerous in his experience, for the proper cases to use this powerful remedy are not of frequent occurrence." SEYMOUR also thinks it might be beneficially employed in proper cases and hands. STEWARD thinks that mental derangement coupled with simple œdema is curable, and Arsenicum might also come in play here.

CASE 6.—A robust man, æt. 32, had suffered for several years with paroxysms of melancholy, which lasted from six to eight days, and had withstood all ordinary remedies.

Symptoms.—By day he had attacks of anxiety as if he had committed some great crime, which drove him from place to place so that it was impossible for him to remain quietly in one spot for a quarter of an hour. He could not control his tears and often wept aloud; avoided his friends, because he fancied that he had injured them in some way, and would gladly ask pardon of every one, because he believed that he had offended them.

Two doses of Arsen. 30, cured him perfectly within four weeks.

Archiv, Vol. 8, part. 2, p. 51.—WEBER.

CASE 7.—A blacksmith, æt. 36, of powerful constitution, after an attack of miliary fever and subsequent cold, fell into a state of melancholy, with anxiety and inclination to suicide.

Symptoms.—Expression indicative of great internal disquiet. He does not know where to go, from restlessness day and night; thinks that he can never be fortunate or happy in his own house, and pesters his family constantly with his fears. Paroxysms of frightful anxiety, attended with heat and redness of the face, and such inclination to commit suicide that he fears to remain alone, and begs his friends not to leave him for fear that he would injure himself.

Bellad. was given without avail, but Arsen. 24, removed the whole mental derangement in a few days.

Annals, Vol. 1, p. 66.—RUCKERT.

CASE 8.—A woman, æt. 65, had suffered for a year with periodical attacks of melancholy.

Symptoms.—Anxiety, burning in the stomach, and retraction of the abdomen. Paroxysms of anxiety drive her out of bed at night, and she roams about groaning; in the evening she has anxiety in the pit of the stomach, with palpitation and flushes of heat, and oppression in the epigastrium. Confusion and tension in the head, bloated face, which is also red and hot, pulse 80, and rather weak than strong. Twisting, gnawing and biting in the stomach, with waterbrash—urgency to urinate, with scanty discharge.

Ars. 30, cured her perfectly in eight days, after an aggravation lasting two days.

Practical Beitrag, Vol. 2, p. 145.—NEUMANN.

REVIEW.—In all three of the above cases we find an *unusually great internal anxiety,* although coupled with very differing physical ailments; also fear of being alone both by day and night, which urges the patient to suicide, although his intellect is otherwise clear; and finally a state similating remorse and the sufferings from a bad conscience, leading one to ask forgiveness.

Dose.—24 and 30, with speedy good effects.

The symptoms undoubtedly point to affection of the organs of *conscientiousness* and *caution.*

4. AURUM.

General Remarks.—*a*) Hahnemann says he has quickly and permanently cured several persons who seriously meditated suicide, of that melancholy in which Gold is indicated.

Chronic Diseases, Vol. 2, p. 18.

b) Not only Aurum, but Nux-vom. will remove the peculiar mental depression, with disgust for life, which leads to suicide.

Hygea, Vol. 2, p. 33.—Ægidi.

c) Both Gold and Arsen. produce sensations of anxiety proceeding from the region of the heart; this symptom, which both have in common, is of importance when we view in connection with the heart-affections which occur in many cases of mental disease. But Aurum is not suitable in the regular and typical occurrence of the symptoms against which Arsen. is so useful; but is indicated where there is decided congestion to the head, certain quite peculiar genital symptoms, &c.

Noack and Trinks with much reason call attention to the state of the genitals common in suicidal monomaniacs, with relation to the action of Gold upon the same organs.

Hygea, Vol. 24, p. 10.—Griesselich.

Vogt tells us that in olden times Aurum was used for its heart-strengthening, vivifying and gladdening powers, Riecke, Dunglison and Dierbach state that the remarkably joyous disposition and loquacity noticed after its use deserve particular mention. Neil and Percy found it to cause general excitement of the nervous system, talkativiness, &c.; and tell us that it was used by the ancients in hypochondria; melancholy and idiocy.

As it also has a specific relation to the syphilitic dyscrasia, while the melancholy occurring after syphilitic gonorrhœa is an extremely disquieting affection, which often leads to suicide, and which is scarcely ever cured by ordinary means, it deserves attention; also in the syphilitic monomania so admirably described by Acton.

Large doses of Aurum are apt to cause obstinate sleeplessness and fatiguing erections; Wendt says, when given in the different forms of dropsy in aged men, it rarely failed to arouse the long-slumbering sexual power. Risneno also alludes to its vis aphrodisiaca, &c.—Hence it may prove homœopathic and curative in melancholy and mental derangement arising from excess, or abuse of sexual power.—PETERS.

CASE 9.—Aurum cured a case of religious melancholy, brought on by stings of conscience, in consequence of misconduct.

Symptoms.—Great anxiety about the heart, fearfulness, weeping, praying, anxious frightful dreams, weakness, emaciation, night sweats, painful menstruation, &c.

Archiv, Vol. 12, part. 3, p. 131.—SEIDEL.

Compare case 107, in which a teacher who naturally had great self-esteem, attempted to strangle himself with a cord after mortification.

REVIEW.—It requires more numerous observations to determine the cases in which Aurum is suitable and what organs of the brain it acts upon, before we can decide positively what kind of disgust of life, with inclination to suicide, it will most readily heal.

5. BARYTA.

GENERAL REMARKS.—The salts of Baryta undoubtedly have the power of depressing the mental powers in such wise as to diminish the understanding. Muriate of Barytes is well known to cause, in scrofulous children, a state which borders closely on idiotcy. This fact should urge us to follow this clue farther, as that form of idiotcy which follows mental derangement is looked upon as incurable, because it is supposed to depend upon profound organic disease, but Baryta, besides its specific relation to idiotcy, also exerts an undoubted influence upon the organic mass. C. H. NEUMANN has found the Muriate of Baryta of the greatest efficacy in that form of mania in which the sexual inclination is much increased; while Baryta-carb. produces analogous effects, viz, increased sexual power, more copious secretion of semen, frequent pollutions, and in females causes premature occurrence of menses, and congestive affections of the sexual organs, and of the sacral region.

6. BELLADONNA.

a) HARTMANN says *Bellad.* is useful in some forms of melancholy, viz., in such as have arisen from disorder of the abdominal organs, and in which spasmodic affections of the throat and the bladder, and gastric derangements occur. He also advises it in melancholy from disappointed love, in which there is excitement of the genital system—also in home-sickness, and loss of memory, and in melancholy during pregnancy, and after confinement.

Still it is more frequently useful in folly and mania.

Archiv, Vol. 2, part. 2, p. 84.

b) *Christison* says that the *Bellad.*-delirium is generally of the extravagant, or of the pleasing kind, sometimes attended with immoderate and incontrollable laughter, or at others with incessant loquacity, and hence would seem to exert a specific action upon the organs of Language and Mirthfulness. *Gray*, the botanist, when poisoned with eight or ten grains of Bellad., experienced a delirium of a strange but not unpleasant character, he wished to be in constant motion, and states that it certainly afforded him an infinite degree of satisfaction to be allowed to walk up and down. The operations of the intellect were very vivid, his thoughts came and went rapidly, and ludicrous and fantastic spectacles were always uppermost in his mind; he was conscious that his language and gestures were extravagant, yet he had neither the will or inclination to control them, as he was in a state of delightful exhilaration. Dr. Barton witnessed a case in which the patient in a quarter of an hour became delirious and insensible, and struggled violently in his unconscious state, so that the combined strength of several men was required to hold him; the stage of delirium was brief, and he soon fell into coma, which was again succeeded in eight or ten hours by violent delirium, the patient being very unmanageable—the mental delusions were for the most part of an agreeable kind, and the prevailing fancy was that he had suddenly become rich and possessed of a splendid mansion. Brit. Jour. Hom. Vol. 6, p. 430.

In another case a lady fell into a delirious state, attempted to bite and strike her attendants, broke into fits of laughter, and gnashed her teeth; her head was hot, face red, looks wild and fierce, tongue dry, abdomen swollen, and pulse small and frequent. Ibid, p. 430. In still another case a boy could not speak at first, but laughed immoderately, and kept grasping at imaginary objects; soon, although laughing continued, his silence was changed into immoderate and incoherent loquacity, with constant bodily motion, &c. Med. Chir. Rev. Vol. 7, p. 233. Leuret, of the Bicetre, noticed in several cases a degree of restlessness and excitement, approaching at times to inordinate gaiety, at others to furious delirium, frequent hallucinations, convulsive crying or laughing, &c.

In another case, a woman æt. 36, took twelve grains of Ext. Bellad. by mistake in the course of six hours; she had illusions of vision, saw everything confused, as if through a fog or smoke, even imagined that she saw things which were not present; a stupid laughter, with merry delirium, soon followed, and were attended with contortions of the extremities, great general debility and coldness.

The old school experience in the use of *Bellad.* is extensive, varied, but not very precise, Mayr in 1817, used it until the fauces became dry and the pupils dilated. Guislain in his Prize Essay on Mental alienation, 1826, says that Murray obtained good effects from it in five grain doses; Muller, of Wurtzburg, saw satisfactory results from it in doses as large as thirty-six grains of powdered root per day, pushed until blindness and vertigo occurred; in this way, among other cases, he cured a woman, æt. 40, affected for a year with furious mania. Münch regarded it as an excellent remedy in melancholy and mania; Frank recommended it in mental alienation with fantastic visions and when accompanied with epilepsy. Seymour thought Bellad. well worthy of trial in mania, especially in that from moral causes and attended with pain and increased sensibility of brain. Millingen found Bellad. more useful than Hyos. or Conium, especially when applied externally by the endermic method, to the epigastric region; very often effectual in reducing excitement.—PETERS.

CASE 10.—A strong, blooming primipara, æt. 20, fell suddenly on the fifth day after delivery into a state of mania, and was treated antiphlogistically for nine days without benefit.

Symptoms.—She talked constantly of every kind of confused and laughable stuff; was much excited, passionate and abusive, sought to destroy everything she could reach, screamed, scolded, spit, struck, laughed and cried. Her husband she damned into the deepest depths of hell, for imagined infidelity to her, &c.

Treatment.—On the fourteenth day after delivery she took Bellad. 3, ten drops in water, a tablespoonful per dose; in two days she was more quiet; on the third day she asked for her child, &c. Bellad. $_{3}$ was continued, two doses per day, and in three weeks she was cured.

Hygea, Vol. 20, p. 223. MAYRHOFER.

CASE 11.—A girl æt. 12, otherwise healthy, was left debilitated after an attack of influenza, then was taken with paralysis of the feet, and finally fell into a state of mania.

Symptoms.—Towards evening she suddenly lost her recollection of every one, screams out aloud, laughs, weeps, talks unconnectedly, at times in a frighted state, at others in despair about death, and the arrangements therefor, believes that she sees strange persons about her who abuse her, and from whom she attempts to escape. She also has twitchings of the face and of all the limbs, wrings her hands and tosses them wildly into the air. In the morning she does not recollect anything that has transpired during the night—she has boring pain in the head and vertigo, so that she cannot raise herself up in bed.

Treatment.—Bellad. $_{3}$, two doses cured her.

Allg. Hom. Zeit. Vol. 13, p. 300. *Bicking.*

CASE 12.—A strong, powerfully built brunette, and blooming girl of 16 years, exhibited in consequence of a long-continued sedentary mode of life, excessive indulgence in reading, and bad mental training, at each access of menstruation traces of wildness and folly, which gradually increased to perfect mania, which recurred repeatedly, in spite of allopathic treatment.

Symptoms.—Babbling, laughing, weeping, scolding, at times she attempted to creep away and hide, at others she fell into paroxysms of rage and spit at those about her, and tore off her clothes. Pulse generally slow, but quickened during the paroxysms; abdomen hard and tense; involuntary urination.

Treatment.—Bellad. 2, one drop every forty-eight hours, cured her entirely and permanently in twenty-four days.

Hygea, Vol. 21, p. 139.—KIESSELBACH.

CASE 13.—A farmer's lad, æt. 17, had been deranged for four weeks.

Symptoms.—Had not slept for five days and nights; spent the night in sitting up, alternately crying and laughing; romanced about soldiers and war, imagined that he was pursued by soldiers, or bulls, and crept away in fear that he should be found. Attempts various foolish things, and goes through the pantomine of shooting; scolds at and strikes his brothers and sisters; frequently walks bent and limping; crowds his hat down over his eyes, eats but little, and does not work at all. His pupils were very much dilated, and his countenance disturbed, yellow and bloated.

Treatment.—Bellad. $\frac{}{30}$, three doses at intervals of eight days cured him.

Archiv, Vol. 12, part. 3, p. 79.—ATTOMYR.

CASE 14.—A sickly woman, æt. 37, had been deranged for six weeks.

Symptoms.—Great restlessness and anxiety, so that she could not remain in one place, in constant bodily motion, so that she cannot remain in bed; talks incessantly of silly stuff, at times jovial, at others gloomy, or shameless, her eyes being in constant motion. At times she smiles to herself, then bursts out into uncontrolled laughter, or sings religious songs, then scolds, or strikes her hands against the walls or windows, or attempts to jump out of the window, spits all about herself and tears her clothes. Coughs up mucus, and has frequent attacks of choking.

Treatment.—Bellad. $\frac{}{15}$, six doses, two or three per day, cured her with the exception of an increased loquacity of an indecent character, which was removed in a few days by Stramon. $\frac{}{6}$.

Allg. Hom. Zeit. Vol. 8, p. 121—ELWERT.

CASE 15.—A man, æt. 28, of powerful build and choleric temper, became deranged without known cause.

Symptoms.—He scolds, riots and attempts to kill his wife, has a frightful, insolent and somewhat anxious look, his eyes glisten and are reddened; his answers are rough, insolent, very abrupt and often threatening. He has œdema of the abdomen and thighs, with scattered red spots.

Treatment.—Bellad. $\frac{}{12}$, one drop cured him of his mania in the course of fourteen days, when Bryon. and China were required to free him from his dropsy.

Archiv, Vol. 19, part. 1, p. 93.—S. Zlartoravich.

CASE 16.—A lad, æt. 12, of delicate and irritable constitution was left with headache and anxious restlessness after an attack of typhoid fever.

Symptoms.—Pressing, stupefying pain in the forehead, especially after mental exertion or emotion; evening restlessness, and anxiety, with unsteady gait. Dreamy sleep, with sudden jerks through the whole body, which causes him to rise up, make anxious motions, cry, scream out complainingly, and attempt to escape. On the following morning he recollects nothing that has transpired.

Treatment.—*Bellad.* $\frac{}{3}$ in repeated but not frequent doses restored him.

Allg. Hom. Ztg. Vol. 13, p. 299.—Bicking.

CASE 17.—A widow, æt. 50, became deranged and was allopathically treated unsuccessfully for a long time.

Symptoms.—She destroys every thing in her reach, riots, raves and spits. With fixed wild looks and dishevelled hair, she utters frightful curses. Her mouth is always covered with froth; she avoids drinking, and when she attempts it she seems to swallow with difficulty.

Treatment.—Pulv. Herb. Bella[illegible] fixed grains, divided into 8 doses, one dose night and mornin[illegible] H[illegible]tored her perfectly.

Annals, Vol. 4, p. 329.—Schu[illegible] ing, a[illegible] ltv.

CASE 18.—A widow, æt. 30, brunette, of a melancholic disposition and high tempered, had been deranged for six years, and was on the point of being placed in an asylum.

Symptoms.—Fearful mistrust of every one, great anxiety day and night, no rest in any place and attempts to escape; her only pleasure is to stare at the sun by day, and the fire at night. She finally escaped into the woods, built herself a large fire and remained there four or five days without food. Always sought to be alone, and fled from all company; whenever she was alone she played ludicrous tricks, and twisted her mouth in all directions—money she threw out of the window; was never disposed to converse, and scarcely returned an answer, unless asked two or three times, and then with great vexation and screaming.

Treatment.—*Bellad.* $\frac{}{30}$, two doses, given in the course of fourteen days restored her completely.

Annals, Vol. 4, p. 340.

CASE 19.—A man, æt. 29, became deranged after great disappointment, and from grief at the death of his sister.

Symptoms.—He calls out constantly the name of his deceased sister, and beats his breast and body with his fist in despair; he strikes at all who approach him, thrusts everything away from him with hands and feet; laments, groans, froths at the mouth; grasps at his throat, and tears off his cravat, as if in danger of suffocation.

Treatment.—One dose of *Bellad.* $\frac{}{30}$, soon restored him to quiet and reason.

Annals, Vol. 4, p. 193.—L. in L.

CASE 20.—An old man had suffered for several years in succession.

Symptoms.—He sees in rapid succession strange figures, houses which are being built before his windows, peacocks which seem to walk about in his garden, &c.; he attempts to observe his visions more accurately with a spy-glass. Anxiety drives him unclothed out of his bed; pulse quick and full; urine scanty and very red.

Treatment.—Bellad. $\frac{}{30}$, two doses cured him speedily.

Practical Communications, Vol. 4, part. 4, p. 223.—THORER.

CASE 21.—A puerperal woman, æt. 25, still nursing her child, was obliged to keep her bed in consequence of intestinal irritation, when she suddenly commenced to talk all kinds of unconnected stuff, with incredible fluency and entire sleeplessness. This was followed by a period of perfect silence, after which she again commenced to sing snatches of disconnected songs, and to grasp at neighboring things.

Treatment—Bellad. $\frac{}{24}$ in water, a table-spoonful every three hours caused the most speedy relief.

Allg. Hom. Zeit. Vol. 37, p. 56.—SOLLIER.

CASE 22.—A man, æt. 34, and another, æt. 55, became deranged from grief and vexation.

Symptoms.—Would not believe that he was sick, would

attend to his business, spoke of much work to be done, complained of men who had injured him; imagined that his wife floated around him, and that he heard her voice proceeding from every object; thought that he was praying with her, and that he must soon die; sleeplessness in consequence of the above illusions. He had a burning miliary eruption upon the chest; felt great lassitude on going up-stairs, his legs felt as heavy as lead; his head was heavy and felt as if it would fall off; darkness before his eyes and vertigo when walking, as if he were drunk. Frequent flushes of heat over the body, with trembling; pulse full, quick and hard; pain in the chest from deep inspiration and cough; noises in the ears, with hardness of hearing; piercing pain in the temples; sensation of icy-coldness upon the temples.

Treatment.— One dose of *Bellad.* cured him.

Jahrb. f. Hom. Hospital, Vol. 1, p. 145, and Vol. 2, p. 120.

CASE 23.—A lad, æt. 20, blond, pale, thin, and easily provoked, suddenly because maniacal on August 31.

Symptoms.—He attempts to destroy every thing near him, or to throw them at his attendants; swallowed his food and drink hastily; pays no attention to any person or question, but screams, hums and runs about, tears his clothes and goes naked; his pupils were contracted and his look wild and fixed. Skin and pulse natural.

Treatment.—Tartar emetic, in emetic doses, did not relieve him. Sept. 2d he took Belladonna-juice, two drops in water; on the 3d and 4th he took a like dose night and morning, and on the 5th he was perfectly restored to his senses, and could be dismissed cured in a few days more.

Allg. Hom. Zeit, Vol. 19, p. 18.—Knorre.

CASE 24.—A woman, æt. 77, previously always healthy, began to be deranged without known cause.

Symptoms.—At first she imagined there was a peculiar vapor in the room, thought that others must notice it also, and wished it to be removed. She felt unhappy, fearful, anxious, and thought she could not be saved. Is timid, easily frightened when any one entered her room, and hid herself. Did not know her own son who stood before her, insisted that he was dead, and could not be convinced to the contrary; did not know her physician, but regarded him as a judge who had been present when she made her will, and hence would not see him again, although she insisted that the right physician should be brought to her. If her friends spoke about indifferent subjects which did not concern her, she would sometimes join in the conversation rationally. She was costive, and had congestion to the head, with flushing of the face.

Treatment.—From May 6, to June 6, she received various doses of Verat., Pulsat., Nux-v., Hyosc. and Sulph., but without visible good effect, except from the Sulph. the action of which was waited for several days. On June 2d, she received *Bellad.* $\overline{4}$, and on the next day she was nearly restored, and recollected every thing she had said during her illness.

Minutes of the L. Society.—Engelhardt.

CASE 25.—A man, æt. 38, suddenly fell into a maniacal state after vexation.

Symptoms.—Face bluish-red, eyes sparkling, pupils dilated; he spat incessantly without excreting much spittle, and had signs of sore throat on swallowing; his forehead was covered with sweat, his limbs cold, his pulse quick and irritable; he talked about the most frantic and disconnected things, and imagined that he saw frightful figures.

Treatment.—*Bellad.* 6, followed by increased excitement, then by a more quiet state, and the frantic paroxysm occurred only every three hours. On the following day he could be liberated, and his whole condition was changed.

Symptoms.—Face paler with but slight redness of cheeks; he assumed a dignified manner, took great pains to speak correctly, broke off a bit of his whip and put it behind his ear for a pen, moved his hands constantly, as in St. Vitus' Dance, spilled his drink involuntarily, and talked constantly of quarrels which had not happened.—Abdomen tense, bowels sluggish.

Treatment.—*Stramonium* 9, after which quiet and sleep at night followed; a remaining sad, almost melancholic mood was cured by Tinct. Hellebor.—Rau, p. 190.

CASE 26.—A boy, æt. 13, became unexpectedly very thoughtful.

Symptoms.—When any one approaches him in the street he is seized with an irresistible inclination to attack and stab him with his pocket-knife ; as he approaches the person, he is seized with great anxiety which hurries him away ; then he runs home and weeps over his conduct.

Treatment.—*Bellad.* 30, followed in eight days by Nux-vom. 30, cured him.

All. Hom. Zeit. Vol. 6, p. 213.—FIELITZ.

Besides, *Bellad.* was also given in cases No' 3, 7, 39, 41, 42, 56, 61, 71, 72, 88, 91, 94, 99, 101, 106.

REVIEW.—In the above cases we notice the following circumstances, with regard to :

a) Age and sex.

In 34 cases, 18 were males, and 16 females. Of the 18 males, 11, and of the 16 females, 9 were benefitted or cured by Bellad.

Of 28 cases, 14 were between 8 and 25 years old.
" " " 17 " " 28 " 77 " "

b) Of the groups of symptoms upon which Bellad. acted *decidedly curatively*, we notice *two principal* groups, and *two lesser* ones.

In the *first* principal form we notice a state of evident *excitement*, attended with rioting, scolding, swearing, attempt at destruction of things and persons. (See cases No. 10, 15, 23, 100, 106.)

In the *second* principal form, we find a state of *dejection ;* the patient exhibits an uneasiness which drives him about, and makes him fearful of even imaginary objects ; is suspicious, fearful, has an inexpressible anxiety, especially about phantoms of the imagination, has fears of death, and is driven to make his escape. (See cases No. 11, 13, 16, 18, 20 and 22.)

In several cases these two principal forms of mania occurred in alternation. (See cases No. 12, 14, 19, 94.)

As a *third* and *lesser* form, we find a silly, indecent behavior, with foolish tricks, laughing, gossipping and imitating. This occurs alone in case No. 100, and either mixed with one or both of the principal forms in cases No. 10, 13, 14, 18.

As a *fourth* and also *lesser* form, we find the predominance or occurrence of fixed ideas ; the patients busy themselves about *dead* persons, (see cases No. 19, 22.)—or regard *well-known* persons as strangers (see No. 24). Still this form never occurs singly, but is always mixed with the first or second principal form.

c) Among the cases in which *Bellad.* was used with *little or no* good effect we notice in :

Case No 100, a restlessness and complaining from fear that he would not be forgiven; in case No. 91, a restlessness which drives the patient away, but without evident anxiety as its cause, (see also cases 72 and 56). We notice anxiety with inclination to suicide, but without urgency to run away in case 7. In case 29 we find a state of excitement, but dependent upon increased self-esteem. Farthermore, *Bellad.* was not useful in case 71, marked by suspicion and anthrophophobia; nor in cases 39 and 41, attended with shameless and lecherous conduct; nor in case No. 42 with visions of animals and convulsive cramps.

d) As regards the *Doses* of Bellad. and their repetition, we find that in thirty cases,

the Herb. Bellad. two grs. in eight doses was used once.
" Tinct. Bellad. two drops in water " " "

Dilut.	2	one dose in 1 case.
"	3	" " " 1 "
"	4	repeated in 3 cases.
"	4	one dose in 1 case.
"	6	" drop, repeated in 1 case.
"	6	" dose in 1 case.
"	12	" " " 1 "
"	15	repeated doses in 2 cases.
"	21	one dose in 1 case.
"	24	in solution, in 1 case.
"	30	one dose in 1 case.
"	30	repeated doses in 5 cases.
"	60	in solution, in 1 case.

Hence we find that the cases in which one dose sufficed are not as numerous as those cases in which repeated doses were required, for only seven cases were cured by one dose, while sixteen cases required a repetition of dose.

The doses varied from quantities of the crude vegetable through the whole scale of dilutions up to the 60th; still the majority, viz., fifteen cases were cured by dilutions lower than the 30th.

If we examine fourteen cases marked by accurate data about sex, age, duration of the disease, rapidity of improvement, in order to determine the relative value of high or low dilutions, we find nothing to lead us to give a preference to one above the other. Equally rapid improvement follows the use of the plant or tinct., as from the 3d, 6th or 30th potency. The right remedy would cure in any dose.

The cures were effected in fourteen cases, in from one to fourteen days in ten cases; and in from fifteen to twenty-four days in four cases; and this happened as well in cases of long-standing as in recent attacks.

e) As regards the *organs* of the brain principally affected in the cases cured by Bellad., we find:

1. Combativeness and destructiveness in an excited state (see 1st form);
2. Caution aroused with depression of combativeness (see 2d form).

N.B. In those cases in which the 1st and 2d forms occurred in alternation we find the above organs in an alternate state of excitement and depression, as is also the case in the 3d and 4th forms to a lesser degree.

In the production of *fixed* ideas we find

3. The organ of *adhesiveness*, and
4. " " " *form* in an abnormal state of excitement or depression or pervertion, so that the patient constantly romances about the dear departed, or mistakes the form of the well known physician for some other, or even does not recognize that of his own son.

7. BRYONIA.

Hartlaub of Reichenau states that when puerperal women feel unhappy and depressed, especially about their property, and imagine without reason, that they can no longer meet their expenses, &c., that *Bryonia* has often proved useful. This experience might lead us to suppose that Bryonia acts upon the organ of *acquisitiveness*.

8. CALCAREA-CARB.

General Remarks.—*a*) That state of despair which occurs in many chronic diseases, which leads the patient to give up all hope of cure, but still does not prevent him from being exceedingly fearful of dying, nor from pestering their friends with constant complaints and lamentations, may often be cured by Calcarea.

Archiv, Vol. 17, part 1, p. 8.—B. in D.

b) Anxiety, shuddering and horror, occurring on the approach of evening; agony occasioned by thinking; agony from hearing of cruelties; paroxysms of despair about ruined health; irritability.

Hahnemann, Chron. Dis. Vol. 2, p. 308.

CASE 27.—A feeble irritable woman, æt. 35, had suffered with melancholy for four years after her last confinement. Pulsat. and Sulph. had been given without benefit.

Symptoms.—Frightful appearances before the eyes and great anxiety about the heart; despairs of her salvation to such a degree that she often wishes to strangle herself; dislikes her children; is fearful of the future and imagines that she will be reduced to poverty; face pale and bloated.

Treatment.—Calc. $\frac{}{30}$ soon cured her, and her menses, which had been suppressed for 2½ months returned again. About the same time she passed a large piece of tape-worm.

Archiv, Vol. 17, part 1. p. 8.—B. in D.

Review.—The absence of hope of recovery, and even despair about it, the want of hope of salvation, &c. point to a depressed state of the organ of hope; while the fear of becoming poor points to an affection of the organ of acquisitiveness.

The presence of tape-worm in this case will certainly be regarded by some as the exciting cause of the disease, which would be regarded as seated in the vegetative sphere, while the mental affection would be regarded as a sympathetic and secondary disorder.

9. CAUSTICUM.

General Remarks.—*a*) Many of the consequences of long-continued grief and care may be cured by Caust.

Archiv, Vol. 17, part 1, p. 8,—B. in D.

b) Melancholy; sorrowful thoughts at night and weeping by day; fearfulness, and want of confidence in the future; hopeless, passionate and irritable.

Hahn. Chron. Dis. Vol. 3, p. 85.

10. CHINA.

The old-school experience with China and Quinine is very large and very loose. Pinel says, melancholy marked by atony and extreme depression is to be remedied by the use of Bark with Opium, of the cure of which he can cite many examples. The success of the justly celebrated Willis and his relatives he thought arose greatly from their decided conviction of the danger of the lancet and debilitating means, and from a thorough reliance on tonic treatment, China being requisite if the irritability proceed from a weak state of the constitution, or occasioned by bloodletting, child-bed or typhus fevers, &c.; it is the more useful in proportion to the quickness of pulse, increase of heat and irritability. Guislain, says, in all ages the success of tonics in some cases has demonstrated the existence of asthenic cases of insanity. Herriae obtained the most happy success in madness with depression from Peruvian bark; Perfect cites different cases in which China was given with success. Reil has proved the excellent effects of it in dementia with the intermittent type. Georget assures us that he has employed China with success in remittent insanity. Castel says, that he has more than once seen insanity yield to China.

CASE 27.—A young woman, æt. 24, deranged for six weeks, until she became inexhaustibly loquacious; spoke on various subjects without the least judgment; she was bled and became furious in consequence; was then leeched and became insupportably gay and loquacious; was then ordered China, and next morning her delirium had almost disappeared and in four weeks she was well.

CASE 28.—A man wandered about without sustenance until his body became wan, eyes dull, pulse very frequent, limbs and face cold, remarkable paleness of tongue, loquacity continual, confused and incoherent; finally the delirium became complete, and he did not speak a rational word. China was given with amelioration in fifteen days and cure in a month.

CASE 29.—A young theologian abandoned himself to study with a sort of fury, and finally became maniacal; various means were used without success, until China was given, when relief and cure soon followed.

Still in a case of mania, the attacks occurring on a fixed day, the delirium lasting six days, and succeeded by perfect sanity, it was given several times without success.

It has been useful when there is loss of appetite, paleness of the tongue and slow digestion. It is particularly useful in most cases of periodical mental alienation, in those from onanism, or complicated by it; in dementia, and especially in that which arises from protracted or badly-treated intermittent fevers. Also in the mental derangement which follows typhoid fevers. BOSTEX found it useful when the paroxysms seemed to have somewhat of an intermittent character. DUNGLISON did not find it to have the same good effects as in other intermittent affections; more useful in long-protracted cases of insanity, when the skin is moist and relaxed, limbs cold, skin shrunk and shrivelled, with a livid and blotchy or a pale and yellow complexion, and feeble circulation.—PETERS.

CASE 30.—A young and powerful man became deranged suddenly, at eleven, A. M. every other day (Tertian type); he became unconscious of his actions, spoke and acted confusedly, in an excited manner, ran to and fro, &c. This state lasted an hour, with gradual increase and diminution, and then ceased without the patient having any distinct recollection of what had occurred.

Treatment.—After the use of China in strong doses the affection ceased after three attacks.

Hygea, Vol. 24, p. 4.—Griesselich.

11. CROCUS.

CASE 31.—A boy, æt. 10, whose father had died suddenly in a lunatic asylum, fell into a feverish state, attended with congestion to the head, and after awaking from sleep exhibited the following appearances.

Symptoms.—He sat up or stood up in bed, and quickly made various strange motions, without knowing what he was about; after such a paroxysm he recovered his senses, but without recollecting what he had been doing. After a period of quiet there soon followed a like attack, again succeeded by a remission, &c. He was beside himself, but soon became conscious and refreshed; his eyes were fixed and glistening; his face red and hot; urine pale and scanty; no desire for food or drink; pulse slow, scarcely sixty per minute.

Treatment.—Tinct. Crocus, twelve drops in four ounces of water, six doses, at intervals of two hours, and then repeated at longer periods. In four days he was quite well.

Schmid, H. A. and G. p. 121.

12. COCCULUS.

General Remarks.—Cocculus in its sphere is as great a spinal remedy as Secale, and manifests this relation by numerous phenomena. Physicians of lunatic asylums should attend to this, and think of Cocculus in the mental affections of irritable and torpid book-worms and house-bodies, of sensitive romance heroines and dreamy moon-struck women, whose menstruation does not proceed as regularly and quietly as the course of the moon.

Mental derangement with vertigo, constant desire to run away, great anxiety, and loquacity has been cured by Baumbach with Cocculus, in doses of one-sixteenth or one-eighth of a grain.

Hygea, Vol. 23, p. 264.—Griesselich.

It was also used in cases No. 94 and 98. In case 94, the patient had lost his decision of character, could not resolve upon any course of conduct, and complained much of stiffness in the joints and limbs.

Treatment.—Cocculus $\frac{}{2}$, one drop night and morning; soon the limbs became more flexible, the patient returned to his employment and took short walks.

Bellad. and Cocc. in alternation completed the cure.

Very little is known of the action of Cocculus, except what

has been derived from the labors of Hahnemann and his disciples. It has been used immemorially in the East, for the purpose of stupefying and taking fish, and is familiarly used for the same purpose in some parts of France, the inhabitants living for one-half the year on fish caught with it. (*Christison.*) In some parts of the world it is used by robbers to intoxicate their victims, and to this form of intoxication the term of *hocussing* is applied. (*Taylor.*) London porter and ale often owe their intoxicating properties to a decoction or extract of Cocculus, which gives an inebriating quality, which passes for strength of liquor. Its action has been compared to that of Nux-vomica and Camphor, and in poisonous doses is said to cause vomiting, vertigo, staggering, trembling, tetanic spasms and coma.—PETERS.

13. CONIUM-MACULATUM.

GENERAL REMARKS.—Dejection, anxiety, discontent, sadness and want of courage.

Hahn. Chron. Dis. Vol. 3, p. 177.

In the case of a robust peasant girl, æt. 20, who had taken a strong decoction of Herb. Conii-maculat. to produce abortion, the patient vomited several times, the expression of countenance was calm, but like a figure of wax, eye immovable and staring, body, limbs cold, with cold sweat on head and forehead, pulse extinct and voice hoarse; her mind was perfectly calm and intellect clear, so that she could tell what she had done; she soon died. Socrates was poisoned with Hemlock, probably Conium, and as is well known, retained his senses to the last. It seems to cause failure of the circulation, coldness of the limbs, lowering of the pulse down to thirty, or less, enormous stagnation of blood in various organs, especially in brain and liver, conversion of all the blood from an arterial to a deeply venous state, diminution of the quantity of fibrine, and consequent production of petechiæ, vibices, &c. From this view of its action it would seem decidedly antipathic to maniacal excitements, and homœopathic to melancholy, hypochondria, &c. Still WOODWARD, of the Worcester Asylum, tells us that Conium is worthy of but little confidence as a means of removing maniacal excitement, but for some forms of melancholy, especially if combined with dyspepsia or neuralgia, it is often very useful; also against melancholy, with disease of stomach, torpor of liver, uneasiness, restlessness and nervous pains.

Cox says that Conium gradually introduced into the system has certainly been of service in some cases by diminishing excitement and irritation and causing sleep; but some systems or cases resist its influence for a length of time, and others are not affected unless administered in enormous doses. Mead says Conium is a more powerful soporific than Opium; in some cases it will fail; has known it to purge, and to constipate. In the McLean Asylum, S. C., Conium is considered a useful medicine; in recent cases is alterative and slightly narcotic, produces calmness after it has been taken some time. Dose seven to eight grains, three times a day. Dr. Woodward, of the Worcester Asylum, regards it as a valuable remedy and useful in some forms of insanity; but as a means of removing maniacal excitement it is worthy of but little confidence; however, for some forms of melancholy, and especially in chronic diseases of the digestive organs, with melancholy or neuralgia, it is often useful; also in cases of melancholy complicated with disease of the stomach and torpor of the liver, attended with uneasiness, restlessness, watchfulness and nervous pains, it often affords great relief and is auxiliary in accomplishing a cure. In any case is useful in large doses only—smallest dose ten grains; largest, two or three or four drachms, three times a day—rarely found any benefit from doses less than fifteen or twenty grains, three or four times a day—unless it produced temporary vertigo, and a heavy dull pain over the eyes or across forehead, thought the dose too small, or the medicine of poor quality.

In Bloomingdale and other Asylums, Conium is given with Iron, when the mucous membranes are disordered, the circulation unequal, secretions depraved, and digestion imperfect, often used in mania after the excitement is subdued, frequently give it in melancholy, and still more frequently in dementia. Kukbude also uses Conium and Iron in the debility of old cases. Fisher did not obtain much benefit from Conium and Iron, except when the secretions were unhealthy, then found it useful in correcting them.—PETERS.

The action of Conium on the brain, and its circulation seems almost antagonistic to that of Bellad.; the latter generally causes delirium and high fever, with active congestion and dilatation of the pupil, while Conium generally causes a torpid condition of the brain so that the patient falls asleep while conversing, great weakness of the intellectual faculties with loss of memory, want of mental energy, unfitness for exertion, confusion of ideas, as if from drowsiness, slow conception, ready forgetfulness, hypochondriacal indifference, aversion to labor, headache with taciturnity and profound melancholy, &c. It rarely causes fever, but is apt to render the pulse slow, even as low as thirty, the skin cool and pale. It does not cause active congestion, but rather a passive stagnation of blood in various organs, especially in the head and liver. It does not often dilate the pupil—still Christison says in some cases all this is reversed, and it may cause frantic delirium, the patient running about the house, knocking against everything, or plunging into the water, under the supposition that he is changed into a goose, &c.—PETERS.

CASE 32.—A strong, previously quite healthy lad, aged 16, became deranged; he was treated allopathically for two years without benefit; his case was peculiar, from his being alternately dejected for ten days and then excited for ten other days.

Symptoms.—During ten days he is silent, dejected and loaded with care, picks his fingers, generally keeps his bed, speaks and answers unwillingly. Vacuity of thought, weakness of memory, and frequently sits as if in a reverie; he eats and drinks; has a movement from the bowels only every three days, but passes urine frequently at night. Is timid, cannot be induced to work, and his sleep is extremely disturbed.

Then for ten other days he is very excited, violent, arbitrary, quarrelsome and scolds readily. Puts on his best clothes, buys unnecessary things, which he then undervalues, or wastes or destroys. Will not work, games, disputes, and will not bear contradiction. He picks his nose constantly, and it bleeds easily.

Treatment.—Several doses of Bellad, were given without effect; then Conium $\frac{}{8}$ was used, two drops per dose, every fourth day. Soon after taking the second dose he was cured, but for precaution sake the remedy was continued for several months in smaller doses and at longer intervals.

General Hom. Journal, Vol. 9, p. 196.—Elwert.

CASE 33.—An intellectual and vivacious lady, with enlargement of her spleen, fell into a melancholic condition every fourteen days.

Symptoms.—Very unhappy state of mind, occurring every fourteen days; she loses all desire to speak, to dress herself, to take food, or to see her children. Great sluggishness of the bowels.

Treatment.—Conium $\frac{}{6}$, one drop twice a day cured her completely.

General Hom. Jour. Vol. 8, p. 198.—Elwert.

REVIEW.—The doses used were Conium $\frac{}{6}$ and $\frac{}{8}$, repeated more or less frequently.

In both cases there was dejection, disinclination to talk and indifference to everything. The alternation of excitement and dejection in case 29 was remarkable, see symptom 866. Dreams full of vexation and fighting.

CANNABIS-INDICA.

This should prove a most important homœopathic remedy; its action throws much light upon mental derangement in general. A marked correspondence may be traced between the phenomena of insanity and those which are induced by the introduction of Alcohol, Opium, Cannabis-indica, Nitrous-oxide, or laughing gas, Agaricus-muscarius, Belladonna, Stramonium, &c., into the system and blood. There can be no doubt that the properties of the blood may be perverted by unnatural changes going on within the system, as well as by the direct introduction of poisonous substances from without. Schœnlein, we believe, was the first to suggest that absolutely narcotic substances were sometimes formed *de novo* in the blood and system; prussic-acid always exists in the saliva; the narcotic properties of Urea are well known; the drowsiness, heaviness, and low spirits produced by bile circulating in the system are familiar. Hence mental derangement is often a blood disease—the presence of a minute portion of any of these substances circulating in the blood, which is passing through the capillaries of the brain, may excite delirium, illusions, fury, or melancholy, &c., &c.

But to return to the action of Cannabis-indica, Moreau found that a small dose generally had no other effect than a moderate exhilaration of the spirits, or at most a tendency to unseasonable laughter; some quickness of pulse, a little slowness of respiration, a general warmth through the body, with the exception of the feet, which are generally cold; the wrists and forearms seem as if loaded with a weight, and movements are performed involuntarily to set them free. At the same time vague muscular sensations of inquietude in the legs are felt, prompting one to continual restlessness, corresponding to what is called the fidgets. A very common feeling is that of the brain boiling over, and lifting the top of the skull like the lid of a tea-kettle. The region of the stomach is very often the seat of similar odd feelings; or the motions of the heart may seem to be performed with unusual violence. Slight or severe twitches of the limbs may take place; there is usually an inclination to lie down, and then the limbs and trunk may be all brought together by this spasmodic action; or the muscles of the face, especially those of the jaw may be effected with these spasmodic twitches and even a temporary state of lock-jaw may supervene. These physical effects of Cannabis-indica are however usually of but short duration; still they often cease only to return again after an interval of variable duration.

"The first result of a dose of Cannabis-indica sufficient to produce the *Fantasia*, as this remarkable condition is termed in the Levant, is usually an intense sensation of happiness; it seems to be really happiness, an entirely mental enjoyment like that of one who hears tidings which fill him with joy, like the miser who is counting his treasures, the gambler who is successful, or the ambitious man who is intoxicated with success. A peculiar state of general exhilaration or joyous excitement, closely analogous to that which is the first result of Cannabis-indica, is often the precursor of an attack of insanity, showing even in the mode of access of the disordered mental state a close correspondence between the two conditions.

"One of the first appreciable effects of the Cannabis is the gradual weakening of that power of controlling and directing the thoughts which is characteristic of the vigorous mind. The person feels himself incapable of fixing his attention upon any subject, his thoughts being continually drawn off by a succession of ideas which force themselves into his mind, without his being able in the least to trace their origin. These speedily oc cupy his attention and present themselves in strange combinations, so as to produce the most fantastic and impossible creations. By a strong effort of the will, the original thread of ideas may still be recovered and the interlopers may be driven away, their remembrance however being preserved, like that of a dream, recalling events long since past."

"Under the full influence of Cannabis one becomes the sport of impressions of the most opposite kind; the course of ideas may be broken by the slightest cause; one is turned by every wind; by a word or a gesture the current of one's thoughts may be successively directed to a multitude of objects, with a rapidity and lucidity which is truly marvellous. The mind becomes exultant in correspondence with the increase of its energy and power. But now it will entirely depend on the circumstances in which we are placed, the objects which strike the eyes, the words which fall on our ears, whether the most lively sensations of gaiety or of sadness shall be produced; or passions of the most opposite character shall be excited, sometimes with extraordinary violence; for irritation may rapidly pass into rage, dislike to hatred and desire for revenge, and the calmest affection to the most transporting passion. Fear may become terror, courage be increased to rashness, which nothing checks and which seems not to be conscious of danger. The most unfounded doubt becomes a certainty, for the mind has a tendency to exaggerate everything, and the slightest impulse carries it along.

"Remarkable illusions of perception as to time and space are apt to occur. Minutes seem hours, and hours are prolonged into years, and at last all idea of time seems obliterated, and the past and present are confounded together." Moreau mentions as an illustration, that on one evening he was traversing the passage of the Opera while under the influence of a moderate dose of Cannabis; he had made but a few steps when it seemed to him as if he had been there two or three hours; and as he advanced, the passage seemed interminable, its extremity seeming to recede as he pressed forwards. In walking along the street, Moreau frequently saw persons and things presenting the same aspect as if he had viewed them through the large end of an opera-glass, that is, diminished in apparent size and therefore suggesting the idea of increased distance. This erroneous perception of space is also one of the effects of the Agaricus-muscarius; a person under its influence is apt to take a jump or stride sufficient to clear the trunk of a tree, when he only wishes to step over a straw or small stick. Such erroneous perceptions are common enough among ordinary lunatics, and become in them the foundation of fixed illusions; whilst in a person intoxicated with Cannabis-indica there is still a consciousness of their deceptive character.

Gaultier, an artist of celebrity, found the slightest deep sound to produce the effect of rolling thunder; his own voice seemed so tremendous that he did not dare to speak out loud for fear of throwing down the walls, or of bursting himself like a bomb; the striking of one or a few clocks seemed to be exaggerated to the noise of more than five hundred striking with a great variety of tones.

It is seldom that the mental derangement caused by Cannabis fixes itself upon any particular train of ideas, and thus gives rise to a settled delusion; for in general one set of ideas chases the other so rapidly, that there is not time for any to engross the attention of the intellect, especially as the patient also preserves a certain degree of self-consciousness. But once MOREAU thought himself poisoned by the friend whom he induced to administer it to him, and persisted in this idea in spite of every proof to the contrary, until it gave way to another more absurd one, viz, that he was dead and about to be buried; still he had consciousness enough to believe that his body only was defunct, his soul having merely quitted it. All this has its counter-part in the different stages of natural insanity; the illusive ideas and erroneous convictions being in the first instance capable of being dissipated by a strong effort of the will, but gradually exerting more and more influence on the general current of thought, and at last acquiring such complete mastery over it, that the reasoning and controlling process can no longer be called into effectual operation.

It would seem to be an antipathic remedy to monomania.—PETERS.

14. CUPRUM-ACETICUM.

General Remarks.—Cuprum is very useful against attacks of anxiety in which the patient cannot control himself, weeps, is in despair, &c. while his body is chilly, the whole being but slightly relieved by external warmth.

Hygea, Vol. 12, p. 122.—Schmid.

CASE 34.—A robust man, æt. 38, had been overpowered for several months by great melancholy and restlessness.

Symptoms.—Invincible dejection has oppressed him for several months and an incessant restlessness annoys him, as if some misfortune were going to happen to him; he weeps easily, and is fearful of losing his reason. Sensation upon the vertex as if some thing like worms were moving in the brain (see Hahn. Chron. Dis., Symptoms 39 and 40). His head was heavy and confused; bowels moved only every three or four days; had difficulty in falling asleep before two, A. M., and was often sleepless.

Treatment.—Seven days after Cuprum $\frac{}{800}$, he was improved, and Sulph. $\frac{}{1200}$ finished the cure.

Gen'l. Hom. Journal, Vol. 34, p. 338.—Croserio.

CASE 35.—A consumptive man fell into paroxysms of anxiety when the lung-disease was checked.

Symptoms.—He was rendered particularly anxious by a fixed idea that he saw police-officers, who intended to deliver him up to justice; this caused him to weep and lament like a child. He imagined that he saw thieves, ghosts and various lifeless things in the room. Some of his disorders he felt and described rightly, but of others he had no or else extremely false notions; he maintained a sitting position, acted like one in despair, had extreme difficulty of breathing, a fearful anxiety and paroxysms of syncope. His pulse during the attacks was variable and weak, and his skin cool and covered with cold sweat.

He was soon cured by Cuprum-acet.

CASE 36.—A student was reduced bodily and mentally to a state of great debility, in consequence of excessive study in preparing for his examination; paroxysms of anxiety were added.

Symptoms.—Pulse weak, but little quickened, and irregular; skin moist and not hot; feet more frequently cold than warm; he has attacks of anxiety which he cannot overcome; his head is dizzy and so painful internally that he fears he will lose his senses; his sleep is disturbed and not refreshing, and full of confused and distressing dreams.

Treatment.—Cured by Cuprum-acet. in three days.—SCHMID.

CASE 37.—A woman about eight days after delivery, fell into a state of anxiety.

Symptoms.—The usually retiring, anxious, timid woman exhibited a remarkable activity in all her thoughts, which were of an anxious character—her eye and expression were generally fixed abstractedly upon one object—she had profuse and debilitating perspirations, and her pulse was quick, weak and irregular. Sometimes when it was supposed that she would be tranquil, she suddenly jumped out of bed, and it required great force to return and keep her there.

Treatment.—She recovered rapidly under the use of Cuprum-acet.—SCHMID.

CASE 38.—After the retrocession of erysipelas of the face, an attack of mania occurred in a woman, and was attended with excessive anxiety.

Symptoms.—Pulsation in the præcordia, and remarkable anxiety, so that she could not control herself. She did not recognize her husband or son; began to talk a great deal of confused stuff, part of which was really ludicrous; then she would sink into a state of apathy, from which however she could be aroused by interesting her. The most violent attacks occurred at night; when she was urged to take medicine she gnashed her teeth and resisted violently.

Treatment.—Bellad. and Hyosc. were used without benefit; but Cuprum in alternation with Stramon. cured her.

Hygea, Vol. 12, p. 120.—SCHMID.

REVIEW.—The deranged states, which were cured by Cuprum, were marked by confused talking, seeing various imaginary things, and erroneous illusions, but invariably attended by anxiety; by restlessness from fear of misfortune, despairing anxiety, with weeping and wailing.

Various decided bodily ailments were associated with the above, viz., irregular pulse, pulsation in pit of stomach, cold sweats, &c.

Like in the *Bellad.*-case No. 24, we find that one patient did not recognize her own husband and son.

Doses.—Schmid used three or four grains of the $\frac{1}{100}$th or 200th of Cuprum dissolved in a tumbler of water, one table-spoonful per dose every quarter, half, one or two hours, according to circumstances. In case 34, Cuprum $\frac{800}{}$ was used.

The anxious state of the patients pointed to an affection of the organ of *Caution;* and the seeing of lifeless figures indicates an increased activity of the organ of *Form.*

Note.—I have always entertained a decided disbelief of the homœopathicity of Cuprum to maniacal affections, but find in five cases of poisoning by copper, observed by Beer of Vienna, that nervous symptoms were present, of which the chief were very severe headache, slight delirium, convulsive movements of the legs, great exhaustion and somnolence, which in three cases amounted to coma, Brit. Journ. Hom. Vol. 1, p. 98. Christison also states that the first symptom is sometimes violent headache, and that in many cases signs of some injury done to the brain are very generally present, while in other instances it would appear that the narcotic symptoms form the commencement, and irritant symptoms the termination of poisoning with Copper.—On Poisons, p. 363. Chapman also used it with benefit in a case of scarlet fever with delirium.—Peters.

15. HEPAR-SULPH.-CALC.

CASE 39.—A man æt. 36, of powerful frame and phlegmatic temperament, having had the itch for half a year, became deranged after taking cold.

Symptoms.—Threatens his relatives, attempts to kill them, to set the house on fire, requires eight men to restrain him. Afterwards sits speechless and motionless in the corner of the room—passes urine and fæces involuntarily—his whole body is covered with an itch-like eruption, with occasional open ulcers.

Treatment.—Hepar-sulph. $_{T}$, cured him in a few days.

Archiv, Vol. 19, part 1, p. 89.—Szatar.

16. HELLEBORUS-NIGER.

General Remarks.—a) Hellebore is most adapted to those states which verge on the boundary line between melancholy and mania; and in actual conditions of depression and debility, in which at times fixed ideas are predominant.

The influence of *Helleb.* seems to irradiate from the abdominal nervous system to the spinal marrow, medulla oblongata, and brain. Hence many sympathetic affections of the brain are cured by it.

Hygea, Vol. 23, p. 262.—GRIESSELICH.

b) From various experience I infer that a primary and principal effect of Helleb., is to produce a kind of stupor, or blunting of the internal consciousness, or a state in which one with good eyesight does not see perfectly, or does not attend to that which he sees; with good hearing does not hear plainly, or does not understand; with good organs of taste, does not taste well; is always, or frequently absent-minded, remembers the past or lately transpired things either not at all, or but indifferently; takes pleasure in nothing; slumbers but lightly, without sleeping soundly or refreshingly; wishes to work, but has not the power, or does not give the necessary attention.

HAHNEMANN, Mat. Med. Pur.—B. 205.

c) GRIESSELICH remarks on the above, that in it we find a condensed description of the state of many melancholic persons; anæsthesia, want of memory, loss of the power of will, and of action are all extremely well marked, and present a marked antagonism to the action of Stramonium and other narcotics.

d) Hellebor.-nig. is very useful in some cases of mental dejection bordering on melancholy, and occurring in females about the time of puberty, either before or shortly after first menstruation, which has again become checked.

KNORRE, General Hom. Journal, Vol. 19, p. 25.

e) Every Homœopathist should read carefully the learned article by Hahnemann, on the Helleborism of the Ancients, see "LESSER WRITINGS, published by RADDE. Hellebore in small doses causes increased secretion of the gastric fluids, of thin bile, more active circulation in the portal system, in the liver and spleen, and it even renders the blood of these parts thinner and more fluid. Although it seems to act most promptly and decidedly upon the gastro-hepatic system, and upon the solar plexus of nerves, still it also promotes in a marked degree the menstrual and hæmorrhoidal discharges; it is apt to cause inflammation of the rectum, and MEAD esteemed it as the most certain emmenagogue. CHRISTISON asserts that in excessive doses, it causes vomiting, followed by delirium, succeeded by violent convulsions; while DIERBACH informs us that it has been used successfully in epilepsy, which passes over into mania, a form of disease regarded as incurable from the time of Hippocrates.—PETERS.

CASE 40.—After typhoid fever, there remained a kind of melancholy in a girl, æt. 20.

Symptoms.—She does not speak a word, is dull and indifferent to external impressions. Sits still upon her bed, apparently sunken in gloomy thought; face pale and distorted; look dull and unsteady; pupils dilated; pulse slow and weak; she eats proffered food, but never desires any; sleep scanty and restless; constant desire to run away, but without wildness of manner; without speaking a word she silently clambers up to the window and attempts to escape through it; whenever she did escape she always made her way towards the river; finally she threw herself into a privy, but was rescued from it.

Helleb. cured her quickly.

KNORRE, General Hom. Jour., Vol. 19, p. 24.

CASE 41.—A maiden, æt. 19, fell after typhoid fever into a dull state, which had lasted five weeks.

Symptoms.—She stares around her fixedly, even when spoken to, with a strange, or stupid, or wild look, and at times grasps at her head; she staggers while walking and hangs down her head; this thoughtless dullness or reverie, with staring at one point, alternates at times with incoherent muttering—constipation.

Treatment.—Ext. Helleb., two grains per day cured her in a few weeks.

General Hom. Journal, Vol. 19, p. 25.—KNORRE.

REVIEW.—The above cases fully substantiate the correctness of the views expressed in the general remarks.

17. HYOSCIAMUS-NIGER.

GENERAL REMARKS.—Hyosciamus is apt to excite erotic hallucinations, and jealousy stands in close connection therewith.

Hygea, Vol. 23, p. 254.—GRIESSELICH.

Dr. SCHNELLER experienced from $1\frac{1}{3}$ grains of the Extract of Hyosciamus, confusion of senses, weakness of sight, and some difficulty of speaking, also a by no means disagreeable state like that of slight intoxication; from two grains, confusion in head, then of sight and hearing, restless sleep, &c.; from three and a half to four grains, dull frontal headache, cloudiness and weakness of sight, with slowness of the pulse; from four and a half to five grains, confusion of head, frontal headache on the left side, dimness of vision, frequent inclination to yawn, and sleepiness; from eleven and one-fourth grains at one dose, giddiness, reticulated vision, frontal headache on right side, and sleepiness. CHRISTISON says, in medicinal doses it induces pleasant sleep, while CHOQUET reports the cases of two soldiers, poisoned with young shoots, who soon became dizzy, stupid, speechless, dull and haggard; their pupils were dilated, and eyes so insensible that the lids did not wink, even when the cornea was touched by the finger; their pulse was small and intermitting; breathing difficult, jaws locked, and mouths distorted by risus sardonicus. PEREIRA says, in persons with great nervous irritability, and too active condition of brain, it frequently causes calmness, and an inclination to sleep, also frequently allays irritations and morbid sensibility of one or the other organ. In one case, a man, æt. 40, was suddenly attacked with severe toothache, and fumigated his mouth with the smoke from the burning seeds of Hyosc.; the pain instantly vanished, but from that moment he became perfectly impotent, and the impotency lasted eight months.—Brit. Jour. of Hom., Vol. 1, p. 412.

Judging from effects similar to the above the antagonistic school have felt themselves justified in using Hyosc. in mental derangement and excitement, but FOUQUIER tells us from his own experience, that it never causes positive sleep, only a greater or less tendency thereto, always attended with headache, painful delirium, feverishness, &c.; CHRISTISON says it causes that singular union of delirium and coma which is usually termed Typhomomania; and that when the prostration and somnolency of this state abates, the delirium becomes extravagant and the patient quite unmanageable. WIBNER cites six cases of poisoning with it; several subjects were delirious, danced about the room like maniacs; one appeared drunk, and another became profoundly comatose. CHRISTISON concludes that it is very apt to cause loss of speech, delirium, commonly of the unmanageable, sometimes of the furious kind, followed by coma, and when the coma passes off the delirium is apt to return for a time. It has caused intense thirst, watchfulness, delirium, depraved vision, and a crowded eruption of dark spots and vesicles like the petechiæ and sudanima of typhus fever, or malignant small-pox. NELIGAN says there are many persons in whom it causes great excitement, headache, and even delirium. VOGT admits that in large doses it causes vertigo, heaviness in the head, sleepiness, confusion of head, and headache, and various traces of commencing distraction of the mind; for the senses commence to deceive one; taste and smell are diminished, noises are heard in the ears, flimmering before the eyes and double vision, &c., occur. CULLEN says in full doses it is more apt to cause delirium than Opium; in many cases it induces turbulent and unrefreshing sleep.—PETERS.

CASE 42.—A lady, æt. 25, of a quiet, peaceable disposition, but readily attacked with epilepsy after violent mental emotions, became deranged on the 5th Sept., after having several epileptic attacks on the fifth day after her second confinement. She was treated allopathically for eight days without benefit.

Symptoms.—Violent paroxysms of rage, maltreated her friends, and tore every thing to pieces; turns of anxiety; then she would sing, whistle, laugh, kiss every one, assumed that she was pregnant, and had labor-pains, &c.

Treatment. — *Bellad.* 30 excited, without benefitting her. *Hyosc.* acted better. Verat. 12 and 15, produced sleep and allayed the most violent symptoms; but from April 16 to May 16, Verat., Acon., Helleb., Stramon. and Bell. were given without permanent benefit, and the following condition remained.

Symptoms.—She is extremely excited, rages when one attempts to restrain her, scolds and strikes every one without regard to person; is talkative, and speaks irrationally; weeping in alternation with joyous mood; anxiety and trembling of the limbs—excessive secretion of milk.

Treatment.—Hyosc. was given again, and her malady was arrested instanter; she was, and remained well.

Annals, Vol. p. 67.—MARTINI and SPOHR.

CASE 43.—A woman æt. 37, given to drink, became deranged.

Symptoms.—Face red, hot; look wild; breathing quick and oppressed; she scolds and swears incessantly, tears the clothes off her body, walks about her room at night, strikes powerfully at those around her, and can scarcely be controlled; will neither eat nor drink.

Treatment.—Hyosc. 2, one drop cured her in twenty-four hours.

Archiv, Vol. 19, part. 1, p. 84.—SZOTAR.

CASE 44.—A maiden, æt. 14, not yet menstruated, became deranged after sleeping in the sun.

Symptoms.—Great lasciviousness in words and actions; quickly becomes enraged and strikes at every one; paroxysms of fearfulness and fright, from fear of an imaginary wolf, and of being burned alive.

Treatment.—Bellad. $\frac{}{60}$ in solution, and Hyosc. $\frac{}{30}$ in solution, followed by Sulphur cured her in six weeks. After taking Hyosc. itching over the whole body especially about the genitals occurred.

New Archiv, Vol. 1, part. 1, p. 80.—HAHNEMANN.

CASE 45.—A youth, æt. 23, showed signs of mental derangement quite unexpectedly in the midst of previously uninterrupted good health.

Symptoms.—Unusual restlessness; piercing fixed look; jerking movements of the head, with staring rapidly first here, then there; face pale; pulse quick, but weak; wishes to get out of the room; sees appearances which frighten him; figures which want to carry him off; fowls which are fastened with chains; a great number of large crabs which are driven into the door; general epileptic convulsions for the first time.

Treatment.—Two doses of Bellad. $\frac{}{30}$, without benefit; then Hyosc. 12, and recovery in eight days.

Practical Observations, Vol. 4, p. 4.—THORER.

CASE 46.—A man, æt. 48, deranged for three weeks and treated allopathically without benefit.

Symptoms.—His cadaverous face has a wild, strange look; he speaks incessantly, mostly about religious things; imagines that he is poisoned, or that his mouth smells badly. Occasionally he scolds or weeps, and says that he hears great noises.

Treatment.—After taking eighteen doses of Hyosc. 2, one

dose night and morning, he again became rational and able to work. The remaining bodily ailments were cured by Sulphur.

General Hom. Journ., Vol. 34, p. 323.—HAUSTEIN.

CASE 47.—An unmarried man became deranged.

Symptoms.—He rages, scolds, sings, and babbles night and day, without eating, drinking or sleeping ; he attempts to escape and breaks the window to effect his object ; required the straight-jacket.

Treatment.—Hyosc. $\frac{}{30}$, one drop. Speedy recovery.

General Hom. Journ., Vol. 39, p. 31.—WEBER.

Besides in these cases Hyosc. was given in cases No. 5, 38, 66, 99, 112, 113.

REVIEW.—The published experience of our school is still too limited to enable us to give positive deductions about the action of Hyosc. in mental diseases.

We see it cure an *excited* state in cases No. 42, 43, 44 and 45 ; and fail in others, viz., No. 66, 112 and 113.

It cures a state of *depression* marked by weeping and sobbing in alternation with laughing, restlessness, fear of imaginary animals in cases No. 44 and 45 ; while in internal anxiety and brooding suspicion, in cases No. 5 and 38, it does not help.

It cures lasciviousness in case No. 44, and leaves shameless ness uncured in case 66.

It removed the inclination to dance, hop, and speak irrationally in cases 42 and 113.

As a general thing the remedy cured when several of the above states occurred in alternation, or in connection with epileptic attacks, or in persons subject thereto.

Doses.—Hyosc. 2 in single and repeated doses.
" 6 in single doses.
" 12 in " "
" 30 in solution and repeated doses.

It is also doubtful upon which organs of the brain Hyosc. acts in particular, still it seems to act upon those of combattiveness and destructiveness, amativeness and caution.

18. IGNATIA.

General Remarks.—Ignatia will rarely or never effect a cure in those who are of an unchangeable disposition, neither disposed to fright or vexation.

Organon, p. 237.—Hahnemann.

CASE 48.—A modest maiden, æt. 20, occasionally exhibited signs of mania after the otherwise regular menstrual flow; finally, she lost all consciousness, and was possessed with various fixed ideas.

Symptoms.—She imagines that she is married and pregnant, is tortured in her conscience by imaginary misdeeds; frequently attempts to escape and drown herself; anxiety and fear of death from congestion to the head and heart; she is only quiet when allowed to lie and to indulge in her fancies, and permitted to give vent to them in a complaining tone; whenever disturbed she screams, strikes, and tears whatever she can reach, and constantly vociferates that "she has neglected her duty, broken her oath, &c." Face distorted and death-like; relish for sour things; it is difficult to get her to eat, and after she has eaten she has stings of conscience about it.

Treatment.—Various remedies, viz., Bellad., Hyosc., Stramonium, Aurum, Platina, Verat. were given without benefit; Gratiola effected some improvement for a time, but was followed by such paroxysms of rage that it was difficult to control her; these subsided and again gave place to the former fixed ideas.

Finally, from the continued use of Ignatia for several weeks, at first in the first, then in the sixth, and finally in the ninth dilution, she was entirely restored. Her menses which had been suppressed during her illness returned again.

Archiv, Vol. 15, part. 3, p. 30, and
Ibid. Vol. 16, part. 2, p. 100.—Gross.

CASE 49.—A maiden, æt. 19, of strong, robust constitution and sanguine temperament, fell into a state of hysteric laughing and crying, which passed over into delirium, and which returned paroxysmally.

Symptoms.—Does not know those about her, speaks to them as to imaginary persons, and calls them by strange names; imagines that she stands upon a fearful heighth, from which she cannot descend.

Treatment.—Two doses of Stramon. 9, followed by Ignat. 8, restored her.

General Hom. Journ., Vol. 17, p. 376.—Gross.

CASE 50.—A youth, æt. 20, of sanguine choleric temperament, active imagination, but otherwise strong and well-conditioned, suffered from undeserved but bitter vexation of spirit; he fell into a gastic fever and subsequent melancholy.

Symptoms.—Head heavy; extreme weakness of memory, forgets every thing except his dreams; hears with difficulty, sees as if through a mist; sits staring quietly before him, constantly thinking of his wrongs, and is unconscious of what transpires around him; wishes to be alone; falls asleep late; restless sleep with starting up in fright, and many dreams; pain in the left hypochondrium (spleen), increased by pressure and slow walking; his hair falls off profusely; face cadaverous and sunken; voice trembling, low and attended with distortion of the facial muscles; does not speak willingly; no desire for food or drink; is quickly satisfied and satiated; always cold especially in the evening; very weak and dejected; walks unsteadily and with great caution; bowels and urine rather free.

Treatment.—Ignat. $\frac{}{12}$, one dose cured him perfectly in the course of fourteen days, after being preceded by a visible aggravation lasting five days.

Archiv, Vol. 10, part. 3, p. 104.—Attomyr.

CASE 51.—A maiden, æt. 20, of sanguine temperament, excessively sensitive to joy and sorrow, fell into a state of melancholy after suppression of her menses.

Symptoms.—Indifferent to every thing previously most dear to her; sits still and weeps, imagines various things, especially that she will become deranged; complains of a sensation and crawling all over, as if her limbs were asleep; the pit of her stomach seems insensible to her; sleep dreamy and not refreshing; menses suppressed for two months.

Treatment.—Ignat. $\frac{}{2}$, repeated daily, cured her in the course of several weeks.

Archiv, Vol. 19, part. 1, p. 56.—Gross.

CASE 52.—A delicate maiden, æt. 17, was attacked with spasms and mental derangement after a fright; she was treated allopathically for fourteen days without benefit.

Symptoms.—Does not think that she can be saved; weeps much; has paroxysms of rage, in which she tears her clothes and can scarcely be held by four strong persons.

Treatment.—*Ignat.* 6, one dose daily, cured her in six days.

Archiv, Vol. 19, part. 3, p. 33.

CASE 53.—A woman, æt. 40, had two attacks daily of the following state.

Symptoms.—Anxiety, restlessness as if she had committed some crime, or feared some great misfortune; is overpowered to such a degree that she can scarcely keep from weeping; oppression of her breathing, which seems to come from her stomach up into her throat; lassitude, inability to work; shyness for all persons; these paroxysms lasted several hours. Loss of appetite, scanty stools, and when most constipated, she was most indisposed.

Treatment.—Ignat. first trit. (2 : 100), ten grains in four oz. of water, taken in five doses in the course of twenty-four hours. The paroxysms returned only on the second and third days, then absented themselves, and she recovered perfectly.

Schmid, H. A. and G. p. 126.

Review.—Ignatia is undoubtedly useful in mental derangement, when single notions become fixed ideas. The patients are quiet when not disturbed in their reveries about themselves or other things, and then are in a dejected state, which rapidly changes to excitement when they are disturbed.

Doses.—The lower preparations were generally used in repeated doses.

The action of *Ignatia* upon the organs of conscientiousness and self-esteem is decidedly evident in the above cases.

19. LACHESIS.

CASE 54.—A youth became deranged from excessive study.

Symptoms.—Extraordinary loquacity, which was quite uncommon for him—carries on incessant prologues in the choicest expressions, but changes rapidly from one subject to another, and treats of the most heterogenous matters. He is proud and suspicious of his friends.

Treatment.—Lachesis $_{30}$ cured him quickly.

Archiv, Vol. 14, part. 1, p. 7.—Gross.

20. LYCOPODIUM.

General Remarks.—It is useful against melancholy, sorrow, anxiety with dolefulness, lachrymose state, and fear of being alone.

Hahnemann, Chron. Dis. Vol. 4.

CASE 55.—A woman, æt. 30, suffering for several years with excessive conscientiousness, received Verat., Ac.-phosph. and Pulsat. without benefit.

Symptoms.—Scrupulous anxiety and conscientiousness, which rob her of all peace of mind; the anxiety occurs regularly every afternoon at 4 o'clock, and lasts until 8 P. M.

Treatment.—Lycopod. $\frac{}{30}$, effected a cure in fourteen days.

Archiv, Vol. 18. part. 2, p. 12.—B. in D.

21. NUX-VOMICA.

General Remarks.—*a*) Nux often proves more useful than Aurum against the peculiar melancholy with disgust for life, which leads to suicide; its good effects are often visible in a few, always in ten days; *dose*, from first to sixth dilution.

Hygea, Vol. 2, p. 33.—Ægidi.

b) It is most suitable in melancholy depending on abdominal derangement; especially when the signs of bodily derangement continue unchanged, notwithstanding the active condition of the mental trouble; or when the depressed state of the ganglionic system occasions a still greater disturbance of the abdominal organs than was present at first.

Hartmann, upon use of Nux-vom. p. 132.

c) There is a remarkable resemblance between the action of Nux-vomica and Strychnine, and that of the electric or galvanic influence; thus it is very apt to cause convulsive motions or twitchings similar to electric shocks, when given in large quantities; also prickling as if from needles, or as if sparks were drawn from the skin, or jerks like those produced by electricity; and if an animal under its full influence be touched, it will experience a commotion similar to that of a strong electric shock. In smaller quantities it produces an increase of the irritability, contractility and tonicity of the motor nerves, muscles and contractile tissues of the parts with which it comes in contact, or to which its influence extends; thus if taken before meals it does not interfere with digestion, but probably increases that peculiar peristaltic movement of the stomach, which has for its object the production of a thorough intermixture of the gastric juice with the alimentary mass. This is a very important part of digestion. The fasciculi composing the muscular wall of the stomach are so disposed as to shorten its diameter in every direction, and by the alternate contraction and relaxation of these muscular bands a great variety of motion is produced in the stomach and its contents, sometimes transversely, at others longitudinally; if these movements be checked or lessened materially it has been found that the food lies still and heavy, and that surface only which is in contact with the walls of the stomach undergoes digestion; the residue of the alimentary mass remains as undigested as when it was first taken into the system.—After a few days' judicious use of Nux the appetite becomes increased, and in some cases extraordinarily great; the stools of those suffering from constipation become more free and easily expelled—but if too great a quantity be used, obstinate constipation from excessive contraction of the bowels ensues, and dyspepsia, from a tetanic rigidity, and want of motion of the stomach. Judiciously used, it facilitates the secretion and excretion of bile; wrongly used, the liver becomes small, hard and contracted, its blood vessels and gall bladder empty, and the spleen is diminished in size and rendered paler. Rightly used, it renders the mind more clear and joyous, and it actions more vivid; improperly used, it induces an altered state of the intellect, marked by excitement like that of intoxication, confusion of mind, restlessness, despondency, love of solitude and darkness, an inclination to keep quiet, but an internal irritation of the sensori-motor apparatus, accompanied with anxiety, oppression and uneasiness, agitates the patient, and frightens him into a state of restless nervous activity. Persons under its full influence become extremely irritable and sensitive to all external impressions, so that the slightest causes will often excite excessive petulance; or they may be restless, dejected, languid, chilly and anxious, with a great tendency to drowsiness.—PETERS.

CASE 56.—A lad, æt. 15, excited by disappointed ambition, began to speak and act in all kinds of strange ways.

Symptoms.—He is abashed, says irrational things and does every thing wrong that he undertakes; complains of heaviness of the head, pain in back and abdomen; feels weak and cannot stand up; face alternately red, then pale, with sharpened features; pulse irritated.

Treatment.—After taking Nux $_{\overline{30}}$, perfect health returned in thirty-six hours

Annals, Vol. 1, p. 50.—C. Hartlaub.

CASE 57.—A weaver's widow, æt. 77, came under treatment on Sept. 21. She had had a shock of palsy one and a half years before, and another ten weeks ago so that she was scarcely able to crawl around. For six weeks she has without other known cause, fallen into an anxious state of mind, with fear of recovery; is weak, chilly, sleepless; has scanty hard stools, but great appetite; urinates often and suddenly, at times involuntarily, which is however an old trouble of hers.

Treatment.—Nux-vom. $_{\overline{30}}$, one-third of a drop.

Result.—Four weeks after she informed me that after taking the powder her appetite was increased excessively, and all other symptoms diminished in proportion, except her urinary trouble, which still remained in a lesser degree.

H. Hartlaub, Private cases.

CASE 58.—A lad, æt. 18, previously always healthy, after suffering for a long time with a decayed tooth had it extracted, and then although free from pain, fell into a state of melancholy, in which he constantly spoke about his tooth. He was treated allopathically for two months, and had an artificial tooth inserted, without benefit to his state of mind.

Symptoms.—Dec. 10, the patient has locked himself up in a room, and only opened it after much entreaty, but immediately took refuge in the farthest corner of the room, on perceiving a physician; eyes cast down, answered but few questions, and constantly spoke about his tooth; all noise and every kind of employment is distasteful to him; he sat about the whole day without employment, weeping and complaining of anxiety; he had some appetite, and his bodily functions were well performed.

Treatment.—Arsen. $_{\overline{30}}$, one dose every evening, for five days without benefit; then Nux-vom. $_{\overline{12}}$, six doses, one to be taken every evening.

Result.—Improvement sat in at once; the anxiety and dejection were entirely gone by Dec. 19, and he commenced to work again. After taking six doses more of Nux, one dose every other day, he was entirely restored.

Records of the L. Society.—Schulz.

N. B.—See *case* 113. Several remedies were required to complete the cure, but Nux removed the following

Symptoms:—Confusion of the head, sensation as if the brain would be pressed asunder; slight movements of the bowels every other day, in place of previous obstinate constipation; morning erections and excessive sexual desire, together with irritability, rudeness, and crossness.

Review.—The most common causes of disorder in the above cases were: mental influences, especially, continuous men tal employment, night watching, &c.; also excessive coffee drinking.

The groups of symptoms against which Nux was used with benefit in the above cases, as well as in cases No. 107, 108, 110, 112, 113, are marked by a depressed state of mind, with self-torture about fixed ideas; the patients torment themselves about injured honor, scruples of conscience, household cares, and speak constantly of one thing. To these are added absurd actions and sexual excitement.

The disorder is present not only in the mind, but various bodily ailments occur in connection.

Doses used.—Nux was used successfully in both high and low dilutions; in single doses, and repeated. In case 108, it was given in alternation with Verat.; in No. 112, between Opium and Stramon.

It seems to act upon the organs of *Amativeness*, Acquisitiveness, Caution, and Conscientiousness.

22. NUX-MOSCHATA.

General Remarks.—This remedy was more used in olden times than at present. Notwithstanding, Helbig's labors, (see Heraklid I.) which have made us well acquainted with both old and new observations about its action, still it has been but little used in the new practice. Its great relation to the activities of the brain are quite remarkable, and it is evidently most indicated when no decided pathologico-anatomical changes are connected with the brain-disorder, and especially in weakness of memory and vision.

Hygea, Vol. 23, p. 256.—Griesselich.

No cures of mental diseases with it have been reported; may our departed colleague's words induce some one to use it in appropriate cases.

23. OPIUM.

General Remarks.—The effects of Opium have so great a similarity with some states of mental derangement, that it must be evident even to the most bigotted, that it cures mental diseases in consequence of its power thus to influence the brains of the healthy.

It requires but a hasty review of the actions of Opium, to become convinced that it acts quite decidedly and peculiarly on the central organ of the nervous system as the source of the mental powers.

Opium produces all the signs of mania; the patient becomes excited, lively, and courageous; a feeling of increased power carries him upwards towards heaven, and heaven seems to descend to him by means of the most pleasant hallucinations and visions; a state of delectable intoxication surrounds the patient with the most fascinating phantasies. All this must be followed by its opposite; dejection follows ecstasy; from misuse of Opium there ensues a state of apathetic idiotcy, with loss of power of will, &c.

Undoubtedly, Opium is most indicated against states of mental excitement and exaltation, and maniacs are more readily cured by it than others, provided it is suited to the whole state of the patient.

Still it may prove useful in states of mental depression; the individuality of the case will decide the matter.

Hygea, Vol. 23, p. 257.—Griesselich.

Note.—According to Wood and Bache, Opium is a stimulant-narcotic, which when taken by a healthy person in a moderate dose, increases the force, fulness, and frequency of the pulse; augments the temperature of the skin, invigorates the muscular system, quickens the senses, animates the spirits, and gives new energy to the intellectual faculties, which it may excite even to intoxication or delirium. In a short time, however, this excitation subsides, a calmness of the corporeal actions, and a delightful placidity of the mind succeed, and the individual insensible to painful impressions, and forgetting all sources of care or anxiety, submits himself to a current of undefined and unconnected, but pleasing fancies; in short, is conscious of no other feeling than that of a quiet and vague enjoyment, and finally in one-half or one hour, all consciousness is lost in sleep. In some persons it produces very peculiar effects, differing from its ordinary actions; thus it may cause even in small quantities, restlessness, headache, and delirium, and even in large doses, it may cause obstinate wakefulness. TROUSSEAU and PIDOUX state that the Opium-sleep may be accompanied or interrupted by painful dreams or reveries, and at times, after it has been used for several days, and its use is then stopped, the patient may be exhausted by the most rebellious sleeplessness, and find it impossible to sleep for several weeks. CHRISTISON says, the effect of a small dose of Opium seems generally to be stimulating in the first instance; the action of the heart and arteries is increased, and a slight sense of fulness is caused in the head. In most persons, the stimulant effect is quite insignificant, still CHRISTISON reports the following experience, repeatedly occurring to a friend of Dr. LEIGH. If in the evening when he felt sleepy, he took thirty drops of Laudanum, he was so enlivened that he could resume his studies; and if when the usual drowsiness again approached, which it did in two hours, he took one hundred drops more, he soon became so much exhilarated, that he was compelled to laugh, sing, and dance, the pulse being full and strong, the temples throbbing violently; but in no long time the customary torpor ensued. By small doses frequently repeated, the stimulus may be kept up for a considerable time in some people, even jaded horsemen and horses may be made to finish fatiguing journeys with great apparent facility, the rider becoming absolutely more active and intelligent. According to VOGT, in the second degree of the action of Opium, there is an enlivening of mental faculties, especially of the passions and imagination, varying according to the character of the individual; the dejected becomes gay; the timid, courageous; the enterprizing, wild and venturesome; the religious becomes a fanatic, or enthusiast; the imaginative are surrounded by numberless beauteous reveries; the lover is lost in sweet dreams, and the gay, dance and sing, &c. According to SCHMID, much depends upon the mental state of the person before taking Opium, if he be melancholic, quarrelsome or enraged, these passions are increased to the highest degree after a slight inebriation from Opium; but if previously contented or gay, it produces an increase of these feelings, and an imperturbable state of dreamy happiness; still the pleasurable feelings are very transitory, and followed by a state of depression and uneasiness, so that the Opium-eater, in order to renew his pleasurable sensations, becomes a very slave to this drug; finally, no refreshing sleep ever visits his eyelids, he never experiences an agreeable dream, everything excites disgust in him, even his Opium, which alone can produce a remission of his sufferings, is taken with repugnance. According to TRINKS, the effects of Opium on the mind, and especially upon the imagination, can hardly be described with words; it is a state of the clearest inward contemplation, which can be carried to the highest degree of clairvoyance, the imagination producing the most delightful and enchanting ideas in quick succession, while the external senses are inactive, and one imagines himself transported from earth to the realms of everlasting bliss. DE QUINCEY, the English Opium-eater, always found Opium to excite or stimulate him for upwards of eight hours; it was a steady, equable glow of pleasure, introducing in his opinion, the most exquisite order, legislation and harmony of the intellectual faculties, communicating serenity and equipoise to all the powers, both active and passive, a healthy restoration to that state which the mind would naturally recover upon the removal of any deep-seated irritation, or pain that had disturbed and quarrelled with the impulses of a heart originally just and good. Opium at first seemed to De Quincey to compose what had been agitated, and to concentrate what had been distracted, to render the diviner part of his nature paramount, to put the moral affections in a state of cloudless serenity, and to shed over all the great light of the majestic intellect; it often led him abroad in delight to public places and theatres, but he admits that these are not the appropriate haunts of the Opium-eater, when in the divinest state incident to his enjoyment. In that state, crowds became an oppression to him, and music even too sensual and gross; he naturally sought solitude and silence as indispensable conditions of those trances or profoundest reveries, which he thought the crown and consummation of what Opium can do for man; it happened more than once that he sat from sunset to sunrise, motionless, and without wishing to move. Ultimately, he took as much as eight thousand drops of Laudanum per day, with the most direful effects, and when he reduced the quantity to one thousand drops, instantaneously as if by magic, the clouds of profoundest melancholy which had rested upon his brain like some black vapors, drew off in one day. Previously, when he lay awake in bed, vast processions passed along in mournful pomp; whatever he did but think of in the darkness, immediately shaped themselves into phantoms of the eye, and were drawn out into insufferable splendor; all these visions were accompanied by deep-seated anxiety and gloomy melancholy, such as are wholly incommunicable by words. He seemed every night to descend into chasms and sunless abysses, depths below depths from which it seemed hopeless that he could ever ascend. Nor did he by waking, feel that he had reascended; the state of gloom which attended these gorgeous spectacles, amounted at least to utter darkness, as of some suicidal despondency. The sense of space, and in the end, the sense of time, were both powerfully affected; buildings, landscapes, &c., were exhibited in proportions so vast, that the bodily eye was not fitted to receive them; space swelled, and was amplified to an extent of unutterable infinity; he seemed to have lived for seventy or one hundred years in one night; the minutest incidents of childhood, or forgotten scenes of later years were often revived; scenes from history or romance, crowds of ladies, festivals, dances passed before his eyes, companies of centurions and roman legions, &c. Dreams of lakes, and silvery expanses of water troubled him, and finally the waters changed their character, from transparent lakes shining like mirrors, they became seas and oceans. Again, a tremendous change, unfolding itself like a scroll through many months, became an abiding torment, and never left him until the winding up of his case. Hitherto, the human face had often mixed up in his dreams, but not despotically, but now what may be called the tyranny of the human face, began to unfold itself; upon the rocking waters of the illusory ocean, the human face began to appear; the sea appeared paved with human faces upturned to heaven; faces imploring, wrathful, despairing, surged upwards by thousands, by myriads, by generations, by centuries, until his agitation was infinite, and his mind tossed and surged with the ocean. Again, his studies of Eastern literature made him tormented by dreams of oriental imagery and mythological torture; tropical heat and sunlight, all creatures, birds, beasts, reptiles, all trees, plants, all usages, appearances and ceremonies common to the East, were crowded into his illusions; he was stared at, hooted at, grinned at, chattered at by monkeys, paroquets and cockatoes; he ran into pagodas, was fixed at the summit, or in secret rooms of temples, for centuries; was transformed into an idol, or priest; was worshipped, or sacrificed; he fled from the wrath of Brahma, and was waylaid by Seeva, or Vishnu, or Isis, &c.; he seemed to have done a deed which the ibis and crocodile trembled at; was buried for a thousand years in stone coffins, with mummies and sphinxes; was kissed by crocodiles; or laid with all unutterable slimy things at the bottom of the Nile. Over every form of delirium, there seemed attached a sense of eternity and infinity, which drove him into an oppression as of madness. The form of the crocodile became as constant as formerly his torture from the human face; he was forced to live with crocodiles; if he escaped, he found himself in Chinese houses with cane tables, sofas, &c., and soon all the feet of the tables and sofas became instinct with life; the abominable head of the crocodile, and his leering eyes looked out at him, multiplied into a thousand repetitions, while he seemed to stand loathing and fascinated, &c., &c. For farther information, the "Confessions" themselves must be consulted—enough has been quoted to give an outline at least, of what may be called *Opium Dream-*, or *Reverie-Insanity.*

On account of the close relation between sleeplessness and insanity, Opium has long been used in the cure of this disease; but of course the experience of different physicians varies. Dr. Woodward says that Opium must be used from a few weeks to some months; that single doses at night are rarely useful, for the system must be kept under the influence of it, in doses repeated every four or six hours. Dr. GALT cured twelve out of fourteen recent cases, with enormous doses of Opium, viz.: from six to twelve grains per dose, two or three times a day, or from one to three grains of morphine, three times a day—he also had Opium mixed with tobacco, smoked in pipes by his patients; he regards his success as unexampled; still in the same year, he cured only fifteen cases of twenty-seven recent admissions, or but little more than one-half. Dr. STRIBLING also gave large doses, viz., one hundred drops of Laudanum every six hours, and cured nineteen cases out of fifty-two new admissions. According to VOGT, in olden times Opium was lauded in mental derangement by VAN SWIETEN, but COX soon proved it to exert a beneficial influence in a few particular cases only, so that justifiable doubts are now indulged against the reputed experience of WENDELSTADT, REIL and others, who claim to have cured mania by large doses of Opium, sufficient to produce sleep. Lately, NEUMANN has advised it in the second period of mental derangement, marked by melancholy rather than frenzy; it is most useful in recent cases not connected with organic changes; in deep-seated cases of hypochondria, hysteria and melancholy, it only affords palliative relief. Dr. WOOD says, want of sleep is the most common cause of insanity, although this in its turn is generally caused by mental emotions; all authors agree that inability to sleep ought never to escape careful observation; excessive watchfulness by day, and restlessness at night, are fraught with danger of insanity to most persons, especially to the already predisposed, and when mental derangement has already occurred, want of sleep is one of its most distressing accompaniments, and contributes greatly to aggravate and sustain insanity, and hence should never be neglected. WOOD says, nothing on the whole is so effectual as Opium; it will often most happily control the maniacal paroxysms, but must be given more freely than in the healthy state of the brain to produce its legitimate effects, viz., quiet and sleep; he has known patients in states of the most violent maniacal excitement, after being put to sleep with Opium, to awake in the morning quite composed and rational; mere nervous irritation, or mental disorder, however violent, is often relieved by it. Still another class of physicians think that narcotics with the insane, generally if not always, act as stimulants, and exercise little or no influence over the sleeplessness of insanity, which they think generally resists all remedies, and only fairly yields when nature fairly tired out by long exertion, sinks exhausted. They would not dare press Opium, Conium or Hyosciamus to the point of producing sleep, as they imagine it would require enough to prove fatal.—PETERS.

CASE 59.—A man fell into a state of mental derangement, with frenzy, from the effects of fright and vexation.

Symptoms.—Great fear of death, and all kinds of fancies annoy him; he sees ghosts and devils, who seek to murder him, in alternation with a comatose state in which he lies unconscious, breathes deeply, and sweats greatly.

Treatment.—*Bellad.* quieted him speedily, but only transiently; Opium cured him quickly.

Archiv, Vol. 5, part. 1, p. 97.—SONNENBERG.

CASE 60.—A man, æt. 84, suffered without known cause, from a peculiar kind of mental derangement.

Symptoms.—He imagined that he no longer lived in his own house and village, but at a place some six miles distant; he stopped all passers by, and wished to go with them to his residence; force he met by force, so that two persons could not prevent him from his purposes; his face glowed from rush of blood to the head, and at times he did not know some of his friends in consequence of a comatose kind of unconsciousness; anxiety, wildness; inclination to sleep without the ability to do so; constipation of several days duration, with meteoritic distension of abdomen; retention of urine from a kind of paralytic condition of bladder; when smoking, he often forgets to draw upon the pipe; with all his disposition to sleep, he had the most active wakefulness. Allopathic treatment had been used in vain.

Treatment.—Opium, one-fourth grain in tincture form, produced quiet night sleep, from which he awaked in full possession of his consciousness.

Annals, Vol. 4, p. 331.—SCHUELER.

CASE 61.—A man, æt. 38, given to onanism since his twelfth year, fell into the extremest despair, on account of his shattered health, followed by perfect idiotic apathy.

Symptoms.—Cannot be induced to rise from his bed, lies quietly there, and pays so little attention to questions, that he must be shaken and pulled to arouse him, when with an expression of perfect mental apathy, he always answers "yes," be it right or wrong; entire want of appetite, no desire for food or drink; whitish coating of tongue; skin moist, pulse normal; urine scanty and high colored, only passed once in twenty-four hours. Attempts to jump out of the bed at times, is refractory and abusive in the evening; at others, can only be made to sit up in bed by much shaking, but cannot be induced to dress himself; must be pushed along; perfect expression of idiocy; trembling of arms and legs.

Treatment—Cold sitz-baths, aided by Sepia and Bellad., were given without effect; then Opium-tinct.-fort, in the proportion of two drops, divided into five powders, was given, one dose every evening, from the 16th Sept. to 10th Oct., when he was perfectly restored.

CASE 62.—A woman, in the climacteric years, of powerful constitution, and subject to nodous gout, fell suddenly into a delirious state during the desquamative stage of erysipelas of face.

Symptoms.—She sits up in bed with disturbed features, pale face, glistening eyes, and dishevelled hair; she speaks incessantly, first in connected, then in an unconnected manner, at times in a low, and others in a loud, strong voice; first she sings, then laughs, or cries, or expresses herself in beautiful or obscene speeches; when she becomes quiet, she either stares fixedly before her, or buries her head under the bed-clothes; she rumples or tears the pillows, so that her hands and arms are in constant activity.

Treatment.—Hyosc. and Stramon. in repeated doses did not help; Morph.-acet. one-sixteenth grain, every two hours, produced quiet in two hours, and the patient awoke the next morning with perfect consciousness.

General Hom. Jour., Vol. 3, part 6, p. 40.—TRINKS.

REVIEW.—Besides in the above cases, Opium was given in cases No. 101 and 112, and relieved the following symptoms, viz. Rapid flow of ideas, sleeplessness, with a kind of stupefaction, (coma vigil,) especially in the evening, and attended with redness of the face and eyes; constipation; speaking confused stuff; pointing at, and fear of imaginary animal forms; anxious starting; jumping up; frenzy, with red face; rigid, glistening, upturned eyes, &c.

The general remarks by GRIESSELICH are corroborated by the individual cases.

Doses.—It was used in the $\frac{}{3}$ dilut.; strong tinct.: and Morph.-acet. one-sixteenth grain, every two hours.

To obtain a clear view of the curative action of such an important medicine as Opium, especially of the organs upon which it acts, it will be necessary to obtain more facts than are included in the above cases. Still the alternations between anxiety, fear and wild excitement, point to the organs of Caution, Destructiveness and Combativeness, being in state of alternating excitement and depression.

24. PETROLEUM.

GENERAL REMARKS.—In anxiety, fearfulness, excited state of mind, scolding, want of memory.

Chron. Diseases, Vol. 4.—HAHNEMANN.

CASE 63.—A plethoric, corpulent man, æt. 50, had been for several months in the following state.

Symptoms.—Irritable, fretful, constantly silent, dejected, close, without pleasure in his previous occupations; heaviness, heat and pain in the head every morning; violent pain in back and sacrum also in the morning; spasmodic eructations; thin, slimy stools, with cutting pains in abdomen; paleness of face, emaciation, profuse night and morning sweats.

Treatment.—Petrol $\frac{}{30}$, one drop daily for several weeks, restored him perfectly.

General Hom. Journ. Vol. 5, p. 306.—KNORRE.

25. PHOSPHOR.

GENERAL REMARKS.—Dejection; fear of being alone; anxiety for the future; disinclination to work.

HAHNEMANN, Chron. Dis. Vol. 5.

CASE 64.—A woman, æt. 49, of choleric sanguine temperament, who had been in an asylum nine years before, on account of mental derangement, had again suffered in like manner for four weeks.

Symptoms.—She destroys whatever she can reach; speaks in a violent, authoritative manner; spits at her attendants; lifts up her clothes without shame, and kisses passionately any one who approaches her; performs foolish actions, and speaks in an unconnected manner; pulse but slightly quickened; tongue whitish; almost sleepless; menses quite scanty, pale and watery.

Treatment.—Acon. Bellad. and Hyosc., were given without benefit; after smelling *Pyosphor* $_{30}$ repeatedly, she was entirely restored in four weeks.

New Archiv, Vol. 2, part. 3, p. 103.—Schmidt.

CASE 65.—A cadet was attacked with frenzied somnambulism and had been treated in an asylum for fourteen months without benefit.

Symptoms.—The paroxysms occur in his sleep and last for two or three hours; he goes about with closed eyes, destroying whatever is in the room; no one dared approach him; when the frenzy is over he lies down, sleeps a few minutes and on waking knows nothing of what has transpired.

Treatment.—Several remedies and magnetism did not benefit him; then Phosphor $_{30}$ was given, one drop morning and evening, and he was cured in fourteen days.

General Hom. Journal, Vol. 16, p. 79.—Hartung.

Review.—In both cases the organ of destructiveness was excited, and in the first case that of amativeness also.

26. PLATINA.

General Remarks.—The timid, silent, and anxious condition which it causes, with fear of death, &c. points to its use in certain forms of melancholy. If to this we add its action upon the uterus, upon the sexual functions, in neuralgia, &c., we can easily divine its adaptation to mental derangement in females, especially in nymphomania and puerperal mania.

CASE 66.—A delicate maiden, æt. 19, who had suffered four years before with eruptions on the head and from fever and ague, had exhibited signs of mental derangement for three years, but for the last half year had menstruated regularly and grown stronger. She had again become deranged for sixteen days.

Symptoms.—She speaks almost incessantly of various things, at times irrationally, at others of things which came before her, of untrueness in love, of her teacher, and of her school-years; she laughed, cried, danced, made faces, gesticulated with her hands, persisted obstinately in her own notions, but without becoming frenzied. Her features were distorted, her eyes fixed, and directed upon one object; she had no desire for food or drink, but devoured whatever was given her in haste.

Treatment.—Ignatia was given without benefit; on the third day she took Platina, which was repeated on the eighth day, after which no sign of derangement occurred until the eighteenth day; but she remained quiet and taciturn; Crocus was given without benefit; on the twenty-ninth day she took Sepia, with improvement on the very next day, and could be dismissed cured on the thirty-sixth day.

Annals of Hom. Hospital, Vol. 2, p. 112.

In another case (see No. 113), Platina relieved the following:

Symptoms.—Griping pain about umbilicus especially in the evening, as if one had drank unfermented beer; notwithstanding frequent urging and pressing in the rectum he did not have a passage every day; was obliged to expel the fæces with much straining; he was forgetful, distracted, often listened attentively to what was said, but in the end knew nothing about it; was dejected, reflective, and had great fear of death; thought himself superior to his wife.

REVIEW.—The organ of *self-esteem* seems to be affected by Platina, as is evident from the cases and symptoms.

27. PULSATILLA.

GENERAL REMARKS.—It is most useful in persons of a bashful, lachrymose disposition, disposed to internal disquiet, and to silent vexation, or at least in those of a mild and yielding temper.

Mat. Med. Pur. Vol. 2, p. 274.—HAHNNEMANN.

CASE 67.—A woman, æt. 45, a-menstrual, had suffered for several weeks with mental derangement from vexation.

Symptoms.—She is in constant anxiety, has palpitations, is afraid of every one, and will be seen by no one, regards every body as her enemies, despairs of every thing, weeps readily, and has no faith in any one. Her face was pale and sallow; her look dull and desponding; she had no appetite, but much thirst; her limbs seemed asleep; she was tired and weak, and could not sleep at night for anxiety and timidity.

Treatment.—Pulsat. $_{12}$, one dose, restored her in a few days.

Annals, Vol. 1, p. 62.—RUECKERT.

CASE 68.—A man, æt. 30, strong, choleric, and inclined to drink.

Symptoms.—Throbbing pain in the brain; dimness of vision as if he were looking through a sieve; when in the dark, or when he closed his eyes every variety of frightful forms appeared to him, and at which he struck as if they were evil spirits, or made the sign of the cross to protect himself.

Treatment.—Pulsat. cured him in ten days.

Archiv, Vol. 19, part. 1, p. 89.—SZTAR.

CASE 69.—A youth, æt. 16, had suffered for ten days with a kind of religious mania.

Symptoms.—Eyes unsteady; lips bluish-red, memory weak; stings of conscience with regard to religion and women; he has violent palpitations whenever he sees a woman, but is filled with anger and disgust for them, so that he must fly in order to keep from injuring them; he regards all women as bad, and thinks that his soul is in danger in their presence; breathing short and oppressed, painful pressure on chest.

Treatment.—He was cured in fourteen days by Pulsat. $_{12}$.

General Hom. Journ. Vol. 13, p. 286.—MALAISE.

CASE 70.—A woman, æt. 40, had suppression of her lochia ten days after her fifth fortunate delivery, and mania set in.

Symptoms.—She is shy and fearful, and looks constantly about her; as often as she sees a man, she hides herself under the bed-clothes, or jumps out of bed and hangs the sheets and quilts over her head; glistening eyes, rigid look; excessive sensitiveness of the uterine region to the slightest pressure; the suppressed lochia returned at the end of eight days.

Treatment.—Eight doses of Pulsat., restored the lochia and perfect health in the course of a week.

CASE 71.—A young woman, æt. 19, naturally, large, strong, active, lively and good natured, became desponding, suspicious and taciturn during the eighth month of the first pregnancy, had disturbed features, and entire sleeplessness.

Symptoms.—She looked about in the yard for her bed; hid herself in a corner to escape a little gray man who wished to tear off her leg.

Treatment.—*Bellad.* $\frac{}{30}$ was given with transient benefit only, but Pulsat. $\frac{}{15}$ quickly and permanently removed the whole trouble.

Archiv, Vol. 9, part. 1, p. 113.—Bethmann.

CASE 72.—A maiden, æt. 18, of sanguine temperament, but who had been chlorotic several years before, and still had not yet menstruated, although she often had various kinds molim. menstrual., became dejected and tired of life after a fit of vexation.

Symptoms.—Frequent frontal headache; sallowness of face, dark rings around the eyes; bitter bad taste in the mouth; disgust for meat and bread; nausea, with pain in stomach, at times vomiting of bilious slimy substances; frequent profuse bleedings from nose; piercing pain in the side when coughing, with expectoration of frothy blood; palpitation, difficult respiration; few and scanty stools; frequent cutting pains in abdomen; heaviness of the legs; feeling as if all the limbs were bruised; swelling of the backs of the feet; anxious dreams; thinks with much pleasure of drowning herself; desponding, and often bursts into tears; dissatisfied with every thing; easily angered; abusive; very fearful, anxious and tired of life.

Treatment.—Pulsat. $\frac{}{15}$ brought on menstruation in a few days, and restored her former hilarity.

Archiv, Vol. 12, part 3, p. 99.—Attomyr.

CASE 73.—A robust woman, æt. 20, of quiet gentle disposition, had suffered for several years after her first confinement, with irregularity of the menses, and anxiety and internal restlessness, so that she did not know what to do.

Symptoms.—Heat and congestion to the face and head; headache, oppression of the heart, and pain in the small of the back; sleepless nights in consequence of great anxiety, and anxious uneasiness in head; does not believe that she can be saved and thinks that her only salvation is in constant prayer.

Treatment.—*Pulsat.* in small doses relieved her in a few days.

Annals, Vol. 2, p. 243.—BETHMANN.

REVIEW.—In all the cases in which Pulsat. was of essential benefit, we find a decided state of depression, a form of melancholy marked by an anxious, scrupulous, lachrymose condition; or the patient sees frightful figures, which frighten him, or believes that he cannot be saved; is tired of life, thinks about drowning, and dislikes society.

The stings of conscience in case 69, when one approaches a female are peculiar and characteristic.

In several cases the mental disease was connected with pregnancy, confinement, or irregular menstruation.

In Case 27, Pulsat. was not beneficial against symptoms which seemed to indicate it, but the mental disorder consisted in an anxious state about her affairs, belief that she must starve, and inclination to run away.

Doses.—In several instances the quantities are unfortunately not mentioned.

The organ of *caution* is the one upon which Pulsat. seems to act most decidedly. Its relations to other organs, such as conscientiousness, hope, marvellousness, &c., can only be settled by more numerous observations.

28. PLUMBUM.

The Lead mental- or cerebral-derangement has been so fully elaborated by TANQUEREL, and the remedy according to homœopathic principles promises so much in the cure of many of the most intractable cases of insanity, that I [PETERS] have deemed it advisable to include Plumbum among the articles here treated of; it being expressly understood that the whole is but a transcript and condensation from TANQUEREL.

"The cerebral lead-disease may occur in a sudden and unforeseen manner, or be announced by some functional trouble of the brain, such as violent headache, either general or partial, and often limited to the forehead; these pains in the head may vary in their nature and intensity, and are generally accompanied by dizziness and sense of intoxication.

"Sometimes it is preceded by wakefulness or by disturbed sleep, agitated and interrupted by dreams and fanciful imaginings ; the unfortunate patients often awake suddenly full of fear, leap from their beds, and escape or injure themselves.

"At other times the approach of the disease is preceded by dimness of sight, tingling in the ears, blindness, squinting, dilatation, or contraction of the pupils ; or by a strange, astonished, dull or pensive look. Some patients have a great fullness or heaviness, with great pain in the orbits of the eyes.

"In another class of patients the moral sensibility is deranged, many have presentiments of sickness, sadness, an extraordinary and causeless uneasiness, or become silent and indifferent to all the objects which surround them. Others become morose and weep without cause, some have their minds agitated, and change their place without ceasing, trying to divert their thoughts, and to remove themselves from the sudden and great terrors which beset them. Some have a stupor, an undefinable uneasiness from embarrassment, and slowness of ideas and motions. About one case in three and a half of lead mental derangement have some of these precursive symptoms ; still, an unusual, strange, astonished, dull or pensive look, taking place suddenly is the most common phenomenon which announces the approach of this disease.

"Lead paralysis precedes the cerebral disease about once in four times ; severe pains in the limbs or lead colic sometimes cease suddenly and the lead mental disease then sets in ; it oftener commences in the night than the day.

"The symptoms of lead mental disease vary very much, delirium, coma, or convulsions may recur separately or combined ;" in short TANQUEREL prefers a mode of describing it similar to that which has been adopted by authors who have written on mental alienation.

1) DELIRIOUS FORM.

This occurred eighteen times in seventy-two cases ; the delirium may be light or profound, partial or general, continued or remittent, and even intermittent, and be accompanied or not by loss of one of the senses. Finally and especially, the delirium may be *tranquil* or *furious*.

A) TRANQUIL DELIRIUM.

"Sometimes the patient seems astonished, his features being at the same time immoveable and his eyes fixed; or he seems absorbed in profound thought, with composed features. TANQUEREL has seen three persons whose eyes were turned upwards, with open mouth and every feature immoveable, as if fallen into a trance.

"Some have a sardonic smile, or laugh without ceasing and without cause; others weep frequently and have an air of sadness and melancholy impressed on the whole person. In many the face is gentle and benevolent, or hard and discontented; some have an air of stupor, with their features weighed down and their eyes fixed and haggard. This state of countenance often varies with prodigious rapidity, so that a single person may offer in a few hours all the varieties of expression first mentioned.

"If they be questioned about the thoughts which they have in connection with so varied a physiognomy, they will answer at random; it will be seen that their words, and consequently their thoughts, are entire strangers to the expression of their countenances. At first the patient may reply like a sane man, and in such a way that one is often in doubt whether there is really any mental disease. But let the physician pursue the conversation, passing rapidly from one idea to another, and the patient will suddenly become wandering, and put together words and phrases without meaning; but soon he returns, especially if aided, to a succession of rational ideas, still by-and-bye the delirium will return again. Sometimes the patient wanders every few moments; at others not for hours, or even for a day, and in the interval is perfectly rational." These variations of physiognomy and speech, and singular union of reasonable and wandering ideas are so frequent that it occurred to TANQUEREL to establish the diagnosis of lead mental disease upon them, and with success.

"Some patients, when questioned, do not reply immediately; they seek for expressions, use one word for another, or again their reply may be correct; they do not always look towards the questioner; sometimes they do not appear to understand what is said to them, and it may be necessary then to speak very loud, to arouse them gently and fix their attention; sometimes they use the same word or words in answer to the most varied questions.

"If left alone they very often speak to themselves, call their neighbors or absent persons; some reply to all that speak, or all that they imagine they hear speak around them. Their speech is very often free and the voice clear; but some murmur unintelligible words between their teeth, or else their voice is so much weakened, that their words cannot be understood. They have periods of entire silence, and some of talking; alternately gay or sad, loquacious or silent, or delirious. The subject of the delirium varies much, and often has no predominant character, still it often has been observed that the same idea returns with several fits of talking, and then the subject of the wandering changes.

"Some patients throw about their arms, uncover themselves, wish to go away, not recognising the place in which they are; leave their own beds to lie in another's; throw themselves against the furniture which they meet, and know but imperfectly the persons around them, although they generally return to their beds with the aid of their keepers, and without resistance.

"Some have a slight trembling of the arms and muscles of the face, find difficulty in using their limbs, or in speaking and stutter.

"Hallucinations of sight and hearing, have been observed in some; many think that they see frightful objects which cause them to leap from their beds; others hear delightful music, which charms away their weariness; one patient imagined that he saw a woman come every morning to provoke him, placing herself sometimes before, sometimes behind him, and saying the most insulting things to him; one day he impatiently seized the poles which supported his curtains, thinking to catch this woman; all this he related with a tone of calm assurance and belief."

B) FURIOUS LEAD DELIRIUM.

"In this variety, the eyes are often wide open, threatening, furious, or haggard; the features contracted, and excitement marks every act of the patient.

"They cry, vociferate, swear, threaten, storm, tear their garments, break the bonds which hold them in bed, run in other rooms, attack the people they meet on their way, try to beat, tear, and bite them, and address them with the grossest invectives. If they are not restrained, they continue to enact the most violent manœuvres; some cast themselves from the windows or throw themselves against the walls or furniture with such violence as to destroy life. If a straight-jacket is put on, their fury is redoubled, they stamp their feet, agitate their limbs, suddenly rise in a convulsive, or tetanic manner, stiffen themselves, and display a strength which can only be overcome by three or four men.

"Once chained, they often grind their teeth, spit at their assistants, call for scissors or knives, tear at their bonds, and exhaust themselves in vain efforts. Constraint agitates and enrages some, who become calm when unbound; sometimes the pain produced by blisters, produces the same excitement. In many, this furious delirium is accompanied by a spasmodic contraction of the muscles of the face, rolling of the eyes, grinding of the jaws, jerking of the tendons, or trembling of the limbs.

"Terrors, visions, and hallucinations, often besiege the minds of these persons; some cry, weep, lament like children, because they imagine they see pistols pointed at their heads to kill them; they supplicate and implore help to remove these causes of despair. Some abuse the nurse, whom they imagine has been sent to poison them, they then may touch the medicine, but suddenly repulse it with great violence. An old soldier thought he saw a regiment of cavalry ready to attack him; some think they have destroyed themselves, by throwing themselves from a more or less elevated place, &c.

"These patients in general talk much, have an incoherent association of words and ideas, and their speech is reprimanding, abrupt, stuttering, and often unintelligible. They may have convulsive agitation of the muscles of the larynx; talking and fury generally return in simultaneous fits; from some minutes to hours, or days and nights may pass in this furious state; then a short calm ensues, but the fury soon returns.

"The face is usually of an earthy yellow, and is sometimes slightly flushed, but has not that warm coloring which is generally remarked in inflammations of the brain. Sometimes the tongue and teeth present appearances which might be thought to indicate typhoid fever; the mouth may become dry, the tongue furred, chapped, or trembling, while blackish sordes cover the teeth and gums; if the pulse be accelerated and irregular, and the body be covered with sweats, it would be easy to mistake this state for that of a grave fever of bad character.

"The delirium may remain incomplete for some hours or days, and then consist only of an illusion of the external senses, and an incoherence of ideas, which produces a singular confusion in the names of persons and places; but as soon as the delirium is completely developed, it proceeds with an incredible irregularity; it exalts and increases, then diminishes in intensity from one moment to another, without any order; there may be remissions marked by a certain lucidness of ideas, but a sudden attack of violent delirium is apt to return. From time to time, the patients are affected with drowsiness, as if asleep, but this somnolent state does not last long, usually after a few minutes or an hour, the delirium returns; the disease is characterized by this alternate delirium and drowsiness; a long duration of somnolency, if it does not become comatose, is of good augury. The whole disease is apt to commence with tranquil delirium; soon fits of fury are added; finally somnolency occurs, and delirium succeeds it at longer or shorter intervals; at length true sleep follows, and the patient is almost restored to reason—from this time on, the tendency to sleep is strong, and almost irresistible; finally he seems merely fatigued, his limbs ache, and he has an expression of surprise."

Enough has been quoted to convince every Homœopathist of the great importance of lead as a remedy against insanity—and DANA's translation of TANQUEREL on Lead-diseases is easily to be obtained by every American and English physician. It only remains for me to add, that Plumbum should be faithfully tried in obstinate and chronic cases of mental derangement; there is literally little or no hope from the ordinary allopathic and homœopathic remedies. The best old school authorities concur in admitting, that in cases of insanity of more than twelve months' standing, the probability of recovery is less than one in four. The mean of recoveries from mental derangement of all ages, is from thirty-three to forty-seven per cent., leaving fifty-three to sixty-seven per cent. to become incurable and chronic—here is a large field for the use of Plumbum. ESQUIREL in 2005 cases, had 604 recover during the first year; 497 during the second year; only 86 in the third year, and only 41 cases in the seven following years, leaving 777 cases, or about 30 per cent., entirely and hopelessly uncured. In March, 1844, in the Hanwell Asylum, of 984 cases, only 30 were regarded as curable. Shall nothing be done for these numerous sufferers?

If there be some or any truth in the homœopathic law, Plumbum should prove useful in some of these chronic intractable cases, especially as no organic disease is generally present in them, for it may be asserted without fear of contradiction, that no pathologist could in nine-tenths of the cases of mental derangement which prove fatal, take upon himself to say whether the person examined had been of sound mind during life, or not.

Again, the Paralysis of the Insane is generally regarded as incurable. Plumbum is also homœopathic here.

Again, Epilepsy is the most common form of convulsions by which the brain manifests the deleterious action exercised upon it by lead. TANQUEREL has observed thirty-six cases of lead epilepsy—the connection between mental derangement and convulsions is well known, and the difficulty of effecting cures in such cases is equally public. WOODWARD says, that "Stramonium is most useful in cases of insanity, coupled with epilepsy; it does not cure, but often the symptoms are greatly diminished in force and frequency by it; in some cases, the epileptic attacks are entirely suspended by it." From the known tendency of Lead to produce paralysis, and its consequent antagonism to convulsions, it has often been a source of astonishment, that old school physicians have not more frequently tried it in convulsive disorders.

Finally, Lead produces a form of idiocy similar to that which succeeds mania or monomania; but lead-idiocy has this peculiarity, that its intensity varies in an extraordinary manner, from moment to moment, from day to day. To-day the patient is careless and indifferent to all that passes around him, lies immovably in his bed, his face dull and without expression; to-morrow he will be bright, pleased, and grateful; but on the third day, this amelioration disappears, and the patient returns to his vegetative life. Hence it might render a fixed idiocy, mobile and transient.

28. RHUS-TOXICODENDRON.

CASE 74.—A maiden, æt. 18, rather short and thick set; somewhat crooked, with the spine bent to the right side, in consequence of a fall, when a child of nine months old.

As a child, and occasionally now, she had eruptions upon the scalp; had had measles, scarlet fever, and small pox; learnt rapidly in school; had not yet menstruated. Three years ago, after a fright, she was taken with heaviness in the forehead, and eight days after, showed signs of mental derangement; did not wish her mother to look at her, was mistrustful, and had a dislike for all company; at times would come in from the street, thinking that everybody looked at her very strangely or curiously; then would sit quite alone; her eyes were dim and sensitive to light.

This kind of attack had occurred three times, had always lasted six weeks, but this time had already continued eight weeks, but without being attended with the affection of the eyes.

Symptoms.—She often weeps without cause, imagines that people talk about her, that she does not earn or deserve anything; acts childishly; heaviness of the head; if she lies with it low she has throbbing in the temple of the side on which she lies; diarrhœa easily excited by cold; cough for eight days, especially on lying down, with piercing pain in epigastrum; coldness of hands and feet; frequent rumbling in the bowels.

Treatment.—*Bellad.* $_{\overline{30}}$ was given for fifteen days without benefit; then Rhus $_{\overline{30}}$, and in six days more, her mother reported her as entirely different, as almost well; she was only somewhat reflective after going to church. During the three months more that she was under observation, she remained quite well.

H. HARTLAUB.—Private cases.

29. SECALE-CORNUT.

GENERAL REMARKS.—The very numerous observations which have been made with Ergot, leave no doubt but that it is a very powerful remedy, which may prove very useful in mental disorders.

Secale is a decided spinal remedy, and may effect great good in mental diseases, when connected with paralysis and paralytic states, intermixed with cramps, especially where corresponding disturbances are found in the sexual system. GUISLAIN regards it as a remedy against nymphomania; it should also be borne in mind in those mental derangements of men which arise from excessive losses of semen, in the melancholy of onanists, and of those who suffer from diurnal pollutions.

Hygea, Vol. 23, p. 263.—GRIESSELICH.

30. SEPIA.

GENERAL REMARKS.—Dejection of spirits, and weeping; melancholy and sadness; anxiety, in the evening in bed; disinclination to labor, indifference towards his family.

HAHNEMANN, Chron. Diseases, Vol. 5.

It was given, but without farther remarks, in cases No. 66, 100, 105, 106.

In case 66, after using Platina, the following state remained:

Symptoms.—She is taciturn, scarcely speaks a word without being aroused to it; sits for hours with her knitting; always answers correctly, but very abruptly.

Treatment.—After taking Sepia, she was better, even on the next day, and was soon completely restored.

31. DATURA-STRAMONIUM.

GENERAL REMARKS.—*a*) I speak from experience when I proclaim the great virtues of Stramonium, when used homœopathically against natural mental diseases, similar to those excited by it.

HAHNEMANN, Mat. Med. Pur. Vol. 3, p. 288.

b) From the effects of Stramonium, the illusions before the eyes always appear *dark* colored, while from the full effects of Bellad., they are always *fiery* and *shining*. Finally, and which I regard as most important, and hitherto too much neglected, the patient under the influence of Bellad., in the majority of instances, is in a *joyous* state of mind; or even when he is depressed, the illusions do not strike him with *fear* and *fright*, as those excited with Stramon., do.

Hygea, Vol. 4, p .115.—KURTZ.

c) The excitement of *fear* is undoubtedly a predominant effect of Stramon.

The remarkable mobility, haste, and precipitancy which is manifest in the Stramonium disease, is worthy of attention; the mental disorder is marked by an unusual agility.

Hygea, Vol. 23, p. 254.—GRIESSELICH.

NOTE.—*d*) A man was induced to drink some wine in which Stramonium seeds were steeped; he was then robbed, and became unconscious for twenty-four hours; he was found wandering in the woods, delirious and incoherent, with staring eyes and oppressed breathing, and was regarded as a madman for some time. In another case, observed by Dr. TRAILL, the patient had a flushed face and glistening eyes, with incoherent speech, so that his friends supposed him to be intoxicated; subsequently he fell into a strain of incessant, unconnected talking, like one demented. Dr. DROSTE, from infusion of 125 seeds, saw delirium followed by fatal coma. DUGUID reports the case of a man who drank a decoction of three thorn-apples; he was seized with great vertigo almost immediately, with stammering, and general torpor for seven hours, from which he aroused in a furious delirium. FRANK saw a man become deranged for eighteen days, after taking a large quantity.

The effects of Stramonium on children, have been more frequently observed. FOWLER saw a little girl, who had swallowed one and one-half drachms of the seeds, become maniacal in less than two hours, with spectral illusions, interrupted by some intervals of lethargic sleep. Another child, besides other symptoms, was remarkable from assuming an attitude and expression as if about to tumble into a fit. VICAT and SWAINE observed furious delirium in two cases. In three children treated by ALIBERT, there was delirium, restlessness, constant incoherent talking, dancing and singing, attended with fever, and flushing of the face. YOUNG witnessed some convulsions in one case. KAAUW BOERHAAVE has reported with great minuteness, the case of a young girl, who was induced by a human fiend to take the powder of Stramonium in coffee, in order to seduce her; the effects were, redness of the face, delirium, nymphomania, loss of speech, fixing of the eyes, tremors, convulsions, and coma. RUST gives a case of a child with spasmodic closing of the eyes and jaws, spasms of the back, and complete coma. Dr. DUFFIN'S child, æt. 2 years, swallowed about 100 seeds without chewing them; she soon became fretful, like a person intoxicated, her face was flushed, pupils dilated, speech incoherent, she had wild spectral illusions, and furious delirium, followed by spasms of the throat, and croupy breathing, coma, with violent spasmodic agitation of the limbs, occasional tetanic convulsions, &c. A girl, æt. 4 years, ate a few seeds; soon had noises in her ears, and sleeplessness; she sang, wept, and spoke confused nonsense incessantly; her eyes were lively; pupils dilated and insensible to light; she snatched continually in the air as if to grasp something; she was unable to stand, her knees knocked together, and she staggered and fell about like one drunk. A boy, aged 5 years, ate more than a drachm of the seeds; in an hour he was much excited, and rather delirious, clinging to the woman who had him on her lap, under the seeming fear of some pressing danger; his pulse was 120, face flushed, eyes brilliant, pupils dilated, and he had convulsive movements of the limbs and neck, with frothing at the mouth. After evacuant treatment, the symptoms were relieved, except the tossing of the limbs, which increased, with great flushing of the face; his skin was intensely red; a state of extreme vigilance succeeded that of terror, and lasted for a day or two. Ten children, from seven to fourteen years of age, ate of the seeds; they all became deranged and furious, and fell into a state of persistent insomnia; at first they had an extreme aversion to liquids, but afterwards drank with avidity. MEIGS observed a girl, æt. 2 years, who had taken a large quantity of the seeds; very soon, singular symptoms set in, viz., gaiety, delirium, hallucinations, disordered vision, redness of the face, more intense than that of the most confluent scarlet fever, &c.

WOOD and BACHE say, that it causes vertigo, headache, dimness or perversion of vision, confusion of thought, delirium, and a kind of intoxication; inclination to sleep is sometimes but not uniformly induced; the delirium is sometimes of the furious, and sometimes of a whimsical character. VOGT asserts that it causes a similar affection of the brain and senses, with the same great congestion towards the head, like that caused by *Bellad.*, but that the Stramonium delirium is much more apt to be attended with spasms. TROUSSEAU and PIDOUX state, that large doses caused vertigo, slight stupor, disordered vision, agitation, spasms, furious or gay, or sad delirium, continual hallucinations, obstinate insomnia, and high fever; the delirium and blindness may last for some days or weeks; the delirium is at times gay, at others sad, but is always accompanied by singular hallucinations, and fantastic visions—hence in old times, Stramonium received the name of *Herbe aux sorciers*, or *Herbe au diable*, and because it was used by pretended magicians to intoxicate, and produce fantastic illusions in those superstitious persons who wished to witness their incantations, or assist at the so-called witches-SABBAT. CHRISTISON says, on account of its intoxicating properties, it was once used extensively in Germany, to cause loss of consciousness and lethargy, preparatory to the commission of various crimes. GMELIN informs us that it was used by prostitutes and thieves to put persons asleep, in order to violate or rob them; by procuresses to take away from their noviciates all sense of natural shame; by old whore-mongers, to seduce young maidens; by criminals, to render their watchers insensible; by false wives, to prevent their husbands from detecting their misdeeds; in short, for exactly the same purposes that gin, whiskey and Opium are used in England and other countries. On account of its specific action on the sexual system, it was also used to cause illusory pleasures in silly lovers, and in the composition of love-philtres. Finally, in the French law annals, there is the record of a band of thieves, called *Endormeurs*, who operated by mixing powdered seeds of Stramonium with tobacco, to be smoked in pipes, with which they plied their victims until stupid and delirious.

It seems very singular in the face of the hot opposition to Homœopathy, that a drug like Stramonium should be used in mental derangement by old school physicians; still it was introduced into general practice by the celebrated STORCK of Vienna, as particularly beneficial in mania; his original recommendation in 1762 was founded upon two cases:

1st CASE.—A young girl, æt. 12, had been deranged for two years; she took one demi-grain of Ext. Stramonium, night and morning, with improvement in the course of three weeks; it was continued for two months more, and the dose very slightly increased; she gradually and perfectly recovered her reason in that time.

2d CASE.—A woman, æt. 40 odd years, had had vertigo for two years, and gradually became deranged, with occasional paroxysms of frenzy. Dose, one grain of Extract, gradually increased to three grains, once a day; decided improvement in four days, and perfect restoration of intelligence in a month. She died some time after, and the brain was found infested with hydatids, yet she had had no return of mania after taking Stramonium.

These cases led STORCK to use the memorable words which so often have given comfort and courage to HAHNEMANN and his disciples: "Si Stramonium turbando mentem adfert insaniam sanis, au non licet experiri, nun insanien tibus et mente captis turbando, mutandoque ideas, et sensorium commune adferret mentem sanam et convulsis tolleret contrario motu convulsiones. See STORCK libell. de Aconito, Stramon. et Hyosciam. VINDOB. WOOD and BACHE say that, subsequent observations have confirmed STORCK's estimate of Stramonium in mania, and that numerous cases are on record, in which benefit has accrued from it. VOGT says it was found useful by STORCK, SCHMALZ and BARTON, especially when the attack of mania was caused by mental influences, and appeared in paroxysms, separated by lucid intervals—said to be more frequently useful than Bellad. TROUSSEAU says, a sufficiently great number of facts confirm the utility of Stramon. against mania; SCHNEIDER slowly cured a lady, æt. 50, with demonomaniac melancholy; also a lady deranged after confinement; BERNARD saw an accidental cure of a chronic mania, also, in a lady after confinement; she took some of the seeds through inadvertence, had all the signs of severe poisoning, and was thus cured. AMELUNG cured four cases of acute mania after the first violence of the symptoms had been subdued by other means. The experience and reasoning of MOREAU of Tours, is similar to that of STORCK and HAHNEMANN, he says he uses it in monomania with hallucinations, because Stramon. causes hallucinations, and imagines that it cures these in the same manner as many local irritating remedies cure irritations of the eye, skin, urethra, &c. BAYLE collected fifty-five cases of mania, treated by STORCK, SCHMALZ, RAZOUX, REEF, MEYER,

OBDELIUS, DURANDE, MARET, BERGIUS, GREDING, SCHNEIDER, BERNARD, and AMELUNG; a considerable majority were either cured or relieved; still PEREIRA thinks that the cases in which it proves of service are very rare, while those in which it will prove injurious, will be found very common; while CULLEN admits that he has not, and doubts if any other person has learned to distinguish the cases in which it is proper to use it. With the hints derived from STORCK, HAHNEMANN, and MOREAU, we add those derived from WOODWARD, of the Worcester Asylum; he says that Stramonium acts favorably in some cases, and disappoints in others, but it is most useful in cases complicated with epilepsy; it may not cure, but often the symptoms will be greatly diminished in severity and frequency, while in some cases, the epileptic attacks will be entirely suspended; still we have seen that VOGT says Stramon. is more apt to cause convulsions than *Bellad.*, and in the cases of poisoning, we have quoted, attacks of convulsions were quite frequent. Again, according to WENDT, *Stramon.* stands in a near specific relation to the nerves of the sexual organs, and in large doses, causes insatiable increase of lust and shameless lasciviousness, which effects may be regarded as characteristic of its action, as that of Phosphor, or Cantharides; still WENDT, who was no homœopathist, found it especially useful in mental diseases, arising from disorder of the sexual functions, from onanism, excess in sexual congress, &c., actually cured a case of nymphomania with it. —PETERS.

CASE 75.—A woman, æt. 62, had been deranged during her confinement with her first child, and had had four more repetitions of mental disease; the last time after an interval of health of six years' duration; eight days before her last sickness she had an attack of chills, which were repeated on the outbreak of the mental disease, six days ago.

Symptoms.—She sits in bed and speaks incessantly and vehemently, sometimes for a quarter of hour at a time; wishes to escape; then she will sit perfectly quiet for three or four hours together; occasionally she supports her head upon her hand, as if she had pain in it; complains of her abdomen; costive; urine passed unvoluntarily at times; sleeps but little; but eats and drinks.

Treatment.—She received two doses of Bellad. $\frac{1}{30}$, one-third of a drop per dose, in the course of forty-eight hours, without evident benefit; the paroxysms of mania became so violent that she was put into a straight-jacket, and required several men to watch her. Then Stramonium was given in like doses, four times, at intervals of four days. The first dose was soon followed by an aggravation lasting three and a half hours, succeeded by perfectly clear, healthy understanding for two hours; the next day, there were several violent paroxsms of no long duration, but interrupted by quiet sleep and lucid intervals; actual complaints about pains in the head and abdomen now occurred, also cough with pain in the epigastrium. After the second dose there only remained hastiness, timidity, anxiety, and timid look. After the third dose, she was able to go out, and several days after the fourth dose no trace of the disease remained.

H. HARTLAUB, Private communications.

CASE 76.—A man, æt. 42, previously affected with Lues, was attacked with erysipelas of the face, after taking cold, and this was succeeded by congestion to the head, obstinate costiveness and mental derangement.

Symptoms.—In the evening he becomes restless, and busies himself with spirits which seem to come to his bed; he grasps after a sword, strikes about him with it, in order to drive a devil out of the room who is seeking to attack him; this conduct lasts the whole night; but early in the morning and during the day he is rational. His face is red, eyes glistening, thirst very great, abdomen moderately distended, and sexual desire much aroused.

Treatment.—Hyosc. was given without benefit; after taking Stramon. he was restored to quiet sleep and to his previous mental powers.

Annals, Vol. 1, p. 230.—TRINKS.

CASE 77.—A man, æt. 26, of sanguine temperament, fell into mania, after a fright.

Symptoms.—He speaks incessantly of incomprehensible and foolish things; first he sits down, then he stands up; or kneels down, and braces himself with great power against the wall; extends his hands alternately, directly before himself, or puts his finger upon his mouth; he tears his clothes, and breaks his bonds with inconceivable rapidity; does not answer questions, and avoids the eyes of others; his pupils were contracted, his eyes dull and sunken.

Treatment.—Stramon. 3 and 6 cured him in three weeks.

Archiv, Vol. 19, part 1. p. 92.—SZTAR.

CASE 78.—A puerperal woman, with natural flow of lochia, and regular state of all her functions, with the exception of an excessive flow of milk, became perfectly deranged; she talked of the most silly and confused stuff, which no one could understand, &c.

Treatment.—Stramon. 9, taken for many days, both night and morning, cured her radically.

General Hom. Journ., Vol. 2. p. 114.—KRETZSHMAR.

CASE 79.—A miss, æt. 30, of delicate frame and timid, desponding nature, became melancholic after a fright.

Symptoms.—She was exceedingly concerned and dejected; believed that she was not worthy of eternal salvation, because she could not accomplish the tasks she undertook in the evening; she wished to have several lights in the room, and begged earnestly that she might not be left alone; her nights were sleepless, and spent in praying and weeping; sometimes she answered questions, at other, she did not speak, but brooded silently, and was frightened by the slightest noise; when urged, she took food; her head and forehead were hot, pupils dilated, pulse weak and quick.

Treatment.—Stramon. 3, at first one drop per dose, night and and morning; then one dose at night only, cured her in fourteen days.

Hygea, Vol. 20, p. 231.—MAYERHOFER.

CASE 80.—A young, volatile man, æt. 22, had already had three attacks of mental derangement, which lasted under allopathic treatment, from five to eight weeks.

Symptoms.—Great bodily restlessness; confusion of memory; alternations of heat of the face and coldness of the body, then anxiety and thirst; frequent flushing of the face, with fixed look; dejection, weeping and fear of death; stuttering and lisping before he could utter a few words; constant coldness of the feet; restless anxious sleep, with wonderful illusions; fear of mad animals and black dogs.

Treatment.—This fourth attack, was cured by Stramon. 15, in the course of twenty-four hours.

Annals, Vol. 3, p. 270.—BETHMANN.

CASE 81.—An emaciated man, æt. 48, awoke from sleep three weeks ago with signs of mania.

Symptoms.—Loud laughing; he makes leaps like those of a rope-dancer, it seemed as if he floated upon the tips of his toes; is irritable like one who has not slept enough.

Treatment.—First Camphor, as antidotal to previous allopathic treatment; then he was cured with Stramon. 3, in four weeks.

Archiv, Vol. 19, part. 1, p. 88.

CASE 82.—A man, æt. 36, had been deranged for several months.

Symptoms.—He imagines that he lies in a vault, confesses, prays, and wishes to be killed; laughs as if he were tickled; wishes to be kissed by every one; accuses his wife of unfaithfulness to him; he scolds, strikes furiously about him, and cannot be held by his watchers; he looks upon his attendants as dogs, and barks at them in order to make himself understood by them; he speaks Jewish-German, which he never did before, and believes that his house is surrounded by wagons full of Jews and geese, who expose their posteriors to him, and thus render him furious. He is pale, eats nothing, and does not sleep; constant twitching of the facial muscles; he pushes his thumbs between his fingers.

Treatment.—Was treated allopathically without avail, and then cured by Stramon. $\frac{}{9}$ in a few days.

Archiv, Vol. 16, part. 2, p. 81.—SCHELLHAMER.

Besides in the above cases, Stramon. was used in cases No. 14, 38, 94, 98, 101, 102, 103, 109 and 110.

An old lady, had restless nights for six weeks, with visions; it seemed as if strange persons entered the room, commenced various indifferent employments, and came so near to her that she became very much frightened and could not stay in bed. Well in six days.—BECKER.

A man of 60, of maniacal family, hypochondriacal for several years, always preceded by great excitement, in which he effected his business with great haste, would not bear contradiction, had no rest, made disturbance and lost his sleep—this state generally lasted two-months, and was then followed by great relaxation, inactivity, grief about his affairs, which were quite brilliant—excitement attended with full quick pulse, strong palpitation and congestion to the head.

Stramonium continued for several weeks, relieved the excitement, and the depression did not follow, he remained well for a year, when a slight renewal was quickly relieved by Stramonium.—SOBERNHEIM.

REVIEW.—Of thirteen cases, treated by Stramon, seven were males and six females, of various ages. Among the causes of the attacks relieved by Stramon. were the puerperal state, in cases No. 75 and 78; previous facial erysipelas in No. 76; and fright in cases 77 and 79.

As to the form of mania cured or relieved by Stramon., that with much excitement is the most common; but attended with scolding and endeavors to destroy, in cases 77 and 82 only; more frequently we find constant talking, preposterous laughing, silly actions, disquiet, inclination to run or go away, but differing from the constant impulse to escape on account of anxiety; visions of spirits and ghosts, and contests with them, or of animals; sexual excitement, the patient wishing to be kissed, and making improper speeches; great muscular activity, hopping and jumping.

A *depressed* state of mind occurred only in cases No. 79 and 80, in the form of dejection, fear of being alone, brooding and feeling unworthy of salvation.

Both these states of excitement and depression occurred in alternation in case No. 75.

Erroneous impressions about oneself, and others occurred in No. 82.

But few physical derangements occurred in connection with the mental disorder.

In several of the cases Bellad, or Veratrum had removed the state of great excitement, after which Stramon. was given with great benefit.

It was useless, or only transiently useful in cases marked by great anxiety, fear, suspicion, and against melancholy from mortified self-esteem. See cases No. 90, 72 and 6.

Of the fourteen cases, five were cured by one dose of Stramon.; nine required repeated doses.

The size of the curative dose varied very much, from the second to the thirtieth potency.

The action of Stramon. extends to several organs of the brain, although but traces of this are to be found in the above cases; it acts upon amativeness; destructiveness; caution; wonder, and imitation.

32. SULPHUR.

General Remarks.—*a*) Against timidity; inconsolableness about every action, which is regarded as wrong; religious fixed ideas; paroxysms of anxiety.

Hahnemann, Chron. Dis., Vol. 5.

b) This much we can assume from what is known of the action of Sulphur, that it will not prove curative against mental disorders originating in the brain—and that it will prove most useful in chronic cases.

Experience has taught many of us that Sulphur is exceedingly useful in chronic affections in which the mental powers are clouded and perverted, without there being actual mental derangement, but much fear of company, despair of recovery, fancies about disease, calamity, care and want; Sulphur seems to unbind the chains of despondency and false fears in which the mind has been cramped.—Griesselich.

CASE 83.—A woman, æt. 40, a brunette, tall, thin and frequently the subject of melancholy, which had increased very much for the last few months, during which her menses had been suppressed.

Symptoms.—Violent headache, severe pressure as if the brain were walled in; eyes dull, face pale, oppression in the epigastric region; stools white and hard; anxious state of mind and fears about her condition; imagined that she must starve, fears the ruin of her household, goes about wringing her hands, and seeks to escape; frequent chills.

Treatment.—Pulsatilla was given without benefit; after taking Sulph. $\frac{}{15}$, the melancholy soon passed away and her menses returned again. Calc. was given to complete the cure.

Annals, Vol. 3, p. 156.—Tietze.

33. TABACUM.

General Remarks.—Whoever studies the effects of Tobacco will not fail to perceive that this drug, almost entirely neglected as it is by physicians of present times, must possess unusual powers in mental diseases, for its relations to the brain are both striking and characteristic.

The Tobacco mental derangement commences with simple hypochondriac mood, increases to melancholy and dejection, passes over into mania in which the patient acts without control, sings, cries and appears almost frenzied.

It is remarkable how deranged persons long for Tobacco; each morsel is a god-send to them.

Hygea, Vol. 23, p. 252.—Griesselich.

34. VERATRUM-ALBUM.

General Remarks.—*a*) The powers possessed by this remedy of benefitting or curing almost one-third of all the deranged confined in asylums, has not been suspected by physicians, because they did not know which particular forms of mental derangement to treat with it.

Mat. Med. Pur., Vol. 3, p. 326.—Hahnemann.

b) It is useful against great restlessness and excitement, screaming and constant laughing in the midst of irrational and mostly incomprehensible talking, fear of strange persons, running about, attempting to escape, &c.

General Hom. Journ., Vol. 19, p. 21.—Knorre.

CASE 84.—A woman, æt. 30, fell into such a state of frenzy, fourteen days after confinement, that she had to be bound.

Symptoms.—She did not sleep, but babbled incessantly; when she heard the clocks strike, or similar noises, she became quite silly, and danced about until she was obliged to keep quiet; slept but little and awoke in fright; wild look, and a peculiar irregular quickness of speech.

Treatment.—Veratrum, at first three doses, and then one per day, cured her; various new symptoms arose during the treatment.

Radmacher, Vol. 10, p. 823.

CASE 85.—A man, æt. 60, of quiet melancholic temperament, had one or two attacks of mental derangement per year; two of his brothers were subject to like attacks.

Symptoms.—He drives all his family out of the house; imagined that the sun turned around the earth; had paroxysms of fear of death, groaning, restlessness and despair; also of confusion and absence of mind, and which led him into the most senseless actions.

Treatment.—Verat. $_{\overline{12}}$, one drop soon restored him to health. —KNORRE.

CASE 86.—A woman, æt. 38, who had had previous attacks of mental derangement, became so bad that she was obliged to be confined.

Symptoms.—Speaks excitedly and incessantly, with unsteady and wild looks and constant smiling face, with alternations of loud laughter; she distorts her face hideously and seeks to keep off all who approach her; does not answer questions, takes refuge behind the table, then laughs and scolds; color of face natural; proferred food she rejects.

Treatment.—Tinct. Verat. from five to twenty or thirty drops given in coffee, restored her in the course of fourteen days.

General Hom. Journ., Vol. 19, p. 21.—KNORRE.

CASE 87.—A case of religious derangement in a farmer, induced in part by hard drinking, and which occurred more severely every other day and was attended with such considerable lameness of the back that he walked with difficulty, was cured by two doses of Veratrum $_{\overline{12}}$, aided by an intermediate dose of Sulph.

General Hom. Journ., Vol. 2, p. 114.—KRETZSMAR.

CASE 88.—A woman, æt. 36, had been for eight days in a state of anxiety and despair, which had not been relieved by allopathic treatment.

Symptoms.—Very red, glowing face; great agony, dejection and despair; she wailed and cried incessantly, but could give no reason for doing so; she did not eat or drink, neither could she sleep.

Treatment.—Veratrum 1st, two drops, divided into four doses, one dose night and morning quieted the patient in twenty-four hours.

Annals, Vol. 4, p. 330.—SCHUELER.

CASE 89.—In mental derangement marked by indecent speeches and lasciviousness, Veratrum often affords the most marked relief. A widow, who had fallen into the above state was quickly cured by Veratrum $\overline{12}$, one drop, after bloodletting, Tart.-emet. and blisters had been used without avail for eight days. She is now married and is quite well.

General Hom. Journ. Vol. 2, p. 113.—KRETZSCHMAR.

CASE 90.—A woman became melancholic after an attack of typhoid fever.

Symptoms.—She is unhappy about the death of her grown up daughter deceased several years ago; reproaches herself that she made her unhappy by the sad tone of her own mind; she attempted to drown herself, but was rescued.

Treatment.—Verat. 6, in repeated doses, soon cured her.

ENGELHARDT, Record. of L. Society.

CASE 91.—A melancholic patient became frenzied, he sang and whistled the most beautiful melodies, of which he knew nothing when he recovered.

Treatment.—Bellad. and Stramon. were given without benefit; but after taking Veratrum 1, one drop every eight hours, he soon improved and recovered.

This led HARTLAUB to remark that Veratrum was the main remedy in the mental derangements of that neighborhood, especially when they verged upon insomnia and mania.

ENGELHARDT, Record of L. Society.

CASE 92.—An old maiden, æt. 32, had suffered for twenty years with an alternately healing and again outbreaking sore upon the left leg; for the last three weeks she had shewn signs of mental derangement. On the 30th August she became frenzied; her pale distorted face, wild threatening look, her dishevelled hair, her grinning, and utterance of almost beastly noises made a dreadful impression upon spectators.

Symptoms.—She struck, bit and spit about her; she constantly moved her head and body to and fro, muttering and groaning all the while; attempted to jump out and run away; alternately she sang in a broken and wild manner, then sank into quiet and hung down her head; she does not understand, or answer questions.

Treatment.—Sept. 5th, she received two drachms of Tinct.

Veratrum, twenty-five drops to be taken per dose, twice a day; this was followed by quiet sleep, desire for food, and she could be released from her bonds; on the 9th Sept., she received fifty drops of Tinct. Veratrum, followed by sound sleep; subsequently she took ten drops, twice a day; she was entirely relieved of her mania but remained taciturn and reserved and finally died of dropsy.

General Hom. Journ., Vol. 19, p. 23.—KNORRE.

Besides, Veratrum was given in cases No. 3, 42, 95, 96, 98, 99, 100, 101. 102.

REVIEW.—Of eighteen cases treated by Veratrum, five were males and thirteen females.

The causes of the mental derangement whenever they were mentioned and whenever the remedy cured without other aid, although very differing, were always of a purely somatic or material nature.

Still but few physical symptoms were met with; sleep however was almost always entirely absent, and food was only taken when urged upon the patient.

As regards the form of mania in which Veratrum was most useful we find first: a state of excitement characterized by rioting, noise-making, laughing, singing, and whistling (see cases No. 42, 84, 86, 91, and 105); or by incessant talking (see cases No. 84 and 86); especially of an indecent character, with sexual excitement (see cases No. 42 and 89); or by senseless actions, (see cases No. 84, 85 and 86).

Second: also a state of depression marked by restlessness, anxiety, despair, imagining an unhappy state, fear of fancied forms (see cases No. 42, 88, 90, 95); and by deficient sexual inclination in case 95.

The religious mania in case 87 has not been accurately described.

These two forms were found in alternation in cases No. 42, 92, 100, 105 and 112.

The Veratrum did *not* prove useful against perverse actions and speeches, with inability to understand questions and the epileptic cramps which occurred in case No. 95; nor against anxiety and reproaches of conscience in case 103; nor in inclination to abuse others in No. 97. Again, in case No. 105, the inclination to destroy was only lessened and changed into loud laughing and active jumping, which were removed by Stramon. The increased state of self-esteem in cases No. 55 and 112 were not removed by Veratrum; while in No. 42, the rage, abuse, desire to run away, and indecent speeches were merely lessened, not removed.

Dose.—In twelve cases, the doses were repeated in nine; in three cases one dose sufficed to effect a cure, from the Tincture down to the fifteenth dilution was the most useful strength; the thirtieth dilution was given without benefit.

Organs of brain.—That of amativeness was excited in some cases and depressed in others; those of destructiveness and combativeness when in a state of excitement were calmed by Veratrum; that of hope was also influenced by it, for we find the unhappy and despairing rendered cheerful.

35. ZINCUM.

General Remarks.—The action of this remedy in brain-fever attended with the violent mental derangement is very striking; it is also homœopathic to dulness of the head, difficult flow of ideas, absence of thought, forgetfulness, dulness of memory, dizziness, drowsiness, manifold pains in the head, paralytic-like oppression of the mental faculties, thoughts of death, disinclination to work, irritability, capriciousness and moroseness.—Griesselich.

CASE 93.—A single woman, æt. 46, a-menstrual for ten months, fell into the following state two months ago, in consequence of vexation and passion.

Symptoms.—She fears that she will fall into hands of justice, because she supposes that it is believed that she has committed some crime. Timid expression; believes that she is watched and followed by her neighbors; that the devil is in pursuit of her, and comes up from under the floor. Restless sleep at times during the day; fever at night, with only one or two hours dreamy sleep; believes that she is about falling down a precipice, and that she is pursued, hence she runs away with all her might. Afterwards she feels exhausted, feeble and inclined to weep. She takes an antipathy to any one who attempts to convince her of her errors. She has headache, heat of the head and face, dusky redness of the cheeks, emaciation of the face. Is dizzy and walks unsteadily; has alternations of moderate heat and coldness of the body; constipation; brick red deposit from the urine. She had already been bled.

Treatment.—Oxide of Zinc, one-sixth grain, per dose, six times every twenty-four hours; with improvement on the second day, and recovery by the eighth; still the remedy was continued for several days longer.—SCHMID.

CASE 94.—RADEMACHER says, that he once cured a deranged girl in five days, with acetate of Zinc.

CHAPTER II.

CASES IN WHICH SEVERAL REMEDIES WERE REQUIRED.

CASE 95.—A woman, æt. 50, formerly always healthy, had been indisposed for four weeks; there was an alteration in her mental state; she often could not recollect herself; was somewhat childish; repeated the same thing several times, and often laughed without cause.

On the 4th of September, at eight, A. M., she was attacked with an apoplectic seizure; she lay quietly upon the bed upon her back, with closed eyes, compressed mouth, very slow and somewhat small pulse, natural warmth of the body without perspiration, appeared constantly in a deep sleep, still she turned over occasionally, and put out her tongue when loudly requested to do so; her tongue was dry and brown, especially in the middle, but was not drawn to one side.

Treatment and Result.—Bellad. was given without effect; two doses of *Arnica* were followed by some vomiting of dark mucus, the tongue became moist, and some perspiration shewed itself; otherwise her condition remained the same. On the following day she was somewhat more conscious; her eyes were constantly open; but frequently spoke quite erroneously, and this wandering of the mind increased towards evening. Thought that her ears were in the wrong place and ought to be cut off; great restlessness, inclination to run away, heat of skin, much perspiration, whiteness of the tongue, constipation.

Bellad. was again given in the evening, but on the next day the following symptoms were present:

Constant inclination to run away; great exhibition of strength, when she was opposed; threw her bed and other things out of the window; spoke a great deal, but always foolishly, with much laughter; if she was spoken to, she appeared to understand nothing, and looked quite stupid; pulse slow, somewhat full; tongue white and dry.

She received *Verat* 30, one-third of a drop per dose; followed by more quiet during the day, but increased restlessness at night, succeeded by violent epileptic-like cramps, lasting about five minutes, recurring every hour for three times, and then every an half hour for six hours.

Symptoms.—At first she fell down suddenly, and commenced to grasp with her fingers; attempted to scream, but could not make a loud noise, but only rattled in the throat, with frothing at the mouth; bent her body backwards; struck out with one arm, and grasped with the other; her legs were quiet; face pale; consciousness lost. Between the paroxysms she was in the same state as the day before, only more languid; but she never entirely recovered her consciousness.

Treatment.—In the afternoon she received Stramonium 30, one-third drop; no more spasms occurred, but she still attempted to escape; this finally subsided and she partially recovered her consciousness. On the next day she had two stools, and was able to attend to her household duties. After the elapse of several days something foolish could be observed in her manner; she laughed while speaking, without cause, turned around her body round and around, &c. But all this subsided in a few days, after the Stramonium had been repeated. She then remained well.—H. HARTLAUB.

CASE 96.—A woman, æt. 33, small in stature and of delicate constitution, had suppression of the menses, and fell into a state of melancholy; her sexual inclinations which had never been very active, now seemed entirely extinct, yet she labored under the fixed idea, that she had been inconstant, and was possessed of the devil.

Treatment.—Sulphur 30, followed by four doses of Verat. 15, one every six days. After the third powder menstruation sat in and lasted for eight days, followed by evident improvement in four weeks. A few doses of Ignat. 2, every forty-eight hours, restored her entirely.

Archiv, Vol. 19, part. 1, p. 48.—GROSS.

CASE 97.—A delicate woman, æt. 30, fell during her confinement, in consequence of fright and vexation, into a state of mental derangement, marked by boundless suspicion and jealousy. She had been treated without benefit for three months, when she was restored by six doses of Ignat. 3 and Hyosc. 2, in alternation, one dose every day.—GROSS.

CASE 98.—A lady, æt. 48, of melancholic sanguine temperament, fell, after an attack of gout into a deep melancholy ; her menses were suppressed and all allopathic means proved useless ; organic disease of the heart was suspected.

Treatment.—She was entirely restored in a few months by Verat. 3 and Bellad. 3, and Coccul. 2 in alternation.

Hygea, Vol. 20, p. 237.—DR. MAYERHOFER.

CASE 99.—A man, æt. 30, delicate and of a phlegmatic temperament, became deranged without any evident cause.

Symptoms.—He believed that he was bankrupt ; had lost his chance of salvation ; saw phantastic shadows and figures, of which he was afraid ; expected evil from every thing and seemed tortured with anxiety.

Treatment.—Several doses of Stramon. were given without benefit ; then excessive anxiety and restlessness were relieved by Bellad. 30 and Aconit. 30. Nux, Bryon. and Verat., finally restored him entirely, after eight days' treatment.—THORER.

CASE 100.—A lady, æt. 32, delicate and sensitive, but choleric became deranged after an attack of nervous fever.

Treatment.—She was quieted and relieved by Verat. 18 in solution, but a state of groaning, crying and sighing remained ; Hyosc. 6 in repeated doses, Opium 3 in solution, and Chamomilla and Sulphur restored her entirely.—DR. GASTFREUND.

CASE 101.—A spinster, æt. 30, suffering with Amenorrhœa, and derangement of the stomach and liver, fell into a melancholic state, from which she was entirely relieved in three months, by Verat., Ignat., Caust., Sepia, Puls., and Cocculus. — RUMMEL.

CASE 102.—A young man, æt. 20, of placid and impressible disposition, fell suddenly into a state of mania.

Symptoms.—He answered no questions; spoke much irrational stuff; tore his clothes; was noisy and destructive; his eyes were red, and he took no food.

Treatment.—Verat. 6, was followed by sleep, and in the morning he asked for food. He had no stool for four days after taking Veratrum, but Opium 9, was followed by a copious discharge. Still he was very suspicious, mistook his physician for an evil spirit. He was finally restored in six weeks by Bellad. 30, Stramon. 6, Verat. 12, and Phos.-ac. 2, given at rather long intervals.—SZTAROV.

CASE 103.—A young man, æt. 18, fell into a kind of mania, after dancing all night and drinking a good deal, during which he became engaged in a quarrel.

Symptoms.—He spoke unconnected stuff about bad treatment and of revenge; spoke to persons by name who were not present; was very restless, brooked no opposition; had gastic derangement from vexation.

Treatment.—Stramon. 6, was followed by some quiet, even by sleep and some appetite; at the end of a few days more he was in the following condition.

Symptoms.—His look was disturbed; face pale and sallow; he sprang up, wrung his hands, complained bitterly that no one would forgive him; sought out dark places, and covered his face with his hands. Bellad. 15 was given, and in three days he was in the following state:

Symptoms.—Dejected look; emptiness in the head; restlessness; inability to collect his thoughts; at night as soon as he shut his eyes, frightful figures appeared to him, he wept, spoke of confused stuff, of being placed in chains and bonds, where neither the sun or moon would shine upon him; that he could not be forgiven; that he had no merciful God.—His urine was pale; skin dry and parched; yawning and shivering; he scratched himself here and there, and an unusual redness appeared at the irritated spot.

Treatment.—Dulcamara 18, one drop, followed by perspiration, and irruption of red spots upon the skin; he no longer spoke irrationally, although his head was still confused, and he had occasional paroxysms of anxiety. Bellad. 24, completed the cure, which required twenty-one days in all.—SPOHR.

CASE 104.—A wealthy countryman, æt. 22, fell, from injudicious treatment in consequence of a suspicion of guilt, into a state of perfect mania, so that he had to be confined. Bellad. 30, three doses, one every day, removed the mania, and quieted the patient very much, so that the straight jacket could be taken off.

Symptoms.—He lay quietly in bed, declared that he was bodily well, but did not know what he was doing at times, and spoke irrationally occasionally.

Treatment.—One dose of Stramon. 9, was given each day, with progressive improvement; then two doses of Nux-v. 3, removed the somatic symptoms; finally a lachrymose condition was relieved by Pulsat.—THORER.

CASE 105.—An active lad, æt. 12, with an extremely irritable nervous system, and who had suffered while an infant with abdominal obstruction and latterly also with congestion to the head, fell into a state of mania. The paroxysms occurred every day, and sat in two hours earlier each time.

Treatment.—Verat. 12, followed by later appearance of the maniacal paroxysms, and shorter duration of them; religious excitement ensued, with declamation of hymns, &c. Verat. was repeated, and on the following day paroxysms of laughing occurred in place of maniacal excitement, with rope-dancer-like agility. These attacks subsided entirely under the use of Stramonium 18;—remaining nervous irritability and constipation were removed by Nux and Lycopod.—FIELITZ.

CASE 106.—A lady, æt. 50, of delicate constitution fell into a state of melancholy after much care and grief, so that she had entirely withdrawn from all society for several years.

Treatment.—She was cured in the course of six months by Ignat., Nux, Arsenicum and Sepia.—THORER.

CASE 107.—A man, æt. 40, tall and thin, had suppressed an attack of itch three years ago, and gradually became deranged.

Treatment.—Nux 4, Verat. 12, Sulph. 6, Psorin 30, Sepia and Carb.-v. 6, were used in effecting the cure.—THORER.

CASE 108.—A lady, æt. 30, got rid of an impetiginous eruption, during her last pregnancy, and then after weaning her child, fell into a melancholic condition, preceded by fright.

Treatment.—Pulsat., Verat. and Bell., at intervals of two days, produced a marked improvement in four weeks; then Arsenicum 30, at intervals of two and four days, and finally Sulphur 6, completed the cure.—THORER.

CASE 109.—A man, æt. 38, had been in a melancholic condition for twelve years in consequence of the unfaithfulness of his wife.

Treatment.—He was entirely cured in three months, by Pulsat. 12, Ignat. 9, Nux 4, Verat. 12, and Arsen. 30 and Calc. 30.—THORER.

CASE 110.—A woman, æt. 30, became deranged after the death of her child.

Treatment.—She was cured in six weeks, with Bellad. 2, Verat. 12, Stramon. and Hyosc. 6.—SZATAR.

CASE 111.—A teacher, æt. 27, who had a great opinion of himself, became deranged after dismissal from his situation.

Treatment.—He was cured in one month by Opium, Nux, Stramon., Hyosc. and Aurum.—SZATAR.

CASE 112.—A learned person, æt. 30, had weakened himself considerally while at the university, by long-continued study, late hours, and coffee drinking. He had scarcely recovered somewhat at home, when in order to forget a disgraceful vexation, he began to apply himself anew to study, and drank large quantities of coffee, in order to keep awake at night. Mental derangement followed, attended with various bodily infirmities.

Treatment.—Nux 30, removed his headache, constipation, excessive lasciviousness and irritability. Verat. 12, only produced transient relief. Ferrum removed the remaining debility, and Platina 3, one-half grain per dose, restored him entirely.—SCHROTER.

GENERAL REVIEW

OF THE TREATMENT OF MENTAL DERANGEMENT.

In the preceding cases, *Bellad.* was administered 32 times; Veratrum, 19 times; Stramonium, 17 times; Hyosc. in 12 cases; Pulsat. in 7; Ignatia and Opium, each 6 times; Cuprum, 5 times; Anacardium, Arsenicum and Nux, each in 3 cases. While Aconite, Aurum, Conium, Helleb., Phosphor and Platina were each used in two cases, and Calc., China, Crocus, Hepar, Lachesis, Lycopod., Petrol., Rhus, Sepia, Sulphur were given each in one case. Besides, Baryta, Bryonia, Causticum, Coccul., Nux-mosch., Secale and Tabacum are recommended in general terms.

In states of *Exaltation* we find: An excited and mild state cured by Opium and Phosphor; (see also GRIESSELICH's remarks on Acon. and Tabac. Raging, shouting, laughing and singing have been removed by Verat.)

Scolding and inclination to destroy, by Hyosc. Ready inclination to anger, to strike, or to tear one's clothes by Stramon.

Mania in the highest degree, with attempts at destruction and murder, by Bellad.

Foolish imaginations, by Anacardium. Great talkativeness, confused talking of complicated things, by Cuprum, Opium and Verat.; when attended with active muscular motions, by Stramon. Talkativeness, with delivery of speeches, by Lachesis. Thoughtless actions by Verat. and Hyosc.; occasionally by Bellad.

Shameful conversation, with sexual excitement, by Veratrum and Stramon.

Religious mania has been cured by Verat. and Aurum. Seeing of ghosts and devils, by Opium and Cuprum; of animals, by Hyosc.

False impressions about one's-self and body, by Stramon. and Anacard.

Among the states of *Depression*, we find : Loss of will, and power to decide upon any action, have been cured by Coccul. and Helleb.

An apathetic state, with dullness, indifference brooding, and stupid expression, by Baryta, Hellebore and Opium.

The most numerous observations and cures have been made in the forms of *melancholy*, from dejection of spirits to the highest degree of anxiety and despair.

Dejection has been cured by Conium and Petrol., with fear of death, by Platina.

Depression of spirits by Stramon. and Sepia.

Anthrophophobia, by Anacard.

Melancholic condition by Aurum, Ignatia, Sepia and Rhus ; when attended with weeping and occurring in connection with pregnancy and confinement, by Pulsat.—with desire for solitude, and fear of coming to want, by Nux and Calcar.

Feeling of being unfortunate, by Veratrum ; when occasioned by child-bed and Misfortune, by Bryonia.

Melancholy from care and grief, by Causticum.

Anxious solicitude and fear of starving, by Sulph. and Calc.

Fear of being alone, by Stramon. ;—of frightful forms and figures, by Pulsat. ;—anxious conscientiousness, by Lycopod.

Anxiety about phantoms of the imagination and constant endeavor to fly from them, by Bellad.

Restlessness and desire to escape, by Stramon. and Helleb., and other remedies.

Despair about shattered health and fear of death, by Calcarea.

Despairing anxiety, with fear of approaching misfortune, attended with complaining and weeping, by Cuprum ;—on account of an unhappy position, by Veratrum.

When the mental derangement assumed the form of *fixed ideas*, we find :

Expectation of approaching death, during child bed, cured by Aconite.

The idea of having committed a crime, with fear of the

officers of justice, by Cuprum and Zinc.—when the physician is mistaken for a police-officer, by Bellad.

The illusion of not being in one's own house, by Opium;—the belief of never being able to be happy more in one's own house, by Arsenicum.

Notions about supposed intentional insults, with scruples of conscience, by Ignat., Nux, and Pulsat.

Fear of not being saved, by Ignat., Sulph., and Calc.

Fear of coming to want, by Bryon, Nux, and Calc.

Notion that one is composed of two persons, by Anacard.

The inclination to *suicide* and disgust for life, require particular attention.

1) *Arsenicum* has cured the inclination to suicide, with clear consciousness, from an internal frightful anxiety; although the patient was not tired of life, but wished to be watched and restrained.

2) *Aurum*, has cured persons who thought seriously of taking their own lives. ÆGIDI says that Nux, not Aurum, will cure the melancholy, with disgust for life, which drives one to commit suicide. Aurum is most useful when there is a state of discontent with one's-self, from supposed bad behavior; or when there is excessive conscientiousness, with anxiety, agony of heart, with longing for death.

3) *Hellebore*, has cured a girl who attempted to drown herself; it is homœopathic when one is tired of life, feels unhappy when he sees others enjoying themselves, and is very anxious.

4) *Nux* is homœopathic when there is anxiety, as if from a bad conscience; or anxiety with palpitation of the heart, driving one to commit suicide; or when one regards his condition as insupportable, so that he would rather die.

5) *Pulsatilla* is homœopathic to disgust for life, with inclination to drown herself; anxiety in the region of the heart, with inclination to commit suicide.

6) *Veratrum* has cured a woman who was about to drown herself on account of her unhappy position.

Forty-six different physicians have furnished the above cases. In twenty-nine cases, doses of the crude drugs or low dilutions were used; while the higher potencies were given in seventy-six cases.

We may infer, that.

1) The organ of *Amativeness* is influenced by Hyosc., Nux, Phosphor, Stramon., and Veratr.
2) That of *Adhesiveness*, by Bellad.
3) *Combativeness*, by Bellad., Hyosc., Op., and Verat.
4) *Destructiveness*, by Bellad., Hyosc., Op., Phosph., Stramon., and Verat.
5) *Acquisitiveness*, by Bryon., Calc., and Nux.
6) *Self-esteem*, by Ignat., and Platina.
7) *Caution*, by Aconite, Arsen., Cuprum, Hyosc., Nux, Op , Puls., and Stramon.
8) *Benevolence*, by Anacardium.
9) *Conscientiousness*, by Arsenicum, Ignat., Nux, and Aurum.
10) *Hope*, by Calc., Verat., and Sulph.
11) *Marvellousness*, by Stramonium.
12) *Imitativeness*, by Stramon.
13) *Form*, by Bellad., Cuprum, and Hyosc.
14) *Causality*, by Anacardium.

APPENDIX.

ON HASCHISCH

This composition is a distillation of the pistils of the Hemp. In one patient it produced dryness of the throat and twitching of the limbs ; the pulse was ninety-six, and face flushed ; his ideas appeared to develop with extreme rapidity ; at one moment he offered the singular phenomenon of a *double man ;* he heard music on one side, and conversation on the other; but this symptom did not continue. His pupils became much dilated, he felt particularly gay and happy wished to be alone in a quiet place; he had great repugnance to speak or move; all faces seemed ridiculous to him. He then moved about, sometimes laughed violently, but suddenly threw himself upon a couch, refused to answer any more questions, and begged to be left alone, and not disturbed in the voluptuous and delicious sensations he experienced ; he had spasmodic movements of limbs and diaphragm ; sighed, moaned, laughed and wept by turns ; pulse increased to one hundred and twenty per minute ; face much flushed. His friends began to feel uneasy, but the experimenter assured them that he did not suffer, but felt happy. He had the most agreeable sensations proceeding from the pit of the stomach ; he seemed in ecstasy, his features bespoke the greatest happiness ; he could not find language to express his feelings ; he would not wish to leave his present condition, he felt so happy. Often said, how much I thank those who gave me that delicious drink. His sense of hearing became exceedingly acute ; he heard very distinctly what was said far off, and in a low voice. In the midst of his ecstasy he neither lost consciousness of persons or things. He felt no distress on the following days, but on the contrary a great sensation of happiness.

Another experimenter, naturally very serious, and who rarely laughed, in two and a half hours after taking Haschisch, suddenly exclaimed that he was delirious, began to sing, took out his pencil and endeavored to write down what he felt; but threw away his paper as his delirium increased; his features became very flexible; he laughed sardonically, his eye was animated, face red, pulse one hundred and twenty, pupils dilated, looked extremely happy, laughed, sang, gesticulated and spoke with great volubility; his ideas followed each other with rapidity; *he was deranged, as in Gay mania.* But in the midst of this abundance, mobility, and variableness of ideas, his naturally serious character and studies obtruded themselves, intermixed with pleasantries, bonmots and puns. His tongue became dry, he spat frequently, his legs became slightly convulsed; his hearing and sight became very acute; he had no notion of time or space, but recognized every one present and answered questions correctly. A multitude of ideas seemed to fill his head, which he could not put in words; expressed his willingness to lose an ear or eye, if he could only have another tongue to make known what he experienced. His pulse fell to ninety, but his delirium still continued; incoherent sentences followed with inconceivable rapidity; when water was given him, he exclaimed that will make the frogs come, who will drink up the liquor. Then the character of his delirium changed: He sat himself in a corner, closed his eyes, talked to himself and seemed inspired; spoke of sciences, gave definitions, then pronounced a few broken words, and immediately recited some twenty very harmonious impromptu and original verses. His countenance expressed gaiety and satisfaction; his skin became very pallid; pulse rose to one hundred. Then left off improvising to speak of foreign countries; described countries and cities which he had visited; but although Haschisch is supposed to cause second sight he could not describe places with which he was unacquainted; he himself finally said that a livelier impulse was given to his ideas, but nothing was added to his knowledge. Finally, the delirium, which had for a long time been confined to a series of ideas, became general again; he sang, laughed, and talked with great vivacity; said he was happy, &c.

Individuals under the influence of Haschisch feel a maniacal exaltation; ideas succeeded each other with rapidity and incoherence; the mind was under the empire of hallucinations and illusions; recollection could be evoked and vivified as if they were real; as in dreams there was a loss of time and space.

An other experimenter saw stars in his plate, and the firmament in the soup dish; turned his face to the wall, talked to himself, and burst into fits of laughter, with eyes flashing and in the highest glee.

A fourth, first saw the pupils of the eyes of his friend sparkle strangely and acquire a most singular turquoise blue color; in a few minutes a general lethargy came over him; his body appeared to dissolve and become transparent; he saw the haschisch which he had eaten distinctly within him, in the form of an emerald, from which thousands of little sparks were emitted; his eyelashes seemed to lengthen indefinitely, twisting themselves like golden threads around little ivory wheels, which whirled about with inconceivable rapidity. Around were figures and scrolls of all colors, arabesques and flowery forms in endless variety, which he could only compare to the variations of the kaleidescope. He still occasionally saw his companions, but they appeared disfigured, half men, half plants; now, with the pensive-air of the ibis, standing on one leg; and, again as ostriches flapping their wings and wearing so strange an appearance that he shook with laughter; and as if to join in the buffoonery of the scene, he tossed up the sofa cushions, catching them as they descended, and twisting them around with all the dexterity of an Indian juggler. One of the gentlemen addressed the experimenter in *Italian*, which the haschisch, by its extraordinary power, delivered to him in *Spanish*.

After some minutes he recovered his calmness, without headache or other unpleasant symptoms, but felt much astonished at what had passed. In a half hour more he again fell under the influence of the haschisch and his visions were still more complicated and extraordinary. Millions of butterflies, whose wings rustled like fans, flew about in the midst of a confused light; gigantic flames with crystal calyces, enormous hollyhocks, gold and silver lilies arose and burst into flowers around him, with a crackling sound like that of a bouquet of fireworks. His hearing was prodigiously developed; he seemed to hear the sound

28

of color, green, red, blue and yellow sounds struck him with perfect distinctness; a glass upset, the creaking of a chair, or a word spoken, however low, vibrated and resounded like rolling thunder; his own voice appeared so loud that he dared not speak for fear of throwing down the walls, or bursting like a bomb; every object gave forth a note of the harmonica or Æolian harp; he seemed to swerve in an ocean of sound. Never before was he bathed in such beatitude; he was so encircled by its waves, so transported from all things earthly, so lost to self, that he comprehended for the first time what might be the existence of elementary spirits, or angels, or souls released from this mortal coil. He was as a sponge in the midst of the sea; every instant waves of happiness washed over him, entering and departing through the pores; for he seemed to have become permeable, even to the smallest capillary vessel; his whole being was filled with the color of the fantastic medium in which he was plunged. Sounds, perfumes and light reached him by multitudes of beams, delicate as hair, and through which he seemed to hear the magnetic current pass.

What is very curious in the intoxicating effects of haschisch, is, that it is not continuous; it comes and goes suddenly; raises you to heaven, and places you again on earth, without any gradual transition; like madness too, it has its lucid intervals. A third attack, the last and strangest terminated the experience of the last experimenter. His sight became doubled; but soon he became completely insane for an hour. All kinds of Pantagonetic dreams passed through his fancy; goat-suckers, storks, stupid geese, unicorns, griffins, nightmares, and the menagerie of monstrous dreams trotted, jumped, flew or glided through the room. He saw horns terminating in foliage; webbed hands; whimsical beings with the feet of the arm-chair for legs, and dial plates for eyeballs; enormous noses danced the Cachuca, mounted on chicken legs. He imagined that he was the parroquet of the Queen of Sheba, and imitated to the best of his ability, the voice and actions of that interesting bird. The visions became so grotesque, that he was seized with a desire to sketch them, which he did with inconceivable rapidity. A friend seated at the piano seemed dressed like a Turk, with a sun painted on the back of his vest; the notes of the piano seemed escaping in the form of guns and spirals, curiously intertwisted. A fancy animal represented a living locomotive, with a swan's neck terminating in the jaws of a serpent, whence issued jets of smoke; two monstrous paws were composed of wheels and pulleys, and each pair of paws had a pair of wings; on the tail of the animal was seated the Mercury of the ancients, confessing himself to be conquered, notwithstanding his heels.—DU BOISMONT.

A

TREATISE

ON THE

INFLAMMATORY AND ORGANIC

DISEASES OF THE BRAIN.

INCLUDING:

IRRITATION, CONGESTION AND INFLAMMATION OF THE BRAIN, AND ITS MEMBRANES, TUBERCULOUS-MENINGITIS, HYDROCEPHALOID DISEASE, HYDROCEPHALUS ATROPHY AND HYPERTROPHY, HYDATIDS, AND CANCER OF THE BRAIN.

ON THE

NATURE AND CAUSES

OF

IRRITATION, CONGESTION, INFLAMMATION, AND DROPSY OF THE BRAIN, AND ITS MEMBRANES.

I.—IRRITATION OF THE BRAIN.

IN CHILDREN.

DR. W. NICKOLL has thus designated a state of brain occurring in children, which appears to hold an intermediate place between hydrocephaloid disease and that of inflammation. It may on the one hand run into inflammation if neglected; and on the other hand is apt, if treated too actively and allopathically, to be followed by symptoms of exhaustion, and of the Hydrocephaloid disease of Gooch and Hall.

In simple irritation of the brain the child is wakeful, scarcely ever sleeping, irritable, highly sensitive to every object of sight and sound; the pupil is in many instances more or less contracted, the limbs are in action, the head tossed about; the child cries without any apparent cause; there is unusual liveliness and animation; it wakes suddenly from sleep, and starts at the least noise when awake; the fists are generally clenched, with the thumbs turned in, and the forearms bent upwards on the arms; and sometimes a degree of opisthotonos is observed, the legs being drawn up, while the head is thrown back. This state of things is usually, though not always, accompanied by increased temperature of the head and of the skin generally, and by an accelerated pulse.

Some children seem to be much more prone than others to this affection, and it is in the nervous, weakly and scrofulous that it is most frequently seen. There is apparently an original difference or excitability of the nervous constitution, which predisposes them to be thrown into this state of Erethism; and when this natural predisposition is not present, defective nourishment, and a debilitated state of the system are apt to induce it. Any long continued irritation of the nervous extremities, particularly of those distributed upon the mucous membranes, may be the exciting cause of this affection; hence, painful dentition, worms, an unhealthy state of the stomach, bowels or liver, or chronic and troublesome eruptions, or sores, or some disease or impurity of the blood, may prove the exciting cause of irritation of the brain or nervous system. When this state obtains, convulsions, it is well known, are apt to occur.

The most deceptive part of the disease is, that the preternatural excitement and mobility of the nervous system is apt to give rise to excitement of the heart and arteries, and determination of blood to the head, from the excited condition of the brain. If the case be regarded as one of active congestion or commencing inflammation of the brain, and treated allopathically and antiphlogistically, irrespective of the peculiar state of the nervous system, exhaustion will speedily follow, and the symptoms of reaction and excitement from loss of blood will be added; if the same treatment be still pursued, the case will soon end fatally, and probably be attended with effusion of water into the ventricles of the brain. If the body be examined after death, the effusion will of course be detected, and will be presumed to have been the cause of death; but the real truth is, in certain states of the nervous system, unpreceded by any great cause of exhaustion, an increased quantity of blood may be thrown to the brain, and give rise to all the symptoms of the first stage of an inflammatory affection, but which cannot be removed by the ordinary allopathic antiphlogistic means, as these will aggravate the original excited condition of the brain and nervous system, inducing new and still more dangerous symptoms, causing the case to terminate fatally, with all the signs of an advanced stage of dropsy of the brain.

In older patients these cases are apt to be attended with

much delirium; WATSON says they seem to be, but are not, cases of Meningitis of any kind. ABERCROMBIE refers to them as instances of a very dangerous modification of inflammation of the brain, which shows only increased vascularity, without any of the other signs or effects of inflammation. WATSON very decidedly asserts that he entertains no doubt whatever, about the nature of these cases, viz.: that they are not examples of inflammation at all, for they neither show the anatomical characters of inflammation, nor do they yield to the remedies for inflammation. In short, they were made to terminate fatally by Abercrombie's outrageous system of extravagant blood-letting. Apoplexy according to Abercrombie, may also arise from exhaustion, and terminate fatally, when treated actively by blood-letting, &c., without any morbid appearance being found in the brain after death, or with appearances so slight as to be altogether inadequate to account for the symptoms, or fatal termination of the case. (See treatise on Apoplexy.) ABERCROMBIE himself admits that in four fatal cases of Apoplexy, all the usual allopathic remedies were used in the most active manner without the least effect in alleviating any of the symptoms, and on inspection after death, either no vestige of disease could be discovered in the brain, or at most there was but slight fulness of the blood-vessels, insufficient to account for death, which was doubtless caused by the too active treatment.

Treatment.—NICHOLLS says that judicious treatment will throw muchl ight on the pathology of these cases. If there be any manifest cause of irritation present, either from teething, or a disordered state of the bowels or liver, and this be removed and the child then placed in as quiescent a state as possible, by excluding it from light and noise, and every source of excitement, giving a dose or two of some sedative, and nourishing but unstimulating diet, and subsequently a gentle tonic, all the symptoms of brain disease will vanish.

The most homœopathic remedies are: Coffea, Cannabis, Thea, Ignatia, Nux. If these fail to afford relief; Conium, Hyosciamus, Opium, Asafœtida, Chamomilla or Valerian may be tried.

COFFEA, THEA and CANNABIS may be used when the attack

has been brought on by excessive and pleasurable excitement, when the child is so excited and lively as to be almost uncontrollable, with sleeplessness, i. e. when the *grey* substance of the brain, and the senses or intellectual faculties are principally aroused, and stimulated.

NUX and IGNATIA are the principal remedies, when the *white* substance of the brain, and the *motor* track and nerves are implicated; when there is a tendency to twitching, starting, &c., especially if the attack has been brought on by a fit of passion, vexation or disappointment.

HYOSCIAMUS and OPIUM are the antagonistic remedies for COFFEA and THEA, and may be used when these remedies seem indicated but fail to afford relief.

CONIUM is the antagonistic remedy for Nux and Ignatia, and may be given when these fail to afford relief.

II.—CONGESTION OF THE BRAIN.

IN CHILDREN.

ACCORDING to WEST, Congestion of the Brain is a very frequent disorder in young children; he quotes Dr. MAUTHNER in proof, who on examining the bodies of 229 children, dead of various diseases, found a congested state of the blood-vessels of the brain, in no less than 186. WEST assumes that the brain in infancy is much more exposed to congestion and irritation, than that of the adult, owing to the far wider variations of which the cerebral circulation is susceptible in early life than subsequently. Nor is the cause of this difficult to discover. The skull of the adult is a complete bony case, and the firm substance of the brain, affords a comparatively unyielding support to the blood-vessels by which it is nourished. The variations in the quantities of blood which the brain of the adult contains, must needs be circumscribed within far narrower limits than in the child, whose cranium, with its membranous fontanelles and unossified sutures, oppose no such obstacle to the admission of an increased quantity of blood, while the soft brain keeps up a much slighter counterpressure on the blood-vessels than is exerted by the comparatively firm parenchyma of the organ in the adult. Hence, if the circulation in the child be disturbed, whether from difficulty in the return of venous blood, as during a paroxysm of whooping cough, or from increased arterial action, as at the onset of a fever, or during the acute inflammation of some more or less distant organ, the brain becomes congested, and delirium, or stupor, or convulsions often announce the severity of the consequent disturbance of its function. The same causes too, which expose the brain to be over-filled with blood, render it possible for it to be drained more completely of its blood, than in the adult. This fact should always be borne in mind, when treating the diseases of infants, for debility, exhausting discharges, and especially excessive allopathic depletion will often quickly induce a bloodless state of the brain, and all the symptoms of Hydrocephaloid disease.

Hence, in the treatment of diseases of children, the physician must be constantly on the watch against congestion of the brain, as a condition which is very likely to come on, in the course of the most various diseases, and of affections even of quite distant organs. But it is not merely as a serious complication of many other diseases, that this congestion of the brain in children deserves notice: its importance depends still more on its constituting the first and curable stage of many diseases of the brain, which, unless arrested at the outset, soon pass beyond the resources of our art.—WEST.

Congestion of the brain may arise from irritation; from the presence in the blood of the poison of some eruptive disease, such as scarlet fever, measles, or small-pox; or the brain may become *actively* congested at the time of teething, or from feverish irritation of the whole system, or from exposure to the sun, or from a blow upon the head, or from the fever of inflammation of some distant organ, such as the lungs, stomach, or bowels, &c. Or a state of *passive* congestion may be induced by some mechanical impediment to the return of blood from the head, such as the general spasmodic compression of the blood-vessels such as occurs in general convulsions, or during a fit of whooping cough; or from the pressure of an overloaded stomach, or liver, or enlarged thymus or bronchial gland. Finally, *passive* congestion, may be merely the result of a languid circulation, arising from debility, or exhaustion, or want of pure air, or of nourishing and sufficient food, such as occurs in diarrhœa or summer complaint, in which the child not only has a great drain upon the system, but either is unable to take or does not receive a sufficient of nourishing food, from a mistaken policy on the part of the physician.

Intense congestion of the brain is not a very unusual consequence of the irritation of the brain and nervous system, from the presence of the poison of some eruptive disease in the system, or from the acceleration and disturbance of the circulation at the outset of the eruptive fevers. Convulsions and apoplectic symptoms then, sometimes, come on suddenly in a child, previously to all appearances, in perfect health, and may even terminate in death in less than twenty-four hours. The brain will be found loaded with blood, but all the other organs of the body are quite healthy. We may be at a loss to account for such sudden and severe symptoms unless measles, scarlet fever or small-pox are prevailing, or some other child in the family or neighborhood is soon after attacked by one or the other of them. That this train of symptoms often arises from the presence of some morbid poison in the blood, is still more evident from the occasional results of repelling eruptive diseases of the scalp. Thus, Golding Bird relieved a child of Porrigo with external applications in three weeks; for a time it appeared in perfect health, but in the act of crying "Papa," it was attacked with a kind of spasm and dropped dead. Dr. Dendy has seen four similar cases, in which death occurred as suddenly, all in the respectable classes.

When congestion of the brain and convulsions precede the eruptive diseases, these symptoms as alarming as they generally are, comparatively seldom end in death; for they generally disappear almost as if by magic, on the appearance of the eruption, except in those few cases in which the quantity of the poison is so great, that it cannot all make its escape upon the surface; or in which the congestion of the brain is kept up by the intensely feverish state of the whole system.

The presence of some irritating substance in the blood, also obtains in those cases in which convulsions, or irritation of the brain arises from suppression of perspiration, scantiness of urine, deficiency of bile or some other secretion.

Another cause may aid in keeping up or increasing the pressure upon the brain in feverish disorders, viz.: an absolute expansion or increase of the volume of the blood; the most marked instance of this is in congestion of the brain from exposure to the heat of the sun, even though the head has not been unprotected from its rays. Of this WEST saw a striking instance in the case of a delicate boy, who when a year old, was taken out by his nurse, during one of the hottest days of summer. He was quite well and cheerful when he left the house, but, after being out for some time, began to breathe hurriedly and irregularly, and his nurse in consequence brought him home. He was restless, fretful and alarmed; his surface generally hot, and his head especially so, the brain pulsating forcibly through the anterior fontanelles; the pulse too rapid to be counted; the respiration hurried, labored and irregular, and there were constant startings of the tendons of the extremities. The child was on the eve of convulsions, but the tepid bath relieved the heat of the skin, and the expansion of the blood, the pulse fell and the twitchings diminished. Light and sound were excluded; he fell asleep and awoke in a few hours refreshed and tranquillized, and on the next morning a little languor was all that remained of an illness which seemed likely to prove so formidable.—WEST. Cooling and soothing remedies are required in almost all cases of irritation, congestion, or expansion of the blood.

Disorders of the nervous system are very frequent during the period of teething. Many of the symptoms which then occur, are the direct result of irritation of the tri-facial nerve, but others are the immediate consequence of congestion of the brain. Febrile disturbance almost always attends upon the process of dentition, and when the circulation is in a state of preternatural excitement, a very slight cause may suffice to overturn its equilibrium, and occasion a greater flow of blood to the brain than the organ is able to bear. Suppression of perspiration, deficiency of bile and scantiness of urine, often occur during dentition and leave the blood overloaded with effete and irritating substances.

According to WEST, congestion of the brain may come on very suddenly, its symptoms being alarming from the first, and such as to call for immediate interference; or general uneasiness, a disordered state of the bowels, which are generally, although not invariably constipated, and feverishness may precede the more serious attack by a few days. The head becomes hot by degrees, the child grows restless and fretful, and seems distressed by light and noise, or sudden motion, while children who are old enough sometimes complain of their head. Usually, too, vomiting occurs repeatedly, a symptom which is not only confirmatory of others, but also may exist before there is any well-marked indication of the head being affected, and when, though the child seems ailing, there is nothing definite about its illness. The degree of fever which attends this condition varies much, and its accessions are irregular; but the pulse is usually much and permanently quickened; and, if the skull be unossified, the anterior fontanelle (or soft spot on the top of the head,) is either tense and prominent, or the brain is seen and felt to beat forcibly through it. The sleep is disturbed, the child often waking with a start, while there is occasional twitching of the muscles of the face, or tendons of the wrist. The child may continue in this state for many days, and then recover its health, with or without medical interference; but, a slight cause will generally suffice to bring back the former indisposition. Striking instances of this are often seen while children are teething; the fever may subside, the head grow cool, and the little patient appears quite well as soon as a tooth has cut through the gum, but the approach of each other tooth to the surface will be attended by a recurrence of the symptoms. Yet, we cannot always reckon on such a favorable result occurring; for the symptoms above mentioned are sometimes the indications of the system generally having begun to suffer from mischief which has been going on for months unnoticed, and which is now about to break out with all the formidable characters of acute dropsy of the brain. Or, should they have no such serious import, yet congestion of the brain is itself a serious and sometimes a fatal malady. Even though on treatment being adopted, the heat of the head may diminish, and the flush and heat of the face grow slighter and less constant, still the countenance may become very heavy and anxious, the indifference to surrounding objects may increase, and the child finally lie in a state of torpor or drowsiness; from which, however, it can at first be aroused to complete consciousness. But after being aroused, it soon subsides into its former drowsiness; the bowels generally continue constipated, and the vomiting seldom ceases, though it is sometimes less frequent than before. The pulse usually becomes smaller than in the first stage, and though there is often irregularity in its frequency, no actual intermission occurs. An attack of convulsions sometimes marks the transition from the first to the second stage; or the child passes without any apparent cause, from its previous torpor into a state of convulsions, which subsiding, leaves the torpor deeper than before. The fits may return and death take place in one of them, or the torpor growing more profound after each convulsive seizure the child at length dies comatose.

The *second* stage, if it may so be called, is usually of short duration, and if relief be not afforded by appropriate treatment, death is seldom delayed beyond forty-eight hours from the first fit, though no graver lesion may be discovered afterwards than a gorged state of the vessels of the brain and its membranes, and perhaps a little clear fluid in the ventricles and below the arachnoid.

Occasionally, death does not so speedily follow these symptoms; but they may continue slightly modified for days, or even weeks, and contrary to all expectation, recovery now and then takes place, especially in very young children, in whom the congestion having relieved itself by a copious effusion of water into the ventricles of the brain, the yielding skull accommodates itself to its increased contents. This chronic dropsy of the brain may even admit of cure.

Treatment.—The principal homœopathic remedies are: Glonoine, Opium, China, Ferrum, Belladonna and Stramonium. If these fail, their antagonistic remedies, Aconite, Digitalis Conium or Veratrum-viride may be used. (See Treatise on Apoplexy.)

INFAMMATION OF THE MEMBRANES OF THE BRAIN.

I.—INFLAMMATION OF THE DURA MATER.

According to Rokitansky, *primary* inflammations of the dura mater to any extent, such, for instance, as would lead to the formation of matter, are of rare occurrence, with the exception of those which are brought on by injury.

On the other hand, inflammations of slight degree, and usually combined with moderate inflammation of the bones of the skull, are frequent. They are characterized by vascularity and rosy-redness of the dura mater, and by softening of its texture; they give rise to interstitial infiltrations of the membrane with the products of inflammation, as well as to exudations upon that surface of it which adjoins the bone; such exudations become organized into loose cellular, or thick fibrous tissues, or at length, especially if there be any attendant inflammation of the bone, into bone; and they bring about a preternatural adhesion to the inner surface of the skull. These patches of inflammation are often widely spread, especially along the sutures; but sometimes they are confined within a smaller compass, so as to form circumscribed islands. Exudations which become converted into bone are generally spread out into a thin layer like that of puerperal osteophyte; they are first spongy, but gradually become compact: sometimes they form a mass of bone which looks as if it had flowed or dropped upon the membrane, and then coagulated; while, not unfrequently there are circumscribed plates or nodules, which, though they in course of time become intimately united to the bone, yet originally adhered firmly to the dura mater.

When the inflammation is more *intense*, and runs a *chronic* course, the dura mater acquires an increase in thickness, sometimes to the extent of three lines, and even more; it becomes indurated and callous, and usually adheres more closely than natural to the bone.

When the inflammation is brought on by injury, or extends to the dura mater from the neighboring tissues, it frequently terminates in the production of pus, and in suppurative degeneration of the membrane. These cases are of great importance, for they are generally secondary to inflammation and suppuration of the bone, or of the neighboring ligamentous structures. They are especially apt to occur in certain localities; thus, the dura mater often inflames, suppurates and sloughs from caries of the bones of the internal ear, and the labyrinth of the ethmoid bone of the nose; from caries of the upper bones of the spine, and suppuration of their ligaments. In the dura mater these processes remain limited and circumscribed, but when they reach the inner membranes of the brain, they usually spread rapidly into general meningitis.

Symptoms.—Inflammation of the dura mater according to WATSON rarely occurs as a spontaneous disease, but is not at all uncommon as a result of external injury. Its symptoms have been excellently well described by POTT: A man receives a blow upon the head; the blow stuns him perhaps at the time, but he presently recovers himself, and remains for a certain period, apparently in perfect health. But after some days he begins to complain; he has pain in his head, is restless, cannot sleep, has a frequent and hard pulse, a hot and dry skin, his face becomes flushed, his eyes red and ferrety; chills, nausea and vomiting supervene, and towards the end, convulsions and delirium. Meanwhile the part of the head which has been struck becomes puffy, tumid and sometimes tender, and if this tumid part of the scalp be cut through, the pericranium beneath is found separated from the skull; and the bone of the skull itself is observed to be altered in color, whiter and drier than the healthy bone; and if a piece of the bone be removed, it is also seen that the dura mater, on the under side of it is detached from the skull, and sometimes smeared with lymph or puriform matter. This is a disease which is often met with by the surgeon.

According to SOUTH and CHELIUS inflammation of the dura mater may be *acute* or *chronic.*

Acute inflammation of the dura mater appears most commonly from the third to the fifth day after the injury; the patient complains of severe oppressive headache, which spreads from the injured part over the whole head; the heat of the head is increased; the pulse is small, compressed and rather hard; the patient is heavy and difficult to arouse; his ideas become unconnected, and quiet delirium comes on; and lastly, when the inflammation proceeds to suppuration, the patient falls into a state of continued stupefaction, from which he cannot be easily aroused; convulsions come on, with continued shivering and irregular pulse; the pupils are wide and fixed; the breathing snoring and slow; the sphincters are paralyzed and finally the patient dies.

On dissection, the dura mater is found reddened, covered with exudations, and separated from the inside of the skull; pus may be found between it and the skull, and at this part the dura mater is often gangrenous.

Chronic inflammation of the dura mater, from injury to the head, often commences only after a long space of time, often after seven or fourteen days, often after a month; it begins with headache, mental and bodily depression, heaviness, unsteady walk, derangement of the stomach, quick pulse; and in its further course a circumscribed painful swelling of the scalp commonly arises at the place of injury; or, if there be a wound, it becomes pale, and secretes a thin, sanious fluid, which sticks fast to the bandages. The pericranium suppurates around the wound, and the inflammation soon runs into exudation of a yellowish, ichorous, purulent fluid, which collects either between the skull and the dura mater, or between the latter and the surface of the brain. The patients sometimes die twelve or eighteen months after the injury. SOUTH has seen several cases of this chronic inflammation, which is always a serious disease, and very difficult to control; often indeed entirely unmanageable under allopathic treatment. The patient then goes on slowly from bad to worse; sometimes with intervals of improvement, and sometimes without, and will frequently live for many months in a constant state of suffering.

According to WATSON the next most frequent cause of inflammation of the dura mater, after injuries of the head, is disease of the internal ear, and of the petrous portion of the temporal bone. Sometimes acute inflammation arises within the tympanum, when there has been no previous disease of the ear: the patient has severe earache; at length a gush of matter comes from the external meatus, but the pain does not cease, as it usually does in such cases; it continues, or even increases in intensity; the patient begins to shiver, becomes dull and drowsy; slight delirium perhaps occurs, and by degrees he sinks into stupor. In some instances no pus issues externally. More commonly symptoms of the same kind supervene upon a chronic discharge of purulent matter from the ear, especially as a sequel of scarlet fever. In some of these cases there is no symptom to mark the extensive mischief going on within the head, except the intense pain; the pulse may not be quickened, the skin may be warm but moist, and there may be neither fever, delirium or convulsions. In other cases, besides the intense pain in the head, there may be vomiting, intolerance of light, slight and transient delirium, a degree of stupor, and slight convulsions.

In some cases, pus is absorbed from the ear, and diffuse inflammation of the veins with terrible consequences in various parts of the body may ensue. In such cases the complaint is marked by pain in the head, fever and chills which intermit; and so regular sometimes are the intermissions that the physician may be led to believe that he has fever and ague to deal with; then pain and swelling of some of the joints may come on, leading to the belief that the case is complicated with rheumatism; but the true and alarming nature of the case will soon become apparent; abscesses form in and about the affected joints, and if they be opened, foul, grumous and dark colored matter will be let out. The patient will generally have more or less fever, with dry parched tongue, rapid and feeble pulse, with more or less diarrhœa.

In short, in these cases the patient has pain in the ear, with discharge of pus from the external meatus, followed by pain in the head coming on with fever and chills, and followed after a short interval by destructive suppuration in several distant parts; all forming a chain of presumptive evidence that the fatal mischief finds its entrance into the head and rest of the system through the porches of the ear.

Although *quotidian* paroxysms of fever have been noticed in several cases, still in one case at least the fever bore a *tertian* type: A young man previously healthy was attacked with fits of shivering, accompanied by pain on the left side of the head; at first the paroxysms were rather irregular; but they soon assumed the form of *tertian* ague, coming on every other day, at about the same hour; the cold fit commencing at noon and lasting about half an hour, followed by a hot fit of somewhat longer duration, and terminating in profuse perspiration. In the intermissions the pain in the head was trifling, there was no thirst or fever, but the patient did not sleep. A tumor formed over the mastoid process, and was opened, giving issue to a quantity of extremely offensive brownish pus, followed by great relief; but in about ten days the pain in the head and ear became very severe, with violent shivering fits many times a day, great thirst, heat of skin, vomiting and delirium; his face was flushed and pulse hard; he soon died.

Suppuration of the tympanum and consequent disease of the bone, are more common in scrofulous persons than in others; and they are more apt to occur as sequelæ of scarlet fever, than in any other way.

Treatment.—The remedies which act principally upon the sero-fibrous tissues are most specific in this disease, viz.: Aconite, Bryonia, Mercurius, Mezereum, Colchicum, &c.

When it arises from a mechanical injury to the head, the treatment may be commenced with *Arnica*, internally and externally; when fever arises, *Aconite* should be used internally, and the Tincture of the Root should be applied freely and repeatedly to the external surface of the head, avoiding the cut or wounded surfaces; if the case progresses steadily, *Mercurius* should be given in alternation with Aconite; if signs of effusion of serum and fibrine from the inflamed membrane arise, Bryonia, Mezereum, Hellebore or Colchicum, should be used in alternation with Mercurius, or the Iodide of Mercury; if the symptoms of purulent exudation arise, Tartar-emetic, or Hepar-sulph., Sabina or Thuya should be given.

INFLAMMATION OF THE ARACHNOID.

ARACHNITIS.

The arachnoid membrane is a shut sack, the *parietal* layer of which is attached to the dura mater, while the *cerebral* or visceral layer is for the most part blended with the pia mater of the brain.

Inflammations of the *parietal* layer of the arachnoid, are on the whole of frequent occurrence; their pathological import, however, is according to ROKITANSKY, mostly subordinate; they are met with, from injuries of the skull, from what is called a phlogistic state of the blood, in pynæmia, in the course of acute eruptive diseases, in Bright's disease, and acute biliary dyscrasia. They are commonly slight in degree; the inner surface of the dura mater is then found streaked with delicate red vessels, and is of a clear rosy tint; it is lined with an exudation, that may be delicate or greyish, and soft like a layer of mucus; or more consistent and membranous, or yellow, loose and pus-like.

In some rarer cases, this inflammation of the *parietal* layer has all the appearance of being primary, and judging from the amount of its products, also severe. These processes usually take place, and furnish their products without being accompanied by any similar disease in the *cerebral* layer: even in the intense primary inflammation, just alluded to, the change which takes place in the cerebral layer is limited to cloudiness and thickening; the false membrane very rarely produces any adhesion between the two surfaces.

Inflammation of the *cerebral* layer of the arachnoid presents peculiar appearances, in respect to the condition of the *pia mater*. We find on the one hand, that, *as arachnitis is not usually fatal in itself*, or at least not in an early stage, it sometimes leaves traces of its existence, in pretty extensive thickenings of the membrane; in free exudations on its surface, which become converted into circumscribed tendinous patches, or diffused false membranes, &c., *whilst very trifling changes are discoverable in the pia mater*, to indicate that an inflammatory process occurred at the same time in it. When, on the other hand, the pia mater is acutely inflamed, and there is profuse exudation into its tissue, the subjacent arachnoid *is in no marked degree affected*, and its surface is entirely without any free exudation. Showing that the inflammations of the two membranes are entirely different and distinct, and that specific remedies must be found to act curatively upon each.

Purulent exudation on the free surface of the arachnoid takes place on the *parietal* layer only when the dura mater is very acutely inflamed in consequence of injury of the skull and caries, proving that remedies which act specifically upon the bones and dura mater, will also probably act specifically in inflammations of the *parietal* layer of the arachnoid; and on the *cerebral* layer, only when a simultaneous acute inflammation of the pia mater also gives rise to an exudation of pus; proving that remedies which act specifically upon the pia mater, will also probably act specifically upon the *cerebral* layer of the arachnoid.

It is remarkable that true tubercular exudations do not occur on the arachnoid; proving that remedies which act specifically upon the arachnoid may prove antidotal to tubercular disease.

Finally, according to ROKITANSKY, on whichever layer of the arachnoid these processes take place, that portion which corresponds to the *convexity* of the hemispheres of the brain is exclusively affected; and in proportion as they approach the base of the brain, (which they occasionally do), the intensity of the inflammation, and the quantity of their products is palpably diminished; again proving that remedies which act specifically upon the upper surface of the brain, and upon the arachnoid are antagonistic, or antidotal to tubercular disease, which acts principally upon the base of the brain, and upon the pia mater.

Symptoms and Treatment.—These are very similar to those of simple inflammation of the pia mater, and cannot be definitely given in the present state of our knowledge.

INFLAMMATION OF THE PIA MATER.

MENINGITIS.

This is the *true meningitis*, and the most important disease of the membranes of the brain. According to Rokitansky it is impossible to depict its general features without distinguishing *two* totally different forms of the disease.

a) *First form.*—This is a true inflammatory affection; it usually extends over the *convexity* of the brain, and diminishes in intensity as it approaches the base. It rarely occurs at the *base* of the brain at all.

The individuals who present this form of disease are generally in the youthful period, the bloom of life; they are usually strong, at any rate they show no trace of the tubercular dyscrasia.

The disease is usually unaccompanied with acute dropsy of the brain; at least the exudations and effusions found in the ventricles are mostly slight; so also, softening of the stomach does not usually accompany or result from it.

Except at its periphery or convexity, the brain is unaltered by it, especially no softening of the brain arises or results from it.

It is a pure inflammatory affection and if any specific remedies against simple inflammation are known in any school of medicine, it ought to be a perfectly manageable disease. In fact Rokitansky says, although this form of meningitis is frequently fatal, yet it often terminates in resolution. A chronic form of it is frequently found in mental disease, especially in cases of secondary imbecility; yet it is frequently acute and even epidemic.

b) *Second form.*—This is the most frequent and fatal disease of the membranes of the brain, especially in children. It occurs according to Rokitansky almost exclusively at the base of the brain, and the peculiar opaline, flocculent, albumino-serous, gelatinous, sero-purulent effusions and exudations which attend it, accumulate especially between the hemispheres of the brain on each side, from the optic commissure in front to the pons, and even over the medulla oblongata behind. From thence they may be traced into the fissure of Sylvius, and the longitudinal fissure of the brain, and so on to the convex surface of the hemispheres; for the fibrino-tuberculous product accumulates along the vascular trunks which run in the fissures, viz.: the arteries and veins of the fissure of Sylvius and Corpus-callosum, and the latter often appear completely enveloped in the exudation.

From these points the inflammation always extends also to the choroid plexuses and the lining membrane of the ventricles, particularly the lateral ventricles, and there gives rise to the effusion and exudation of similar products, from which a distinct purulent sediment is often deposited; hence it is almost always combined with acute dropsy of the brain; and very often it is also associated with softening of the stomach.

The brain itself is always in a state of acute œdema, or serous infiltration, with hydrocephalic swelling. At those parts where the disease is most intense, and particularly in the fissures of Sylvius, the convolutions of the brain, especially at the superficial parts, become the seat of red, or yellow softening.

The subjects of this form of the disease are mostly children, although it is also frequent at later periods of life. The individuals who are attacked with it are generally persons already suffering with the tuberculous dyscrasia, or those in whom tubercle is actually deposited.

The base of the brain is the chief seat of this form of tuberculosis; from thence it extends towards and over the hemispheres; it is rare to find the convex surface of the brain the principal seat of its development.—Rokitansky.

It is the most frequent and fatal disease of the head; as it is generally associated with the deposit of tubercles in other, and often many other organs, with extensive dropsy and softening of the brain, and with decided softening of the stomach, there is almost necessarily scarcely any chance of recovery.

Symptoms of primary meningitis.—This disease is most frequent in persons from the age of sixteen to forty-five years; next, in children from five and a half to eleven years; it is very rare in infants, and more common in males than females. It is most frequently caused by exposure to the sun, by excessive intellectual labor, by intemperance in drinking, and by depressing mental emotions; in children it is most common during dentition, or from suppression of eruptions of the scalp.

In the simple, *primary* form of the disease, the *pain in the head* is always very prominent, and sets in at the very beginning of the attack; it is violent and continued, with more or less severe exacerbations; it often obliges the patient to cry out; it is complained of spontaneously and unceasingly; the patient insists that his disease is solely in his head, can point to the exact seat of it, and complains of it until he falls into a state of unconsciousness.

The *intelligence* is very quickly involved in the great majority of cases; there is great mental agitation, soon followed by active delirium, which is sometimes violent, or even furious. The patients are apt to get out of bed, and attempt to jump out of the window, &c. This is soon followed by somnolence, which alternates at first with the delirium, but finally settles into a profound coma, or complete loss of consciousness.

The *eyes* are sensitive to light, the pupils are almost always dilated, but at times they are contracted or irregular; they finally become immoveable, and in some cases vision is entirely abolished; squinting is also frequently observed, especially in children.

The *nerves of motion* do not ordinarily present any peculiar symptoms, especially in the early stages of the disease, except that the patient is apt to totter and fall if he attempts to rise; at a later stage, however, we often notice stiffness of the limbs, or spasmodic contractions, or even convulsions; but these symptoms are not constant. Towards the end of the attack, subsultus, carphologia, and convulsive movements are generally present. It is rare that we observe partial stiffness of one limb, or paralysis; when these are present, there generally is a simultaneous affection of the brain itself.

Sometimes *the nerves of sensation* are blunted, either throughout the whole body, or in more or less extensive parts; at times, however, there is an increase of sensibility, at least for a time.

The countenance is generally animated, the eyes haggard and brilliant; there are frequent alterations of color, from red to violet, and thence to pallor, more or less intense. Sometimes the features are contracted and grimacing, at others they are relaxed. The eyes often express astonishment, fright or fury; at others they seem dull, glassy, and without expression; at times they are prominent, at others sunken. An unintelligent smile often flits over the features. The nostrils are generally dry; the lips pale and parched.

Of the symptoms of the *digestive organs*, the *vomitings* are without doubt the most remarkable; they are generally bilious, and often abundant; they often cease on the second or third day of the attack, but sometimes persist to the end, although they may intermit for a time, to be renewed again. The *tongue* is generally dry, often red, or covered with various kinds of coating. *Constipation* is also one of the most constant symptoms; it generally sets in from the beginning, and may even precede the other phenomena.

The *breathing* is generally remarkably irregular.

Fever is always well marked, the pulse is quick and hard at first; afterwards it becomes small and irregular. The skin is hot and remarkably dry.

Secondary meningitis occurs during the course of some other disease, especially typhoid fever; the headache is apt to be not very well marked; the vomitings are often absent; the most remarkable symptoms are the softness, and irregularity of the pulse and respiration, the paleness and expression of anxiety upon the face, and the extreme agitation which precedes the delirium.

The *course* of the disease is onwards, and although there are some exacerbations, yet the remissions are not as notable as in tubercular meningitis. The *duration* of the disease is very short; it does not last longer than from three to nine or eleven days.

Diagnosis.—Inflammation of the pia mater may be mistaken for tubercular meningitis, or for typhoid fever. But in tubercular meningitis there are generally preceding signs of ill-health, or of tubercular disease; the symptoms of inflammation of the pia mater set in more suddenly, are more severe from the onset, and persist more actively; the headache is more violent, also the heat of the head, redness of the face and intolerance of light; the delirium is also more intense; the vomitings are more frequent and abundant; the fever more severe and constant. The symptoms progress more rapidly and regularly.

It may be distinguished from typhoid fever by the less frequent vomiting, more frequent pains in and distension of the bowels, with diarrhœa, which are so characteristic of the latter disease; enlargement of the spleen may also be distinguished by percussion; bleeding from the nose and ringing in the ears, the rose colored spots, sudamina, the regularity of the pulse and breathing, and absence of rigidity or paralysis of the limbs will also serve to distinguish the two diseases.

Treatment.—If the symptoms of arachnitis or meningitis begin to show themselves, or even if the disease be fully developed we may begin the treatment with *Aconite;* it acts specifically upon the serous and fibrous membranes, and is thought to be homœopathic to all acute inflammations, while physicians of the dominant school suppose it to be as antipathic to all acute inflammations and congestions as Digitalis or Veratrum-viride. According to KREUSSLER it is not a question of fever or no fever, for an acute inflammation of the brain as well as of the meningeal membranes requires the use of Aconite, from the commencement of the disease until the period when essential changes develop the full characters of the affection. He says it is always safe to commence the treatment with a few doses of Aconite, even if it be possible to discern the homœopathicity of another and apparently more specific remedy from the very beginning of the attack.

Dose.—Of course, in so serious a disease, the remedy should be used promptly and thoroughly; it should be given not only internally, but also applied externally, and that right freely. I have been in the habit of applying the Tincture of the *Root* of Aconite, over a large portion of the scalp, every 2, 4, 6 or 8 hours, according to the severity of the symptoms. The Tincture of the *Plant* may be given in repeated doses, every $\frac{1}{4}$, $\frac{1}{2}$, 1 or 2 hours, in acute and rapid cases; every 2, 4 or 6 hours, in sub-acute and slighter attacks.*

If the case progress, so that it is probable that exudations of plastic lymph or sero-fibrous effusions have already commenced to take place, then *Bryonia* and *Mercurius* are the most important remedies; if there be much vomiting with obstinate constipation, great heat of head and much fever, one or two full

* The dilutions and pellets are probably not useful in cases of meningitis of any kind.

doses of *Mercurius* may be given so as to bring about free action upon the bowels. Small doses of *Tartar-emetic* may also serve to allay the irritability of the stomach, to moderate the fever, tend to produce perspiration and aid the action upon the bowels; but they must not be continued long, or else too great prostration may be produced. The Tartar-emetic must be quickly changed to alternate doses of *Bryonia*, and small but repeated doses of Mercurius. If Mercurius be at all indicated it may also be allowable to apply a weak solution or ointment upon the scalp, in the immediate neighborhood of the seat of the disease.

If it becomes apparent that a large effusion of serum, has taken place from the inflamed membranes, *Helleborus*, *Digitalis*, *Kali-hydriodicum*, and *Mercurius-iodatus*, become the principal remedies. If Hellebore and Digitalis, either singly or in alternation fail to produce an alleviation of the symptoms, Kali-hydriodicum may be applied over the whole of the scalp in solution, or in the form of an ointment, and frequently repeated small doses may be given internally. If these also fail, Iodide of Mercury may be applied in the form of an ointment over the scalp, and small doses of this, or of Mercurius-corrosivus may be given internally.

If an almost entire suppression of urine occur, *Cantharides* will prove the most homœopathic remedy. It is far more homœopathic to inflammations of the membranes of the brain than either Belladonna, Stramonium or Hyosciamus, which only produce congestion, rarely inflammation of these parts. *Cantharides* has caused congestion of the vessels of the brain; thickening of the arachnoid of the brain, but especially of the cerebellum, which is covered with a very thick layer of lymph, while a large quantity of serum has been found at the base of the brain. As the suppression of urine in arachnitis and meningitis, does not depend upon an inflammation of the kidneys, but upon a torpid or semi-paralytic state of these organs from pressure upon the brain, *Cantharides* which acts far more specifically upon the kidneys, than upon the brain or its membranes, may arouse the former organs from their torpor, and bring on a secretion of urine which may relieve the pressure upon the brain; at the same time it will not exert an injurious or too irritating effect upon the brain or its membranes, as the stage in which it is most indicated, and hence is most useful, is that in which the profuse exudation of fibrine and copious effusion of serum from the meninges of the brain has brought about a resolution of the inflammatory congestion of these organs, and left them in a state of torpor from over-exertion and secretion, which will not bear debilitating remedies, and may tolerate exciting or stimulating ones; the depressed state of the general system when copious effusion has taken place, marked by sopor with complete insensibility to external impressions, with a small feeble and intermitting pulse, coldness and clamminess of the skin, calls for the use of stimulants, and Cantharides may prove the best, from its specific relation to the seat and nature of the disease, and its marked power over the secretion of the kidneys, which it is so important to restore. If the case be not absolutely hopeless, and the internal use of Cantharides does not produce the desired effect, and the physician and parents are willing to inflict some suffering in the hope of saving life, which might otherwise be lost, a blister of Cantharides may also be applied to the back of the neck, or even to the scalp. But such an extreme and severe measure should only be used in cases of pure or simple arachnitis, or meningitis; if it be at all probable that *tubercular meningitis* be present, all temptations to severe and active measures should be steadily rejected by the physician, whose sole endeavors in such almost invariably hopeless cases, should be directed towards soothing and allaying any and every painful symptom of the case; narcotic remedies, such as Belladonna, Conium, Hyosciamus, Opium, or Stramonium, or Cannabis-indica, or Chloroform should be used freely and without hesitation. To save life is next to impossible; to allay suffering is both possible and imperatively demanded.

It may be allowable to mention here that Dr. HAHN has succeeded several times with the cold affusion, in arousing and curing children, after the supervention of complete coma. He has also succeeded in 14 cases, after the patients were in an apparently hopeless state of coma, with frictions of the scalp, with Tartar-emetic ointment repeated every two hours, until pustulation was established; it is a severe measure and occasionally induces gangrene of the scalp, yet it is perhaps allowable in the advanced stages of simple inflammatory meningitis.

TUBERCULAR MENINGITIS.

IN CHILDREN.

This is one of the most common diseases of the brain or its appendages in children. It is by far the most common cause of so-called acute- or sub-acute dropsy of the brain, and furnishes a satisfactory reason why this disease is so frequently fatal under every variety of treatment, at the same time that it renders it self-evident that any physician or class of physicians who pretend to cure the majority of their cases of dropsy of the brain, are either self-deceived, or are absolute impostors.

Green says that at least one-fourth of all the diseases of the brain in children are tubercular in their nature; Becquerel in 30 cases of meningitis, found tubercular granulations in the membranes of the brain in no less than 28; Jackson found them in 4 cases out of 6; Green discovered them in 56 cases out of 60; Rilliet and Barthez in 29 cases out of 33; Bouchut in 6 cases out of 9. Hence in 138 cases of so called acute hydrocephalus, tubercles were found in no less than 123 instances. Hence it is evident that until within a few years, tubercular meningitis, simple acute meningitis, independent of tubercularization, and simple dropsical effusion within the cavity of the skull, independent of inflammation have been confounded together under the single term of hydrocephalus or water on the brain.

Symptoms.—Unlike acute simple meningitis there is more or less of a premonitory stage. According to West, in the first or premonitory stage there are many indications of cerebral congestion, coupled with general febrile disturbance; and presenting exacerbations and remissions at irregular periods. The child becomes gloomy, pettish and slow in its movements, and is but little pleased with its usual amusements. Or, at other times its spirits are very variable; it will sometimes cease suddenly in the midst of its play, and run to hide its head in its mother's lap, putting its hand to its head, and complaining of headache, or saying merely that it is tired or sleepy, and wants to go to bed. Sometimes, too, it turns giddy, as may be known, not so much from its complaint of dizziness, as from its suddenly standing still, gazing around for a moment as if lost, and then either beginning to cry at the strange sensation, or seeming to awake from a reverie, and at once returning to its play. The infant in its nurse's arms betrays the same sensation by a sudden look of alarm, a momentary cry, and a hasty clinging to its nurse. If the child can walk, it may be observed to drag one leg, halting in its gait, though but slightly, and seldom so much at one time as at another, so that both the parents and the physician may be disposed to attribute it to an ungainly habit which the child has contracted. The *appetite* is usually bad, though sometimes very variable, and the child, when apparently busy at play, may all at once throw down its toys and beg for food; then refuse what is offered, or taking a hasty bite, may seem to nauseate the half-tasted morsel, may open its mouth stretch out its tongue, and heave as if about to vomit. The *thirst* is seldom considerable, and sometimes there is an actual aversion to drink as well as to food, apparently from its exciting or increasing the nausea. The *stomach*, however, seldom rejects everything, but the same food that occasions sickness at one time is retained at another. Sometimes the child vomits only after taking food; at other times, even when the stomach is empty, it brings up some greenish phlegm, without much effort, and with no relief. These attacks of vomiting seldom occur oftener than two or three times a day, but they may return for several days together, the child's head probably growing heavier, and its headache more severe. The *bowels* are generally constipated from the first; the evacuations are usually scanty, sometimes pale, often of different colors, almost always deficient in bile, frequently mud-colored and very offensive. The abdomen is seldom full or distended, but the child sometimes complains of pain in the belly, which may be tender to pressure. The *tongue* is not dry, generally rather red at the tip and edges, coated with white fur in the centre, which becomes yellowish towards the root; occasionally WEST has seen it very moist, and uniformly coated with a thin white fur. The *skin* is harsh, but there is no great heat of surface. The *nostrils* are dry; the *eyes* lustreless; the *pulse* accelerated, but seldom exceeding 120 in children of four years old and upwards, not full and strong, but often unequal in the force and duration of its beat.

The child is apt to be drowsy, and will sometimes want to be put to bed two or three times in the day; but it is restless, sleeps badly, grinds its teeth in its sleep, lies with its eyes partially open, awakes with the slightest noise, or even starts up in alarm without any apparent cause. At night, too, the existence of intolerance of light is often first noticed in consequence of the child's complaints about the presence of the candle in the room.

West truly says, that we must not expect to find all these symptoms in every case, neither indeed, when present are they persistent, but the child's condition is very apt to vary greatly in the course of a few minutes; cheerfulness alternating with depression, and sound sleep being now and then enjoyed in the midst of the unrefreshing dozes of the night.

Hartmann says, the precursory stage does not offer any of the characteristic symptoms of acute dropsy of the brain. Thus the child, which was previously able to run about with ease, has an unsteady vaccillating gait; he raises his feet high from the floor, or is liable to fall on the level ground, even in the room. This unsteadiness communicates itself to the whole body. We observe, moreover, a sudden change of disposition; in the place of the former cheerfulness and lightness of heart, the child is apt to become morose and peevish. On moving the head suddenly, or raising it from the recumbent posture, vertigo or a sense of stupefaction is experienced. In some cases the secretion of urine is scanty, in others it is turbid, flocculent or opalescent. Some authors number a fine, dry, colorless eruption on the outer side of the upper arm, on the cheeks and lips among the precursory symptoms of dropsy of the brain.

Besides these symptoms there are others which are more or less characteristic; such as a loss of the previous blooming appearance; restless sleep during which the child is apt to moan, groan, start up as in a fright, alternations of creeping chills and flushes of heat; a pulse of the ordinary rapidity, but one which intermits at times, or beats irregularly or more feebly.

If many of these symptoms be present, the physician should be led to suspect the impending approach of dropsy of the brain and to watch the development of the symptoms with anxious and redoubled attention. If the child be descended from scrofulous or consumptive parents it may already be too late to save life; the tuberculous dyscrasia may already be so fully developed, or the blood be already so fully overloaded with tubercular matter, or the capillary vessels may have lost their power and function of forming or separating healthy materials from the blood, that it will be impossible to prevent the formation and deposition of tubercle in the membranes of the brain, or even in many other organs. Still the trial must be made, late though it be. But in order to treat the tuberculous tendency or dyscrasia with the faintest hope of success, we must first understand, thoroughly understand, of what tubercle consists, and what it really is.

TUBERCULOSIS.

TUBERCLE.

THE physical description of tubercle is well known to every physician, the *chemical* is not so. According to HASSE, who drew his conclusions from numerous analyses carefully compiled by CERRUTTI and VOGEL, the organic component parts of tubercle are principally *Caseine*, with some fat, and a little albumen. According to PREUSS the animal portion of tubercle is principally made up of *Caseine*, with some fat in the form of Cholesterine, and a trifle of Phymatine. GÜTERBOCK found much *Caseine*, some Albumen, Phymatine and fat.

Less accurate observers, such as THENARD, found Albumen in excess; while HECHT and SCHARLAU, who probably did not separate the cellular and other tissues, or products of inflammation found intermixed with the surrounding tubercular masses, found nearly equal proportions of Gelatine, Albumen and Fibrine, in their analyses of tubercular substance.

ANCELL, justly says, if we admit that tubercle is a definite chemical compound, which is very probable, still this compound must be subject to changes and to admixture with numerous extraneous and accidental materials, as with those composing the tissues in which the tubercle is deposited, and which by pressure and otherwise, become disintegrated and blended with the essential constituents of tubercle, or with the products of inflammation, such as coagulable lymph, or fibrine, or pus from inflammation of the substance of the tuberculous organ, or with mucus or pus from the mucous membrane of the lungs, or with blood itself. It is always difficult, and frequently impossible, for the chemist to separate these different products, or to estimate their proportions. Tubercle must also, from the same causes, exhibit differences, according to the nature of the tissue in which it is seated. Still, he says, chemical analysis leaves no doubt that tubercle contains a protein compound as an essential constituent, which appears to bear a close analogy to, if it be not identically *Caseine.* Tubercle has a decidedly cheesy appearance to the naked eye, and tuberculous pus resembles a mixture of soft cheese and water both in color and consistence. ANCELL repeats that the *caseous* quality of tubercle and scrofulous pus indicates the presence of a nitrogenous compound of a caseous nature in the liquor tuberculi, showing that from the liquor sanguinis of tuberculous blood a caseous blastema is exuded, differing from the ordinary healthy blastema. Its caseous quality renders it unfit to nourish the tissues, and gives it a tendency to solidification.

Another large class of medical chemists think that tubercle is essentially *albuminous* in its nature. Thus HECHT found in crude tubercle: Fibrine 30 parts; Albumen 23; Gelatine 27; water and loss, 27. BOUDET found: Caseine, Gelatine and a considerable quantity of Cholesterine; when tuberculous substance was treated with cold water it yielded: Albumen, a substance resembling Caseine, and a fibrinous residue. GÜTERBOCK found: Pyine, Phymatine, Albumen and fat. SCHARLAU, Albumen, Gelatine, Fibrine, fat and water. VOGEL, Fibrine, Albumen and Caseine, with fat, a material analagous to Pyine, &c. GLOVER, Pyine, Albumen, (but no Caseine,) fat, &c. L'HERETIER found softened tubercle to consist of Albumen, very soft Fibrine, fatty matter and lime.

It is easy to account for many of these discrepancies; thus PREUSS in the most complete chemical analyses of crude tubercular pulmonary substance which has yet been furnished, found Gelatine in the residue of the pulmonary tissue, which he carefully separated from the tuberculous substance, but none in tubercle itself. If other chemists had been equally careful, they probably would not have found much or any Gelatine in tuberculous matter. Again, ANCELL says that Pyine is by no means a constant constituent of tubercle; it is a trit-oxide of Protein, the result of inflammatory action on tuberculous blood resulting in the super-oxidation of the Protein compounds, such as Caseine, or possibly Albumen or Fibrine, which make up the bulk of tubercle. The Fibrine is also probably the result of inflammation, hence, we can easily narrow down the two essential constituents of tubercle to Caseine and Albumen.

Caseine and Albumen are analagous substances; both are compounds of Protein; Albumen consists of 10 atoms of Protein, 2 atoms of Sulphur and 1 of Phosphor.; while Caseine consists of 10 atoms of Protein, 1 of Sulphur and none of Phosphor. Hence it is very easy for careless or not very expert chemists to mistake one for the other.

TUBERCULOUS BLOOD.

As tubercle is evidently derived from the blood, we have next to examine the character of the blood in tuberculous subjects. According to ANCELL tuberculous blood is defective in vital properties; the red globules are *deficient* in number and defective in structure; the globulin, hæmatin and iron are all *deficient*.

The *serum* of the blood is vitiated in quality, the water, Albumen and lime are in *excess*, and the Albumen also defective in quality. Caseine does not exist normally in the blood, and hence the defect in the Albumen may consist in its tendency to be converted into Caseine.

The Fibrine is rather deficient in quantity and defective in quality, the fats probably deficient; the alkaline and earthy salts, especially the chlorides and phosphates of Soda and Potassa decidedly deficient.

DIETETIC TREATMENT OF THE TUBERCULOUS DYSCRASIA.

Hence the indications for the improvement of the quality of tuberculous blood, are: 1st, to increase the quantity of iron, fat, alkaline- and earthy-salts and Fibrine, and to improve the quality of the latter; 2d, to diminish the quantity of water, lime and Albumen, and improve the quality of the latter.

As blood is formed from the food by the processes of digestion, chymification, chylification and sanguinification, tuberculous blood may be produced from improper food, by a peculiar form of indigestion, or by a defect in sanguinification in the lungs or other parts of the body.

In the first place vegetable Albumen, according to MULDER is perfectly identical with animal Albumen, and hence it is probable that the whole quantity of Albumen required for the purposes of the body is delivered to it already formed, and does not require to be elaborated by the processes of digestion or sanguinification. Great care should be exercised in the selection of the albuminous articles of food for consumptive persons, that they be of the best quality; as there is already a tendency to excess of Albumen in tuberculous subjects, articles of food should be selected which contain comparatively little of already formed Albumen. According to PROUT the following quantities of Albumen are found in the subjoined animal substances.

East India Isinglass, - -	7.2 to 13.5	per cent.
White of Egg, - - - - -	15.5	"
Yolk " - - - - - -	17.47	"
Liver of Ox, - - - - -	20.19	"
Sweetbread, - - - - -	14.00	"
Caviare, - - - - - -	31.00	"

Hence the above articles are more or less objectionable in the diet of scrofulous, tuberculous or consumptive persons.

The muscle of	Beef	contains only,	- 2.2	per cent.
"	Mutton	"	- 2.6	"
"	Venison	"	- 2.3	"
"	Veal	"	2.6 to 3.2	"
"	Chicken	"	- 3.0	"
"	Fish	"	4.4 to 5.2	"
"	Pigeon	"	- 4.5	"

Hence, beef, mutton, venison and chicken form the best animal food for tuberculous subjects.

Again, as the Fibrine of the blood is defective and deficient, articles of food which contain much Fibrine should be selected.

The muscle of	Beef	contains	20 per cent.	of Fibrine.
"	Mutton	"	22 "	"
"	Chicken	"	20 "	"

The muscle of	Veal contains	19 per cent.	of Fibrine.	
"	Pork "	19	"	"
"	Fish " from	13 to 15	"	"
"	Sweetbread, only	8	"	"

Again, articles which contain Caseine should be avoided in the diet of tuberculous persons—milk, curds and cheese are objectionable, cream and whey are allowable. Asses' milk is the least objectionable as it contains only 1.82 per cent. of Caseine, while cows' milk contains as much as 4.48. The milk of cows fed on hay, turnips and potatoes contains only 3.3 per cent. of Caseine, and is perhaps less injurious than some other kinds.

Vegetable Caseine is chiefly found in the leguminous seeds, such as beans, peas, lentils, &c., hence these may have to be avoided.

Vegetable Albumen is present in considerable quantity in most vegetable juices, such as the juices of carrots, turnips, cabbages, cauliflowers, asparagus, &c.—Potatoes contain far less Protein and Albumen than any other vegetable substance used for food,—only 1 per cent.

Vegetable Fibrine is most abundant in the seeds of the cereal grasses, such as wheat, rye, barley, oats, maize, rice; it also exists in buckwheat; the juice of grapes is especially rich in it, &c.

As the fat is deficient in the tuberculous dyscrasia, the oily alimentary principles should be used.

Filberts contain	- - -	60	per cent.	of oil.
Walnuts "	- - - -	50	"	"
Olive seeds	- - -	54	"	"
Cocoa and Earth-nuts	- -	47	"	"
Almonds "	- - - -	46	"	"
Maize "	- - - -	9	"	"
Dates "	- - only	.02	"	"
Yolk of Eggs	- - -	28.75	"	"
Ordinary meat, with cellular tissue		14.3	"	"
Liver of Ox	- - only	3.89	"	"
Caviare	- - "	4.3	"	"
Cow's Milk	- - "	3.13	"	"
Asses "	- "	.11	"	"

Butter and olive oil, fats, meats and marrow may be used, suet puddings, salmon, herrings and eels abound in oil, chocolate and cocoa, hashes, stews and broths contain much fat. As the fixed oils and fats are difficult and slow of digestion many physicians may consider them objectionable. It is well known that in many delicate persons fat does not become properly chymified. It floats on the contents of the stomach in the form of an oily pellicle, becoming odorous, and sometimes highly rancid, and in this state excites heartburn, most disagreeable nausea, and eructations, or at times actual vomiting. These effects are owing to the development of volatile fatty acids, and may be prevented by the use of alkaline and earthy salts, such as the chlorides and phosphates of Soda and Potassa which are also required to make up the deficiency of them, which has been shown to be present in the blood of tuberculous subjects.

As the *Iron* of the blood is also deficient, a certain quantity must be supplied to the system.

TUBERCULOUS INDIGESTION.

Such is the theoretically correct system of diet in tuberculous dyscrasia and affections; but it is very evident that healthy animal or vegetable Caseine or Albumen will not be converted into tuberculous Caseine and Albumen if all the functions of digestion and sanguinification be perfectly and healthily performed. According to BENNETT, many observing physicians have not failed to notice that tubercular disease is ushered in with a bad or capricious appetite, a furred or morbidly clean tongue, *unusual acidity of the stomach* and bowels, loss of appetite, constipation alternating with diarrhœa, and a variety of symptoms denominated dyspeptic, or referable to a deranged state of the digestive organs. It is probable that tuberculosis is a disease of the primary digestion, causing, 1st, impoverishment of the blood; 2d, local exudations from the bloodvessels presenting the characters of tuberculous exudation; and third the consequent softening, ulcerations and destructive results which distinguish it. BENNETT also asserts that further observations show, that circumstances which remove the malassimilation of food frequently check further tubercular exudations, while those which previously existed become abortive, and that occasionally more extensive excavations may heal up and cicatrize.

A healthy nutrition of the body cannot proceed without a proper admixture and proportion of the albuminous and oleaginous elements. This may be inferred from the physiological experiments of Tiedemann, Gmelin, Leuret, Lassaigne, Magendie and others; from an observation of the constituents of milk, (caseine, butter and sugar,) the natural food of young mammiferous animals; from a knowledge of the contents of the egg, (albumen and oil,) which constitute the source from which all the tissues of oviparous animals are formed before the shell is broken; and from all that we know of the principles contained in the food of adult animals.

The peculiarity of tuberculosis, however, is that an excess of acidity exists in the alimentary canal, whereby the albuminous constituents of the food are rendered easily soluble, whilst the alkaline secretions of the saliva and of the pancreatic juice are more than neutralized, and rendered incapable either of transforming the carbonaceous constituents of vegetable food into oil, or of so preparing fatty matters introduced into the system, as will render them easily assimilable. In consequence, more albuminous than fatty matters enter the blood, and the necessary waste of structure is supplied by the absorption of the adipose tissues of the body. Hence the emaciation which characterizes tubercular disease; hence also, as the fatty matters introduced into the stomach are not digested and assimilated, but are simply taken up into the vena porta and carried to the liver, the fatty liver which occurs so frequently in the tuberculous dyscrasia. In the meanwhile local congestions occur in various parts, leading to an exudation containing a super-abundance of albumen; which in its turn being deficient in the necessary proportion of fatty matter to form elementary molecules, remain abortive and form tuberculous corpuscules.

To improve the faulty nutrition which originates and keeps up the tubercular disease it is of all things important, therefore, to cause a larger quantity of fatty matter to be assimilated. The use of alkalies or other solvents or digestives of oil are all-important, although a mere increase in the amount, or even quality of the food will often accomplish this. The treatment practised some years ago by Dr. STEWART, which consisted in freely administering beef-steaks and porter, and causing exercise to be taken in the open air, excited considerable attention from its success. BENNETT has been informed, that in some parts of America the cure consists in living on the bone-marrow of the buffalo, and that the consumptive patient gets so strong in this way, that he is at length able to hunt down the animal on the prairies. All kinds of food, rich in fat, will not unfrequently produce the same effects, and hence the value long attributed to milk, especially ass's milk, the produce of the dairy, as cream and butter, fat bacon, caviare, &c.

But, in order that such substances should be digested or assimilated, solvents of fat (alkalies) must be used, if the powers of the stomach and alimentary canal have undergone any great diminution. Unless this precaution be used, it will be found in many cases that the patient is unable to tolerate such kind of food, and that it either lies undigested in the stomach, or is sooner or later vomited.

Children born of tuberculous mothers should be weaned early; unless a perfectly healthy and robust wet-nurse can be procured it is better to feed them with diluted or undiluted cream.

FULLY DEVELOPED TUBERCULOUS MENINGITIS

Is marked by three important symptoms, viz.: by *headache*, *vomiting* and *constipation*, to which is added in the great majority of cases, some acceleration of the pulse; the intelligence may remain perfect, showing that the brain itself is not yet involved; the strength may not be greatly diminished, nor the appetite entirely lost, and the thirst may be moderate. These symptoms usually last but two or three days before others make their appearance, showing that the attack is confirmed. In some few instances, however, the precursory symptoms last, with irregular intermissions, for several weeks. In some cases the invasion may be preceded for three months by occasional cough, irregular attacks of fever, progressive emaciation, paleness, languor alternating with extreme irritability, disinclination to take exercise, and during the latter part of the time by partial lameness, and in fact by all the signs of general tubercular disease. In other cases the invasion may be preceded for several months by frequent complaints of intense headache, especially after taking active exercise, and by unusual languor, and by no other symptoms; there may be long intervals of health, and the child then be taken down suddenly.

According to MEIGS, *headache* is a nearly invariable symptom in children old enough to describe their sensations, and is therefore very important. In infants its presence is to be inferred when the child frequently carries its hands to various parts of the head, and presses strongly against it, and when the head is constantly rolled from side to side. It is usually referred to a point just over one or both brows; in other cases it extends over the whole head. It is commonly severe so that the child, when old enough, complains of it spontaneously; they may even cry frequently and bitterly, beg to have the doctor sent for, and submit willingly to any remedy suggested for its relief. It is thought that the acute, shrill cry of the disease depends upon the acuteness of this pain. It usually lasts throughout the first stage, and ceases only as the delirium and coma of the second stage come on.

As long as the membranes of the brain are alone involved the headache is not attended with delirium. In truth, the intellectual faculties remain undisturbed in the majority of cases during the first few days; and this fact, which is so contrary to what is generally supposed, is apt to mislead the physician in his opinion and treatment of the case; he is generally too apt to give remedies which act more specifically upon the brain, than upon its membranes.

I trust that it has been rendered evident that a correct system of diet is as necessary in tuberculosis as in diabetes or adiposis. There is frequently time sufficient to make the trial, for the healthy and robust are comparatively seldom attacked by dropsy of the brain, and in many instances the evidences of declining health, precede for weeks or months the real premonitory symptoms of the disease. We often observe a gradual decay of the child's strength and wasting of its flesh, it becomes subject to irregular febrile attacks, coughs a little, loses its appetite, its bowels are almost always disordered, and generally constipated, it makes frequent vague complaints of pains in its limbs, or of weariness or headache.

Medical treatment.—HARTMANN correctly states that one of the most homœopathic remedies for the precursory stage of tubercular meningitis is *Pulsatilla;* it corresponds more especially to the derangement of the stomach, to the inability to digest rich and fatty food, to the gradually failing health, loss of flesh and ill-conditioned look, to the tottering gait, the vertigo, and deranged secretion of urine, to the headache, nausea and vomiting. Still it is not positively known to have a specific curative relation to the albuminous or tuberculous dyscrasia.

Hepar-sulphur. deserves great attention when the albuminous excess, or dyscrasia is fully developed, at least, according to SOBERNHEIM it renders the pulse softer and slower, the blood darker and *decidedly deficient in albumen;* its powers in this respect are so decided that HARTWIG asserts, in half an hour after taking Hepar-sulph. in massive doses, the blood of horses will be found from three-fourths to four-fifths deficient in albumen. When small doses fail, the following prescription may be used:

Hepar-sulphuris,	grs. 18.
Cocoa Butter,	drachms 2.
White Sugar,	" 3.
Oil of Almonds,	ounce ½.

One or more tea-spoonsful per dose.

This prescription will meet many of the requirements in the tuberculous dyscrasia, viz.: the alkaline, oleaginous and anti-albuminous treatment. BUSCH of Strasburg, has cured several cases of confirmed tubercular consumption, with Aconite in the first stage, and Hepar-sulphuris in the subsequent periods. Prof. BANG, of Copenhagen, has had similar good fortune; also Dr. HAREL DE TANCREL.

Treatment of the headache.—If fever and other symptoms of inflammation be present, *Aconite* will be the most important remedy. It may be given internally in the usual doses; besides, as the seat of the disease is at the base of the brain, Aconitine ointment, (from 1 to 4 grains to the half ounce of simple cerate,) may be rubbed behind and below the ears, and on the back of the neck where it joins the head; or Tincture of the Root may be applied freely in the same localities, every two, four or six hours, according to the severity of the symptoms. In simple acute meningitis these remedies should be applied to the top of the head.

The next most important remedy is *Belladonna* or *Stramonium;* they may be given internally; and the Extracts or Tinctures may be used externally, as directed for Aconite.

If these fail to afford relief, Hyosciamus or Opium may be used both internally and externally; as soon as the physician is decided in his opinion that the case is one of Tubercular Meningitis, and hence almost necessarily hopeless, his principal endeavors should be directed towards soothing the sufferings of the patient.

But *Glonoine* should be tried faithfully before palliative remedies are given; especially when there is violent congestion to the head, throbbing in the forehead, temples and vertex, violent beating of the carotids, redness of the face, quickness of the pulse, &c.

Vomiting is the next most important diagnostic symptom, and almost a constant one; Barrier found it absent in only 15 cases out of 80, or in less than a fifth. It generally makes its appearance on the first day, rarely later than the second or third, and lasts two or three days, and sometimes longer; it may, however, last ten or twelve days; the matters ejected consist of food, mucus and bile in various proportions; it is commonly repeated two or three times a day. The vomiting is often, although not always, of a peculiar character, viz.: projectile, i. e. it occurs without much or any nausea, and the contents of the stomach are propelled suddenly with great force, often to the distance of several feet from the person of the patient. The vomiting may arise from irritation of the Pneumogastric nerve at the base of the brain; or from commencing disease in the Corpus-striatum, (see treatise on headaches, p. xiv.); or from gelatinous softening of the stomach.

Treatment of the vomiting.—This may subside under the use of Aconite or Belladonna. If these fail, *Cuprum* or *Zin-*

cum are best suited to the peculiar spasmodic vomiting, attended with little nausea. Zincum is also supposed to exert a specific action on the brain, (see treatise on Mental Derangement, p. xxiv.) and HARTMANN says it is very useful in the first stages of the disease, when the children become irritable in the evening, are somewhat delirious during their sleep, but become more quiet after midnight, and are quite bright again towards morning; also when the bowels are costive, violent headache sets in, the eyes become sensitive to light, the nose dry, retching, vomiting and insatiable appetite occur, the urine becomes scanty, turbid and loam-colored, with evening fever, frequent pulse, heat and anxiety, and twitchings of the muscles. Zinc has also a well-established reputation against many subacute and chronic inflammations, many nervous and spasmodic affections, such as asthma, St. Vitus' dance, epilepsy, convulsions of children, constipation, flatulence, &c.

In vomiting from softening of the stomach, *Kreosote* is the best remedy.

Constipation is said to be even a more important symptom than vomiting; according to BARRIER it is absent in only 7 cases out of 87; it generally persists obstinately for several days; and sometimes is not present at the very beginning of the disease, but sets in soon afterwards. It generally depends upon the disease at the base of the brain, more especially seated in the Corpora-quadrigemina, (see treatise on headaches, p. xiv.)

Treatment.—In children predisposed to dropsy of the brain, the condition of the bowels must be most carefully watched, constipation must not be allowed to exist even for a day, and the least indication of gastric disorder must be regarded as a serious matter. If constipation has already been present for several days before the physician is called in, some simple but efficient purgative or injective medicine should be given at once. When this has been done, Zincum and Opium will probably keep them regular; at least Dr. STRONG, (allopathic physician) ably advocates the use of Zinc and Opium in flatulence, and in constipation. WEST thinks that the value of purgatives in the treatment of ordinary hydrocephalus can scarcely be overrated; but he says that they must be given so as not merely to obtain free action of the bowels, but to maintain it for some days. In tubercular meningitis any very harsh and active measures for this purpose are entirely misplaced and useless.

The *urine* is scanty, frequently turbid and cloudy in the first stage; afterwards it may deposit a chalk-like sediment, and finally it is passed involuntarily. Other authors say that it is apt to be of a deep amber hue, of high specific gravity, sometimes milky depositing a slimy sediment, and it is apt to smell offensively after being passed and to cause pain in the urethra. In simple meningitis or phrenitis, the urine is of a dark-brown or porter-color, containing an excess of urea and less of lithates; the sediment is generally reddish or reddish-brown.

Again hydrocephalus has been known to commence and proceed to the last stage with scarcely any other symptom than slight fever, with little or no pain in the head, but a constant and nearly ineffectual desire to pass urine; in one case not above a gill of urine was passed in twenty-four hours for five days, and no other symptom of consequence was present. MONRO and EBERLEE have observed such cases.

On the other hand GUERSENT observed five cases in which the profuse secretion of urine was quite remarkable, and in these tubercles were found in the kidneys in every case.

Treatment of the urinary disorder.—Many physicians think that the peculiar milky urine, with chalk-like or slimy sediment indicate an endeavor on the part of nature to drain off some noxious substance from the blood: if this be the case, *Phosphoric-acid* will prove the most homœopathic remedy to milky urine, with gelatinous lumps, or appearing as if flour were stirred in it. This remedy is also indicated against softening of the stomach.

Carbo-vegetabilis, and *Iodine* when the urine is thick and milky.

Chin.-sulph., when there are slimy flocculi, and a clay-colored greasy sediment.

Tart.-emet., when it is pale, with a flour-like sediment.

Rhus-tox., pale urine with a snow-white sediment.

Zincum, when it is turbid and clay-colored.

Muriatic-acid, when it is white and turbid like milk when passed.

China, when it is white and turbid, with a white sediment.

Graphite, when it is turbid, with a white sediment.

Dulcamara, when it is turbid and white.

Mercurius, when it is turbid as if stirred with flour; or clear at first, and then becomes white as if mixed with chalk, with burning in the urethra.

Zincum, yellow urine, depositing whitish flocculi.

Some physicians think it very important that there should be a free flow of urine, and erroneously suppose that the brain is safe as long as the kidneys act freely, (see above).

Among the brain remedies, Belladonna produces a free flow of urine. Dr. H. M. Gray thinks that it exerts a tremendous diuretic power; is confident that its power over the secretion of urine is very great, as he passed three pints of urine in the course of an hour, attended with slight strangury, while under its influence.

Cantharides is perhaps the most homœopathic remedy to meningitis, and its action upon the kidneys is well-known; it is most indicated when the urine is full of mucus, with flocculi and filaments, or mixed with sand or clots of blood.

Arnica, when clear urine soon becomes white and turbid.

Zincum has already been alluded to.

If these remedies fail Digitalis and hydrodate of Potash will almost certainly produce a free flow of urine, but that will very often not ward off a fatal termination.

The next most important symptoms are observed in the *pulse* and *respiration;* they do not accord; the pulse is apt to be rapid at first and the respiration disproportionably slow; irregularity of breathing is often noticed by an attentive observer, long before there is any irregularity of the pulse; one, two or three respirations may be taken at equal intervals, but the breathing is apt to be quite superficial, the upper ribs only slightly rising and falling, but then there comes a full deep inspiration, very often attended with a sigh: again, there are one, two, three or four, superficial inspirations followed by a deep loud one. At other times the inspiration is quick, hurried and convulsive, followed by a marked increase in the duration of expiration and the period of repose; the inspiration is considerably shortened and a deep prolonged sighing often supervenes, and considerably diminishes the amount of respiratory movements.

In the *first* stage the pulse is much accelerated, full but compressible, with a perceptible variation in the rythm of the artery, and in the regularity of the strokes; the pulse sometimes beating as quick during one-third of a given time as it had previously done during the former two-thirds; thus, in a pulse of 140, one-half, or 70 strokes may be performed in 40 seconds, and the other 70 in 20 seconds. This is often noticed before there is any intermittence noticed. Then some slight intermission will be noticed every 7th, 17th or 20th stroke; finally the pulse will begin to change its character, one or two strokes in quick succession being soft, weak and fluttering.

In the *second* stage the pulse becomes slow, labored, intermitting and irregular, but is easily quickened by motion or mental disturbance to double its previous amount of pulsations. If the pulse beat only 60, 80 or 90 per minute, we may be certain that life will last for some days; but as soon as a new acceleration ensues, death will occur in two or three, or at most in five or six days. In the second quickening of the pulse it generally rises to 112 or 120 on the first day, and will be from 140 to 160 on the very day of death, it increases in frequency up to death.

The pulse always begins to become slow after the headache and vomiting have lasted sometime, and before somnolency sets in; it falls from 120 or 140, to 80 or even as low as 54.

These alterations in the breathing and pulsations are doubtless produced by irritation, followed by pressure upon the parvagum at the base of the brain.

Treatment.—Mercurius-corrosivus is indicated when the breathing is difficult and irregular.

Belladonna, when the respiration is natural at times, at others almost extinct; also when it is labored, irregular, sometimes hurried, at others slow.

Opium, when the inspirations are slow, long or sighing; or the breathing is irregular and suffocative; or deep and strong, followed by difficult and feeble breaths.

Stramonium, when the inspirations are slow, followed by sudden expirations, with frequent sighing.

Camphor, when the breathing is slow and deep.

Laurocerasus and *Hydrocyanic-acid*, when it is slow, moaning and rattling.

Iodine and *Spongia*, when it is slow and deep, as after exhaustion.

Aconite, when it is slow during sleep.

Nitric-acid, when slow and feeble, with wheezing.

Scilla, when it is slow and heavy.

Lobelia-inflata, when there is an inclination to sigh.

As regards the *Pulse:*

Belladonna is indicated when it is quick and strong, or slow and full.

Aconite, when it is slow irregular and intermitting.

Opium, when slow and full, afterwards becoming weak.

Stramonium, when irregular, frequent, quick; intermittent, tremulous and weak.

Laurocerasus, when irregular, slow, down to 30.

Digitalis, when irregular and small; irregular and unequal, or slow; very slow, down to 35 or 40; intermitting and slow.

Agaricus, when it is unequal, slow, feeble and intermitting.

Hyosciamus, irregular and weak; intermittent, small and quick; falling from 80 to 59.

Cuprum, irregular, small and contracted.

Conium, unequal in strength and quickness.

Secale, irregular, at times slow and full, then small and contracted; intermittent, slow and small.

Tartar-emetic, irregular and weak; slow, down to 50.

Tobacco, slow, small and intermitting; down to 45, and very weak.

Mercurius, irregular and small; feeble, slow and tremulous.

Plumbum, irregular, first quick, then slow; sluggish and intermittent.

Phos. and *Nitric-acid*, irregular and intermittent.

Muriatic-acid, intermitting every 3d beat.

Hellebore, slow and very small.

Cough.—A slight false cough which partly resembles a suppressed effort to vomit, and not unlike the morning liver cough of drunkards, is not unfrequent in all three stages. When it occurs in conjunction with the peculiar breathing before described, it is supposed to be a sign of effusion in the ventricles. It may depend upon irritation of the pneumo-gastric nerve at the base of the brain; or upon the deposit of miliary tubercles.

Treatment.—It is stated that nothing will relieve it; but Conium is often a useful remedy.

Retraction of the abdomen is a valuable diagnostic sign; it usually occurs about the sixth day; the belly becomes depressed at its centre and takes on the form of a boat; it is almost a constant symptom, and does not arise from the constipation, as it is equally present when diarrhœa sets in; it is almost peculiar to this disease of the brain.

Treatment.—Plumbum and Zincum are the most homœopathic remedies, although Nux, Ignatia, Angustura, Alumina and Colocynth may seem to be indicated.

I have been in the habit of placing great stress upon the presence of *stiff neck*, occurring every afternoon or evening, and disappearing in the morning. It probably arises from irritation at the base of the brain, near the origin of the twelfth pair of nerves, as this supplies the muscles of the nape of the neck and shoulders. If this symptom occur in a person born of tuberculous or consumptive parents, and is attended with headache, fever, vomiting, constipation and signs of irritation of the brain, it always excites our liveliest apprehensions as to the result.

Treatment.—Zincum and Plumbum are the best remedies.

The *precursory* stage above alluded to is of variable duration, but on the average does not exceed four or five days. When the second stage sets in, the nature of the affection becomes very apparent. The child no longer has intervals of cheerfulness, nor attempts to sit up, but wishes to be left quiet in bed, and the face assumes a permanent expression of anxiety and suffering. The eyes are often kept closed, and the eyelids are knit, the child endeavoring to shut out the light from its morbidly sensitive retina. The skin continues dry, the face is sometimes flushed, and the head often hot; and though these two symptoms vary much in their duration, coming and going without any evident cause, yet there is a permanently increased pulsation of the carotids, and if the skull be not ossified, the brain may be seen and felt forcibly beating through the anterior fontanelle. The child is now very averse to being disturbed, and often lies in a drowsy condition, unless spoken to; when old enough to answer, it usually complains of its head, or of weariness or sleepiness. Its replies are génerally rational but short; and if it needs anything, it asks in as few words as possible, in a quick, pettish manner, and shows much irritability, if not at once attended to. At other times it lies with its face turned from the light, either quite quiet, or moaning in a low tone of voice, and now and then uttering a short, sharp, lamentable cry, which is regarded as characteristic of the disease, and hence termed the *cry hydrencephalique*. To this, however, there are exceptions, and children sometimes scream out with the intensity of the pain. As night comes on, there is almost always a distinct exacerbation of the symptoms, and the quiet of the day is frequently succeeded by a noisy and excited state, in which vociferous cries about the head alternate with delirium. At times, however, an increase of restlessness is the only difference from the state of stupor in which the child lay during the day. At the commencement of this stage the pulse is quickened, sometimes very much so. The child sometimes keeps its eyes so firmly closed that we can scarcely see the state of its pupils. Usually they are not much affected, but sometimes one is more dilated and acts more sluggishly than the other; or, in other cases squinting exists, though perhaps in a very slight degree, or confined to one eye. It is seldom that vomiting continues beyond the commencement of this stage, but its cessation is not followed by any desire either for food or drink. The bowels usually become even more constipated than they were before, and the evacuations continue quite as unnatural, while all flatus disappears from the intestines, and the abdomen thus acquires that shrunken form on which much stress has been laid by some writers, as characteristic of dropsy of the brain.—West.

Treatment.—In this stage Mercury and purgatives are generally given freely and barbarously by allopathic physicians. But the most efficient allopathic remedies are a few small doses of Mercury or Proto-iodide of Mercury, followed by Hydriodate of Potash internally, aided by the free and frequent application of Hydriodate of Potash ointment over the whole of the head, and back of the neck. In desperate cases Dr. HAHN has several times succeeded in arousing the child with the cold effusion, after the supervention of complete coma. Friction of the scalp with Tartar-emetic ointment, repeated every two hours until pustulation was established, enabled Dr. HAHN to save fourteen cases, when in an apparently hopeless state of coma; even in tuberculous meningitis cures were obtained in several cases by the Tartar-emetic frictions under the most unpromising circumstances.

The *third* stage commences when the brain itself becomes involved and becomes softened. The transition is sometimes effected very gradually by the deepening of the state of drowsiness, till it amounts to a stupor, from which it is impossible to arouse the child. At other times, the stupor comes on very suddenly, immediately after an attack of convulsions. These convulsions usually affect one side much more than the other, and after the fit has passed off, one side is generally found partially or completely paralyzed, while the child makes constant automatic movements with the other, carrying the hand to the head, and alternately flexing and extending the leg. The side which is the most affected during the fit, is generally, though not invariably the most palsied afterwards. When the third stage is fully established, the child lies upon its back in a state of complete insensibility, with one leg stretched out, the other drawn up towards the abdomen. The tremulous hands are either employed in picking the lips or nose until the blood comes, or one hand is kept on the genitals, while the other is rubbing the face or head. The head is at one moment hot, and the face flushed, and then the heat disappears and the flush fades, though usually there is an increase of heat about the back of the head. Sometimes the skin will be dry, at others though the extremities are cold, a profuse sweat will break out on some part of the body, or on the head. The pulse becomes regular again, but grows smaller and more rapid until it can only be counted at the heart. The eyelids close only partially; there is some squinting; light is no longer unpleasant, for the dilated pupils are motionless. The child now often makes automatic movements with the mouth as if chewing, or as though endeavoring to swallow something, and it generally happens, that although sensibility is quite extinguished, the little patient will still swallow anything that is put into its mouth, and the power of deglutition is in most cases one of the very last to be abolished.—WEST.

Many of these symptoms are sometimes very stupidly regarded as signs of worm disease, and Cina and Spigelia or other worm remedies are administered. But these are signs of softening of the brain, and cannot be removed by any remedies, although Zincum, Plumbum, Nux and Arsenicum are the most appropriate medicines.

An attack of convulsions now sometimes puts an end to the painful scene; but often the child lives on for days, though wasted to a skeleton, and its features so changed by suffering that those persons who had seen it but a short time before would now scarcely recognize it. The head often becomes retracted, and the child bores the back of its head into the pillow; the eyelids are wide open, and the eyes are turned upwards, so as to conceal three-fourths of the iris beneath the upper lid, while the countenance is still further disfigured by a horrible squint, or by a constant rolling of the eyes. The pupils are now fixed and glassy, the white of the eye is extremely bloodshot, and their surface besmeared with a copious secretion from the meibomian glands, which collects in their corners. One arm and leg are stiff and motionless; the other in constant spasmodic movement, while the hands are often clenched, and the wrists bent upon the forearm. Subsultus and spasmodic twitchings of the face are common. Cold clammy sweats break out, the breathing is labored, swallowing becomes difficult, and the child almost chokes with the effort to swallow, or lets the fluid run out at the corners of the mouth. It is uncertain how long this condition may endure; sometimes many days will pass, during which death is hourly expected and earnestly prayed for, to put an end to the patient's sufferings.

Treatment.—In this stage, palliatives only should be used, such as Opium, Conium, Hyosciamus, Cannabis-indica, Chloroform, Ether, &c. In some instances I have applied anodyne fomentations to the head, and used anodyne inhalations after the little patient was unable to swallow.

TUBERCULOUS MENINGITIS.

IN YOUTHS AND ADULTS.

Dr. KENNEDY, of Dublin, has seen about 30 cases in the course of nine years; and thinks that it is more common in females than males, in the proportion of 2 to 1. Of 80 cases of tubercular meningitis observed by GUERSENT, 33 were over 15 years of age; and of 12 cases by JACKSON, 7 were adults. Of 10 cases, 6 were in females, aged 27, 20, 28, 28, 26 and 23 respectively; and 4 in males, aged 22, 20, 21 and 24.

According to KENNEDY, in the majority of cases the disease commences with the symptoms of a mild, continued or remittent fever, which goes on without change for 10, 12 or 14 days. It occasionally begins by a distinct complaint of the head, the patient still being able to go about.

When it commences with fever, the symptoms are usually very mild; there is some quickness of the pulse, heat of skin, furred tongue and headache. The case seems to go on favorably, remedies seem to avail, and the patient may even be pronounced convalescent; or the symptoms may become so slight that the tongue is scarcely furred, some appetite may be present, and the patient may sleep well at night.

When the disease commences by fever, the first sign of anything going wrong commonly takes place at night; a marked increase of fever may then be observed, the tongue becomes more furred, the skin feverish and the pulse rises to near 100. KENNEDY has sometimes been led to suspect the serious nature of the case, by the nurse casually stating that on the previous night the patient had not slept so well, had talked in her sleep, or awakened with a scream; these symptoms may return for four or five nights in succession, and yet the patient seem comparatively well during the day.

Alterations in the movements or expression of the eye, are often among the earliest signs, pointing to coming trouble. Squinting may occur, and yet be so slight as to be doubted or disputed, or it may be intermitting, i. e., present at one moment and absent the next; or else it only occurs when the patient is left to herself, but disappearing the moment she is spoken to;

these slight changes may occur in one or both eyes, and are better observed at a little distance. One eyeball may be almost immovable, and yet it is easy to overlook this; or one pupil may be somewhat larger than the other; neither are dilated, but they differ in size. Sometimes the eyelids have a tendency to droop, and this ptosis may be most marked in one eye. These eye symptoms are among the most constant and important signs.

At times the first symptom is vomiting, occurring most frequently in the morning; it may happen one or more times, but never takes the prominent part it does in the hydrocephalus of childhood.

The head is now more apt to be complained of; perhaps there may be pain, only when the patient coughs; as a rule it is referred to the forehead over the eyes, but sometimes extends to the whole head.

This state may continue for four or five days when the symptoms will become more serious; the patient is apt to wander a little while awake, generally towards evening, but only momentarily, as she is quite herself again when spoken to. The countenance is also apt to become heavy, as if she were inclined to doze.

The next sign which attracts attention is the pulse; in the course of 24 hours it may fall remarkably, viz.: from 100 or 108 to 60, 55 or even 48. After the lapse of 48 hours more it begins to rise again, often getting up to 130 or 140, and now the case progresses rapidly; the patient becomes obtuse, difficult to rouse, and the signs of confirmed dropsy of the brain are soon added.

In the advanced stages it is very common to find the patient's hand applied to the head, and the brows strongly knit, even in sleep. In some cases the patient will sing the same tune all night, or may grit her teeth with a degree of violence almost insupportable. The entire duration of these cases is about three weeks; the disease seems to run in families, several members, young and adult being affected; three-fourths of the patients have naturally a heavy aspect; their faces are apt to be large in proportion to their heads, the lips to be large, and the skin rather coarse. In fact if a mild remittent fever occur in a young person, especially in a girl about fifteen years old, born of scrofulous or consumptive parents, and slight brain symptoms show themselves, be upon your guard.

Treatment.—See Tuberculous Meningitis of Children.

HYDROCEPHALOID DISEASE.

THIS is a most frequent and often fatal affection, though if rightly treated it is a very manageable one. It is especially common in this country, where infantile diarrhœa and summer-complaint occur frequently and severely, and blood-letting and other reducing treatment are resorted to so commonly, quickly producing that state of general exhaustion which leads to a train of symptoms about the head, closely resembling those of dropsy of the brain. According to WEST, hydrocephaloid disease is that condition which is induced when the brain is somewhat suddenly deprived of its usual supply of blood. Even in the adult a profuse loss of blood is often followed by an extremely severe headache, and by various other brain-symptoms; while in the child, whose brain needs a proportionably larger quantity of blood for the due performance of its functions, the symptoms that follow its excessive loss are of a corresponding gravity; often indeed they present a striking similarity to those which betoken inflammation, or dropsy of the brain. MARSHALL HALL even says that in young children, bleeding, purging and giving calomel enough, in any disease, will bring it on.

Again, there is no disorder in which the two conditions of considerable sympathetic disturbance of the brain, coupled with rapid exhaustion of the vital power, are so completely fulfilled as in infantile diarrhœa, and summer-complaint, and in no other affections do we meet with such frequent or such well-marked instances of the supervention of the hydrocephaloid disease.

Symptoms.—This affection may be divided into two stages: the first, that of irritability; the second, that of torpor. These two stages resemble in many of their symptoms the first and second stages of dropsy of the brain.

In the first stage the infant becomes restless, irritable and *feverish;* the face is flushed, the surface hot, and the pulse frequent; there is an undue sensitiveness of the nerves of feeling, and the little patient starts on being touched, or from any sudden noise; there are sighing and moaning during sleep, and screaming; the bowels are apt to be flatulent and loose, and the evacuations are mucous and disordered.—M. HALL.

If the affection arises from the exhaustion caused by diarrhœa, and if from an erroneous notion as to the nature of this disease, nourishment and cordials be not given, or if the diarrhœa be allowed to continue, or be kept up by medicines, the exhaustion which ensues is apt to lead to a different train of symptoms:

The *second* stage then sets in: the countenance becomes pale, and the cheeks cool or cold; the eyelids are half closed; the eyes are fixed, and unattracted by any object placed before them; the pupils unmoved on the approach of light; the breathing from being quick becomes irregular and sighing; the voice becomes husky, and there is sometimes a husky, teazing cough; and eventually, if the strength of the little patient continues to decline, there is a rattling in the breathing, and the feet become cold.

Again, according to WEST, under no circumstances are mistakes more easily committed, and never are their results more mischievous, than when primary and real congestion of the brain has been somewhat over-treated allopathically, and the consequent symptoms of exhaustion are supposed to be those of advancing disease of the brain. In such a case, however, it would usually be observed that great faintness had been induced by the profuse depletion, and that the quiet which succeeded it was that of exhaustion, as much as of mitigated suffering; the fontanelle sunk below the level of the bones of the skull, instead of being tense and pulsating; the cool surface, and the pulse presenting no other characters than those of frequency and feebleness, would all point to the real nature of the case. To deplete further under such circumstances would be to destroy the patient; food is needed, not physic; the sunken powers of life must be rallied, and as strength returns the functions of the brain will again go on harmoniously.

The early stages of inflammation of the lungs, are also often attended with so much sympathetic disturbance of the brain, as to throw the other symptoms into the back-ground. The child may vomit, refers all its sufferings to the head, and possibly have an attack of convulsions almost at the onset. The routine allopathist will naturally assume the case to be one of congestion of the brain, and treat it accordingly with free local depletion; the next day the indications of disordered breathing are more apparent, and more leeches are applied to the chest. The urgency of the symptoms may be relieved by these means, or at least the child may seem to suffer less; but soon the restlessness of exhaustion comes on, and then follow the soporose condition and the apparent coma; if the antiphlogistic treatment is resumed to arrest this imaginary dropsy of the brain, the little patient will die.

Treatment.—A large number of cases of hydrocephaloid disease are not only caused, but absolutely killed by allopathic treatment, while a proportionately large number will die under purely homœopathic treatment: for as WEST truly says, food and stimulants are required, not medicine. Although the diagnosis of this affection is sometimes attended with difficulty, the rules for its prevention and cure are happily very simple. Bearing in mind the possible supervention of hydrocephaloid disease, an infant should never be kept from the breast, nor a young child put upon spare diet for several days without the most absolute necessity. Especial attention must be paid to the food of young children, if the disease from which they suffer be diarrhœa, or some other which interferes directly with their nutrition; if the child be given nothing more nutritious than barley-water in small quantities, because the irritability of the stomach which results from weakness, seems to be the indication of disease in the brain, the restlessness will before long alternate with coma, and the child will die either comatose, or in convulsions. The irritability of the stomach is best overcome by giving nourishment in extremely small quantities, as a desert-spoonful of ass's milk, or equal parts of milk and barley-water for an infant, or of strong veal tea, for an older child, given little by little, every half hour. If the exhaustion be very great, and a state analagous to stupor impending, a hot mustard bath is sometimes very serviceable in rousing the child, while, at the same time, a few drops of Spirits of Hartshorn, or 5 to 15 drops of Brandy may be given every few hours. It is desirable, however, to suspend the use of the more powerful direct stimulants as soon as it can safely be done, though a nutritious diet will be necessary for some time.—WEST.

WASTING OF THE BRAIN.—(ATROPHY.)

IN CHILDREN.

SMALLNESS of the brain sometimes occurs in consequence of a premature closure of the sutures and fontanelles. Such cases are apt to be attended with frequently recurring convulsions; loss of taste, so that the child cannot distinguish between what is nice and what is nasty, swallowing all things with the same readiness; the body and limbs may seem well nourished and well formed, yet the patient cannot stand or use his limbs properly; the urine and fæces are apt to be passed involuntarily and unconsciously; and gradually every glimmering of understanding will disappear.

Treatment.—These cases are generally quite hopeless; Phosphoric-acid in full doses may do some good.

According to WEST those cases are of much higher practical importance in which the brain of the child wastes or grows smaller during long-continued ill-health. The scalp will usually be found pale, thin and bloodless, the fontanelles sunken, and the process of ossification of the skull unusually tardy; fluid will be found effused into the sac of the arachnoid and the subjacent pia-mater; the substance of the brain is pale and its texture firmer than usual.

The important point about such cases is, that brain symptoms and frequently recurring convulsions may be observed in a child whose brain is not absolutely diseased, but merely too feeble and too wasted to perform its functions.

Treatment.—In infants who have been exhausted and wasted by previous illness, the physician must not interpose too hastily with remedies directed against a supposed brain-disease, but pursue a tonic and nourishing plan of treatment. Iodide of Potash may be used internally and externally to remove the fluid effused, and may possibly have some effect upon the hardening of the brain, although *Plumbum* is the most homœopathic remedy.

Partial atrophy will be marked by symptoms most decided in particular parts, or on one or the other side of the body.

IN ADULTS.

According to ROKITANSKY this disease is also common in old age, and is within certain limits a natural process of shrinking or decay; it becomes, however, a pathological condition even in old age, if it proceed to a very great extent, and still more if it come on prematurely at an early period of life.

The *grey* substance of the brain is apt to become of a dirty, or rusty brown color, running into yeast yellow; its consistence may be natural or distinctly softer than usual. The *white* substance loses its clear color and becomes of a dirty white; it is denser too than natural, and is sometimes as tough as leather. The vacuum within the skull, produced by the shrinking of the brain, is filled up chiefly by a clear colorless serum; the vessels of the pia-mater become enlarged and varicose.

It leads to congestions of the brain, or *Hyperæmia ex-vacuo*, causing transient or protracted attacks which simulate apoplexy, and are so frequent in old age; or to actual apoplexy, with hæmorrhage within the brain; or to œdema of the brain.

Treatment.—Iodide of Baryta, Plumbum, and Iodide of Iron are the principal remedies.

ENLARGEMENT OF THE BRAIN.

HYPERTROPHY.

ACCORDING to ROKITANSKY enlargement of the brain is sometimes congenital and is then often combined with dropsy of the brain; still it more usually comes on after birth, and is almost exclusively confined to the period of childhood. It is occasionally met with about the time of puberty, and sometimes, although exceedingly rarely, even in manhood.

It is the *white* substance of the brain which is increased in volume; it is always dazzling white, and remarkably pale and bloodless, showing that it is not caused by congestion. When it comes on in childhood, and at puberty, it is combined with general enlargement of the lymphatic glands and partial obliteration of the thymus; it is also apt to be attended with rickets and feeble muscular development.

Its course is generally chronic, but not unfrequently it is

somewhat acute; the cause of the acute symptoms when they occur, is a rapid and tumultuous addition to the bulk of the brain; this only takes place in some instances.

The majority of cases of enlargement of the brain which have fallen under WEST'S notice in London, occurred in infants about six or eight months old. Their history has usually been, that without any definite illness, they had lost their appetite, and grown by degrees dull and apathetic, though restless and uneasy. Notwithstanding the general apathy, this restlessness is often very considerable, though it does not show itself in cries, as much as in a state of general uneasiness, and in frequent startings from sleep. Short gleams of cheerfulness occur when the children are awake, but these are usually very transient. The head seems too heavy to be borne, and even when its size is not much greater than natural, it hangs backwards, or to one side, as if the muscles were too weak to support it. If placed in its cot, a child who is thus affected, bores with its occiput in the pillow, while its head is almost constantly in a profuse perspiration. Convulsions sometimes occur without any evident cause, but threatenings of their attack are much more frequent than their actual occurrence, the child awaking suddenly with a start, and a peculiar cry, like that of spasmodic croup, the surface turning livid, and the respiration becoming difficult for a few moments, and the symptoms then subsiding of their own accord. Such attacks may issue in general convulsions, which may terminate fatally; but infants thus affected do not by any means invariably die of the cerebral disorder, but, being weakly, they are often cut off by the first malady that attacks them.

If life be prolonged the child loses flesh, and looks out of health, while enlargement of the wrists and ankles, shows the connection between this disease and rickets; a connection which becomes more evident in the second and third years of life. When the child survives infancy, or when as occasionally happens the symptoms of enlargement of the brain do not come on until dentition has been in a great measure accomplished, convulsions are of very rare occurrence. Complaints of headache, however, are frequent and severe; and, though drowsy in the daytime the child generally rests ill at night, and often awakes crying and alarmed. Besides these symptoms, too, the child has occasional attacks of feverishness, with great increase of headache and giddiness, which last for a few hours or a day, and then subside of their own accord, while it grows by degrees more and more dull and listless, and its mental powers become obviously impaired.

It happens in some cases, that, as the child grows older, these symptoms become less and less severe, the health improves, the ricketty deformity of the limbs gradually disappears and the infant who had excited so much solicitude becomes at length a healthy child.

Chronic dropsy of the brain is the only affection with which enlargement of the brain is liable to be confounded. The diagnosis between the two affections is often by no means easy, though it is of much importance with reference to the treatment.

The symptoms of chronic dropsy of the brain generally come on earlier, and soon grow much more serious than those of enlargement of the brain, and the disturbance of the brain is throughout much more marked in chronic hydrocephalus than in hypertrophy. Convulsions, sopor and restlessness attend the early stages of chronic hydrocephalus, while spasmodic affections of the respiration are among the earliest indications of enlargement of the brain.

The form and size of the head, too, present peculiarities by which we may often distinguish between the two conditions; both diseases are attended with enlargement of the head, and in both the ossification of the skull is very tardy, but the head does not attain so large a size in hypertrophy of the brain, neither are the fontanelles and sutures so widely open.

The skull also presents some remarkable peculiarities; the head not only shows no tendency to assume the rounded form characteristic of chronic hydrocephalus, but its enlargement is first apparent at the occiput, and the bulging of the hind-head continues especially striking.

The forehead may, in the course of time become prominent and overhanging, but the eye remains deep sunk in its socket, for no change takes place in the direction of the orbitar plates, such as is produced by the pressure of fluid within the brain, and which gives to the eye that unnatural prominence, and that peculiar downward direction which are so striking in cases of chronic hydrocephalus.

In chronic dropsy of the brain the anterior fontanelle is tense and prominent, owing to the pressure of the fluid within, but when the brain is enlarged, there is no prominence but an actual depression in this situation. WEST has more than once observed this condition in a remarkable degree, the depression not being limited to the anterior fontanelle, but being also observable at all the sutures.

When enlargement of the brain occurs in the adult, the symptoms that arise are in a great measure due to the compression which the organ undergoes from its bony case being too small to contain it. The symptoms are of course exceedingly obscure. —MAUTHNER and WEST.

Treatment.—Vinum-ferri, Ferro-citrate of Quinine, Iodides of Iron and Potash and Cod-liver Oil, have been used most frequently and successfully. Agaricus, Calc.-phos., Kali-carb., Mezereum and Rhododendron are the principal homœopathic remedies.

Daphne-indica is suitable when there is a sensation as if the outer part of the brain were inflamed and striking against the skull.

Sulphur, *Staphysagria* and *Stannum* when there is pain as if the brain were beating against the skull, or a painful pressing of the brain against the skull and occipital bones, in the evening, even after going to bed.

Chelidonium when there is a pressing in the brain, as if the skull were too narrow, and the brain would be pressed out of the eyes, nose or ears.

Baryta and *Conium* when the head seems too full as if it would burst; especially in both frontal eminences and in the orbits.

HYDROCEPHALUS.

DROPSY OF THE BRAIN.

In by far the greater number of cases the fluid collects in the interior of the brain, constituting what is called *internal* hydrocephalus in contra-distinction to other cases in which the fluid is contained in the sac of the arachnoid, and to which the name of *external* hydrocephalus has been given.

INTERNAL HYDROCEPHALUS.

The internal membrane of the ventricles of the brain is composed of a very delicate continuation of the arachnoid and pia-mater, and a layer of epithelium. The most frequent and important diseases to which it is liable, have, from one most striking characteristic which they present, viz.: an excessive accumulation of fluid, been included together under the title of hydrocephalus.

The disease may be acute or chronic, inflammatory, or non-inflammatory.

In the *acute inflammatory* form, a turbid fluid is found in the ventricles, composed of serum and lymph or pus; the lining membrane of the ventricles becomes dull, opaque, softened and even diffluent, so that shreds of it often appear in the inflammatory effusion in the ventricles.

The substance of the brain is in a state of acute œdema, and infiltrated to such a degree that it seems as if it were in a state of watery softening; hence the brain itself is swollen and actually increased in volume, so that its convolutions are forced against the skull and flattened.

It is very apt to be associated with tubercular meningitis.—Rokitansky.

In the *acute non-inflammatory form*, a clear, colorless, serous fluid, varying in quantity from one or two to six ounces, is found in the ventricles. Although the disease is often acute, it cannot be admitted to be inflammatory; it arises from congestions of various kinds, viz.: such as are connected with the development of the brain in childhood, or those produced by chronic eruptions on the scalp, by the irritation of morbid growths within the skull, &c.; or it may be occasioned, too, by the congestions which follow concussion of the brain, or mechanical obstructions of the heart, chronic catarrh of the lungs, or bronchi, &c., &c. The result of these congestions is an excessive effusion of serum, first from the lining membrane of the ventricles, and then into the brain itself. It is frequently associated with enlargement of the whole system of lymphatic glands, and of the follicular apparatus of the intestinal mucous membrane; with enlargement of the thymus gland, with chronic catarrh of the bronchi, and with rickets.—Rokitansky.

CHRONIC HYDROCEPHALUS.

According to Rokitansky this disease may be divided into three varieties, viz.: 1st, into congenital hydrocephalus; 2d, that which commences at various periods after birth, but generally during the first six months; and 3d, hydrocephalus occasioned by a vacuum within the skull, from atrophy of the brain.

According to West, in the majority of cases the disease is not a mere passive dropsy, but is the consequence of a slow kind of inflammation of the arachnoid, especially of that lining the ventricles, which may have existed during fœtal life, or not have attacked the child until after its birth.

In 50 cases collected by West, some symptoms of it were observed in 46 instances before the child was six months old; in 12 of these the disease was congenital; and in 19 more, the malady was established before the child was three months old.

Symptoms.—The *early* symptoms vary; when it is congenital, indications of disturbance of the brain are generally apparent from the infant's birth; these are sometimes serious, such as convulsions, recurring almost daily; or slight, consisting of nothing more than squinting, or strange rolling of the eyes. The size of the head generally attracts attention before long, and causes importance to be attached to symptoms which otherwise might have given rise to but little anxiety. In some instances, however, the increased size of the head is not very obvious until the child is a few weeks old, although well-marked symptoms of mischief in the brain existed from its birth; enlargement of the head, in fact, is by no means invariably the first indication of chronic hydrocephalus. According to WEST in 12 cases out of 45, fits returning frequently, had existed for some weeks before the head was observed to increase in size; in 6 instances the enlargement of the head succeeded to an attack resembling acute dropsy of the brain; and in 4 other examples, it had been preceded by some well-marked indications of mischief in the brain; in the remaining 23 cases, out of 50, no distinct brain-symptoms preceded the enlargement of the head.

In whatever way the disease begins, the child's health will have been noticed to be failing for some time, although the cause of its illness may not be apparent; impairment of the processes of nutrition is sure to be among its earliest symptoms. The child may nurse or feed well, and indeed may seem eager for food, but still it loses both flesh and strength; and often, although the head has not yet attained any disproportionate size, the child is unable to support it, either losing the power it had once possessed, or never attaining that which, with its increasing age it ought to acquire; the bowels are generally constipated, but diarrhœa often comes on for a day or two, and the evacuations are almost always unhealthy. In short, in the primary symptoms there is but little to distinguish the case from any other in which a young infant is imperfectly nourished; even, although occasional attacks of heat of head may be observed, attended with pulsation or tension of the anterior fontanelle, attended with crying and restlessness, alternating with a drowsy condition by day and restless nights, still these symptoms occur frequently enough from transient causes: they acquire a more marked significance, if coupled with an unusually open state of the fontanelles and sutures, even if no marked enlargement of the head be yet perceptible.

By and by, however, the increased size of the head grows very manifest, and the child's physiognomy soon assumes the distinguishing features of chronic hydrocephalus; the sutures become wider, the fontanelles increase in size, and the head assumes a globular shape. But the greatest increase in the size of the head is effected by the enlargement of the anterior fontanelle, and by the widening of the sagittal suture. The forehead is projected forwards; the orbitar plates of the frontal bone are driven by the accumulating fluid from a horizontal into an oblique direction, and sometimes indeed they become nearly perpendicular, when by contracting the orbits they give to the eyeballs that unnatural prominence and that peculiar downward direction which constitutes one of the most remarkable features in cases of chronic hydrocephalus. In hypertrophy of the brain the back of the head is much larger than the front.—WEST.

The symptoms of disturbance of the brain that attend the advance of the disease differ much in severity; sometimes there is little but uneasiness and restlessness, aggravated at intervals when the head grows hot and the fontanelle grows tense; in other cases, convulsions occur frequently, from very slight, or no evident causes; in another set of cases, spasmodic attacks of difficult breathing, attended with a crowing sound in inspiration are apt to occur, even before there is much enlargement of the head.—WEST.

Treatment.—WAHLE says that Hellebor.-nig., Arsenicum and Sulphur are the principal remedies; he has often effected radical cures even in congenital hydrocephalus. He always commenced the treatment with Hellebore, and persisted in its use for eight or ten days. Against the spasms, Sulphur 30, was the most efficient remedy, all other seemingly appropriate remedies were useless. Aconite 30, was most useful against mental disturbances.

The treatment of GÖLIS of Vienna, was to have the head shaved, or hair cut close, and one or two drachms of the mild mercurial ointment rubbed daily into the scalp; the head to be constantly covered with a flannel cap, and $\frac{1}{4}$, or $\frac{1}{2}$ grain of calomel to be given twice daily, unless diarrhœa comes on. This plan requires perseverance for thirty to forty days. Hydriodate of Potash is safer and perhaps more efficient.

Methodical compression of the head with strips of adhesive plaster has been used successfully; and 18 cases out of 63, or 2 cases out of 7 are said to have been radically cured by puncture of the cranium and evacuation of the fluid.

CASE 1.—A rhachitic child, aged 3 years, had swollen joints, was unable to walk, even when supported, and finally became affected with full developed chronic hydrocephalus; the sutures were widely separated; the child lay upon its back, covered with a sticky perspiration, it had constant fever, grasped at its head, became unconscious and passed its evacuations involuntarily.

Treatment.—Calc.-c. 30, one dose every week; in five weeks the dropsy of the head seemed removed and the enlargement of the joints lessened. By the continued use of Calc. the child gradually recovered perfectly.—IVANOVICH.

CASE 2.—A boy, aged 14 months, was attacked with inflammation of the brain which terminated in dropsy; spasmodic and paralytic affections ensued, and finally the child lay unconscious with all the usual signs of hydrocephalus.

Treatment.—The patient was entirely restored in the course of ten weeks by Bell., Bryon., Merc., Hell., Hyosc. and Sulph. —MALY.

CASE 3.—A boy, aged 1 year, had a very large and heavy head, with widely open fontanelles; the eyes projected over the edge of the orbits; there was strabismus; almost entire absence of all human expression; the child only made grunting and beastly sounds; the skin hung loose upon the emaciated hands and feet; the abdomen was much bloated; there was offensive diarrhœa intermixed with hard masses of fæces; involuntary discharge of urine and fæces; spasms and opisthotonos; canine appetite.

Treatment and Result.—From Jan. 6 to Nov. 18, the child received Calc. 200 and Sulph. 200, in alternation every ten or fourteen days, with constant improvement; the spasms lessened, the teeth came through, the eyes retreated into their sockets, the expression became human and pleasant, it improved in body and began to walk and speak.—BREDENOLL.

CASE 4.—A boy aged 3 years, had already suffered for two years with signs of hydrocephalus; his head was large, and inclined to fall forwards; the fontanelles were very large, the forehead projecting, the eyes sunken, the pupils dilated, face earthy and bloated; there was constant dribbling of water from the mouth; the teeth were small and imperfect; the limbs weak and unable to support the body; greedy desire for food.

Treatment.—Five doses of Bellad. 30, ½ drop doses, were given in the course of sixteen days, with evident signs of improvement. A feverish attack with aggravation of all the symptoms, was then relieved by Acon., followed by 2 doses of Bellad., without further benefit to the principal disease; hence 9 doses of Merc.-viv. 6, were given, 1 dose every three or four days, with remarkable relief from all the symptoms. The paralytic weakness of the limbs was removed by 2 doses of Phosph. 30 and China 6. Finally the child was perfectly restored.—SCHWARZ.

CASE 5.—A boy, aged 3 years, was attacked with dropsy of the head. Bellad., Hepar. and Conium diminished the great size of the head.

Sometime after he fell in the water, after which he could no longer stand upon his feet, nor move himself, nor speak, or eat; while drinking he pressed his tongue against the hard palate, so that one-half of the fluid ran out of the mouth again.

Treatment.—Hyosc. 18, 1 dose every night and morning removed this state in three days.—HARTUNG.

REVIEW.—*Calcarea* was used in 2 cases, in the 30th and 300th potencies; the latter in alternation with Sulphur.

Belladonna effected most in case 4, but was also useful in cases 2 and 5.

WAHLE calls particular attention to Hellebore, Sulphur and Arsenicum.

Mercurius was very useful in case 4.

The general paralytic state in case 5, was evidently in close connection with the previous state of the brain and was soon cured by *Hyosciamus*.

EXTERNAL HYDROCEPHALUS.

In this disease according to HOWSHIP the patient seems always disposed to doze, yet its senses are awake to the lightest and least impression; the peculiar symptom is that of being at one and the same time light-headed, yet perfectly sensible; the patient speaking incoherently to himself, yet if spoken to answering clearly and rationally. This peculiar state is supposed to occur only when there is an abundant serous effusion between the membranes, and none in the ventricles of the brain.

Treatment of Hydrocephalus.—*Aconite* is supposed to be homœopathic to congestion of the brain only.

Aethusa-cynapium to congestion of the brain and its sinuses.

Ammonium-mur. is homœopathic to atrophy and collapse of the brain.

Arsenicum, to inflammation of the membranes and substance of the brain, serous effusion into the ventricles.

Belladonna, to excessive congestion of the brain.

Bismuth, to serous effusion, here and there between the convolutions of the brain, and in the ventricles.

Bromine, to venous congestion and considerable redness of the pia-mater.

Brucea-antidysenterica, to great congestion of the left hemisphere of the brain and cerebellum, with effusion of a considerable quantity of serum into the ventricles.

Camphor, to violent congestion and inflammation of the membranes and substance of the brain, with softening.

Cannabis-sativa, to congestion and extravasation upon the arachnoid, clear serous effusion in the convolutions of the brain, throughout and into the lateral ventricles, with some softening of the brain.

Cantharides, to congestion of the brain, particularly of the cerebellum, which is covered with a thick layer of exuded lymph, attended with an effusion of a quantity of serum at the base of the skull.

Chininum-sulphuricum, to congestion of the brain and spinal marrow, red and white softening of the medullary substance, with effusion of serum.

Cicuta-virosa, against meningeal apoplexy, induration of the brain, serous effusion in one of the ventricles, and dark red fluid at the base of the skull.

Colocynth, against congestion of the surface of the brain, and inflammation of the pia-mater.

Conium, when there is a considerable quantity of water in the ventricles of the brain.

Digitalis, when the membranes of the brain are strongly injected.

Gratiola, when there is a fiery-red injection of the pia-mater.

Helleborus, when there is *no* fluid in the ventricles of the brain, but the superficial veins are filled with black blood, and the pia-mater is considerably injected, the brain being softened and withering, or atrophied.

Hydrocyanic-acid, when the brain and its membranes are congested, with extravasation of blood, (true apoplexy,) with effusion of serum at the base of the skull; congestion of the walls of the ventricles.

Hyosciamus, when the brain is congested and the ventricles empty.

Laurocerasus, when the upper surface of the brain is congested, and also the inner vessels of the ventricles.

Nux-vomica, softening of the brain and spinal marrow, congestion of the cortical substance and pons varolii.

Oleander, when the ventricles of the brain contain a small quantity of reddish fluid, and the superficial vessels of the brain are tinged with blood.

Opium, when there is congestion and extravasation of blood, in and upon the brain; softening of the brain so that it was almost impossible to distinguish the medullary from the cortical substance; extravasation of serum at the base of the brain and in the ventricles.

Oxalic-acid, when there is effusion under the arachnoid.

Phosphorus, when there is a wide-spread and thick accumulation of yellowish-white, opalescent exudation (plastic lymph,) between the pia-mater and arachnoid, by means of which these two membranes are glued together, (meningitis).

Plumbum, when there is a considerable flatness (atrophy) of the convolutions of the brain, with paleness and softness of the parenchyma, brown clear serum in the middle ventricle, unusual softness or hardness of the substance of the brain, with clear serum at the base of the skull.

Secale, when the vessels of the brain are empty.

ACUTE AND GENERAL INFLAMMATION OF THE BRAIN.

IN ADULTS.

According to WATSON, acute inflammation does sometimes appear to invade at once the whole of the parts that are lodged within the skull, or, beginning in one part, it extends rapidly to all the rest. This disease as it occurs in adults presents two periods, which are marked by different symptoms, and are in most instances distinctly observable. In the first period, what are called symptoms of excitement predominate; in the second period those symptoms appear which are comprised under the term collapse. Sometimes these two periods instead of following each other are more or less mixed and confounded. But the distinction is real and requires to be attended to.—WATSON.

Period of excitement.—The symptoms are pain in the head, often intense and deeply seated, or extending over a large part of it; a sense of constriction across the forehead; throbbing of the temporal arteries; flushing of the face; injection of the eyes, which have a wild and brilliant look; contraction of the pupils; unusual sensitiveness to external impressions, amounting frequently to impatience of light and sound; violent delirium; want of sleep; paroxysms of general convulsions; a parched and dry skin; a frequent and hard pulse; white tongue; thirst; nausea and vomiting; constipation.

Modes in which the disease commences.—The attack may come on in three or four different ways:

1st. Sometimes there is a sudden alteration of manner, and the patient, complaining probably of his head, becomes all at once and furiously delirious; fever is also lighted up.

2d. In other cases the first thing noticed is nausea and vomiting, which may soon cease, or continue for several days, or even throughout the whole course of the disease. Great quantities of yellow, bitter, bilious fluid are brought up, and whatever is introduced into the stomach, even a small quantity of the most simple drink is immediately rejected. With this state of matters there is generally much constipation, and the bowels refuse to act except under the influence of strong purgatives. It is very easy to mistake these cases for attacks of sick-headache, bilious derangement, &c., &c.—WATSON.

3d. Another set of cases of acute inflammation of the brain, commences with paroxysms of general convulsions, such as often usher in an attack of meningitis. This symptom according to ANDRAL is a much more certain sign of inflammation of the brain, than the occurrence of active delirium, and WATSON quite agrees with him in so thinking.

WATSON supposes that the cases which are characterized by early and fierce delirium are cases in which the inflammatory action has invaded the whole of the brain and its membranes simultaneously. It is more probable that a large portion of the *grey* substance of the brain is principally inflamed. He also assumes that when nausea and vomiting are the earliest symptoms, the inflammation has taken its point of departure in the cerebral pulp; in the substance of the brain. The seat of the disease is, however, doubtless in the corpora-quadrigemina and striata, (see Treatise on Headaches, p. xiv.) Finally, he guesses that when the attack comes on with a sudden fit of convulsion, the inflammation has commenced in the pia-mater or arachnoid. It is more apt to be located in the *white* substance of the brain.

Simple inflammation of the brain proper, without any simultaneous affection of the membranes, has been fully considered in the chapter on red or inflammatory softening of the brain, (see Treatise on Apoplexy, p. 143.)

Period of collapse.—The first or acute stage lasts for a variable period, i. e. from one-half to two days or more, and then it is succeeded by the second stage, or that of collapse. The patient then ceases to complain of headache; instead of being excited or wildly delirious, he mutters indistinctly, and falls into a state of stupor, from which it is difficult, and at length impossible to arouse him. His vision and hearing are no longer painfully acute; squinting and double vision are not uncommon; and the pupil, from having been contracted to the size of a pin's point, becomes first oscillating, then widely dilated, and ultimately motionless. Twitchings of the muscles and startings of the tendons take the place of convulsions, although some of the limbs may be agitated with tremors, or become powerless and palsied. The face becomes ghastly and cadaverous; cold sweats break out; the sphincters relax; finally the coma becomes profound and life ceases.—WATSON.

Treatment.—In this disease, which is too often fatal under any mode of treatment, a mere symptomatic homœopathic procedure is ruinous. If too much attention be paid to the management of the delirium, convulsions or vomitings, the inflammation will progress rapidly and unchecked. *Aconite* should be used freely, internally and externally; if this fails *Veratrum-viride* may be used. In some cases *Opium* and *Aconite* should be given in alternation. As soon as exudation takes place, Mercurius, Hydriodate of Potash and Phosphor. are the principal remedies.

ABSCESS OF THE BRAIN.

According to VALLEIX it is much more rare to find a perfectly circumscribed abscess than a diffuse softening with suppuration.

The causes of this affection are very similar to those of inflammatory softening, such as external violence in young and vigorous subjects, absorption of pus in consequence of operations on distant parts, and especially from the suppression of chronic discharges from the ear.

Symptoms.—The most important one is *headache*, the pain of which is acute, persistent, and causes constant complaints from the patient, who almost always presses his head with his hand, contracts his brows, and assumes the strangest positions in the hope of escaping his agony. After the disease has lasted a certain length of time the pain subsides and even disappears.

The *intelligence* may be disordered in various ways; sometimes there is an active, more frequently a quiet delirium; at other times there is a marked dulness of the intellect, and the patient has an obtuse manner, does not answer questions, but continues to complain of his head. This hebitude generally follows after previous delirium and agitation.

On the *motor* side, we may observe convulsions, epileptiform attacks, or rigidity; or there may be paralysis more or less complete, or merely a weakness and sluggishness of every movement, similar to the hebetude of the brain. The paralysis does not ordinarily set in suddenly, but sometimes it succeeds soon after the convulsions. The *sensibility* is not always diminished unless there is simultaneous paralysis.

Sometimes there is *fever*, with heat of skin, acceleration of pulse, redness of the face, &c.; in other cases there is none.

Vomiting and constipation are far from being constantly present; the respiration is not apt to be affected.

It is supposed that the symptoms of abscess of the brain from external violence are the most decided and acute, and that paralysis promptly follows the agitation and delirium. Abscess from disease of the bones of the skull, has less severe and urgent symptoms; while that which arises from suppression of a discharge from the ear, follows a slow and insidious course, with but few prominent symptoms.

When the abscess is seated in the *grey* substance of the convolutions, the delirium and agitation are the most marked symptoms; when it is located in the *grey* portions of the interior of the brain, rigidity of the limbs and convulsions are the most prominent symptoms; paralysis is most common when the disease is in the *white* substance; general paralysis occurs when the collection of pus is in the annular protuberance; when the abscess is in one hemisphere of the brain or cerebellum, the paralysis will be on the opposite side.—VALLEIX.

Treatment.—The truly homœopathic remedies against suppurative inflammation are Tartar-emetic, Cantharides, Rhus, Sabina and Phosphor. The solvents of the pus globules are: Kali-carb. and Baryta-muriatica.

HYDATIDS IN THE BRAIN.

There are several varieties:

1st. The *hydatids spuria* is merely a hydropic primordial cell; it is more frequently met with than the other varieties and may be found in almost every part of the brain.

Symptoms.—The pain in the head they cause is constant; in true hydatids it is intermittent. They are apt to be attended with loss of sensation, dulness of intellect and loss of memory.

2d. *Acephalocysts*, are very rare; of 21 specimens presented to Klencke for examination, only 3 were genuine; they are generally of the size of a lentil or pea, of an opaline color, and contain a mass of microscopic cells.

Symptoms.—These vary much; generally there is headache, but not more severe than in some other diseases.

If they are developed in the póns, fornix, crura-cerebri, hemispheres of the cerebellum, or base of the medulla-oblongata, or if they compress these structures, they induce peculiar affections of the muscular system, ending ultimately in epilepsy.

When confined to the cerebral hemispheres they cause stupor only, or headache, or in extreme cases, apoplexy.

If the acephalocysts be numerous, the respiration is apt to be slow; if they are seated in the corpus callosum the pulse is generally slow; if in the pes-hippocampi the pulse may be quickened.

If seated in the thalami-optici and crura-cerebri, they are apt to be attended with hallucinations, flashes of light before the eyes, or blindness.

If in the corpora-striata, or quadrigenema, we are apt to find spasms of the stomach, spasmodic colic, or paralysis of the colon.

If the cerebellum be implicated, there generally is paralysis of the bowels or bladder, with abolition of the sexual functions.

3d. The presence of *polycephalus* causes the rotary disease in sheep. In man it causes headache, rotation, loss of memory, and insensibility to light.

4th. The *cysticerus*, and also the polycephalus are apt to cause periodic headaches, owing to the greater or less active movements of the parasites; every motion of the neck, or the crown of hooks around it causes irritation of the brain.

Treatment.—Many of the symptoms produced by these parasites are relieved in a remarkable manner by brandy, for alcohol acts as a poison, especially upon the cysterceri and converts them into a torpid mass.

Nitrate of silver has relieved many of the gastric affections, also the trembling of the hands and convulsive action of the eyelids, &c.

Nux-vomica and Secale are supposed to exert a beneficial action upon them.

TUBERCLES OF THE BRAIN.

Under this head we do not refer to cases in which tubercle is present merely in the membranes of the brain, producing that granular appearance which has been alluded to when treating of tubercular meningitis, but to separate and independent deposits of tubercular matter into the substance of the brain itself.

Tubercles of the brain though exceedingly rare in the adult, are not very uncommon in the child: thus, while LOUIS met with only 1 case of tubercle in the brains of 117 adults who died of tubercular disease, RILLIET and BARTHEZ found it 37 times in 312 cases of fatal tubercular disease in children.

WEST knows of no instance in which tubercle was limited to the brain in childhood, for if present there it always existed in other viscera, especially in the bronchial glands and lungs, shewing that it is but one of the results of that general cachexia which may show itself in any of the various forms of scrofulous or consumptive disease. This fact is very important in forming an opinion as to the nature of various local diseases of the brain; for softening of the brain, or abscess, or tubercles, hydatids or cancer, do not disclose their precise nature by any peculiar symptoms, or succession of symptoms. They all, sooner or later disturb the functions of the brain, and they may all disturb them very nearly after the same fashion. But we may judge sometimes, from other circumstances, that the disease is of this or that character; thus, if we find scrofulous or cancerous disease in other parts of the body, we may safely infer that the symptoms which denote disease of the brain, are caused by scrofulous or cancerous tumors there situated; but from the symptoms themselves, we can only learn that there is some morbid condition of the brain.—WATSON.

According to ROKITANSKY the number of tubercles in the brain is usually small; one or two being met with in most cases, and more rarely, three, four, five or a few more; some extremely rare exceptions do occur in which twenty or more are found. When they are but few, each separate tubercle acquires a considerable size, the most usual size is that of a hazel or walnut; when they are more numerous, no single one often is found much larger than a hemp-seed or pea, although I have seen at least twenty in one child's brain, and none less than a hazel-nut in size. Tubercles of the brain are also peculiar in not being generally aggregated together, but separated widely apart.

Every part of the brain is occasionally the seat of tubercle. They are very common in the brain itself, and less so in the cerebellum; they are rarely found in the pons, and still less so in the medulla-oblongata. As a general rule they are deposited in or near the *grey* substance, hence near the surface of the brain, or in the grey portions of the corpora striata or optic thalami. The corpus callosum, fornix, septum lucidum, and crura scarcely ever contain any.—ROKITANSKY.

Its most frequent combination is with tuberculosis of the absorbent glands; and next in frequency with tubercle in the lungs.

When seated near the surface of the brain, they may cause tuberculous inflammation of the membranes, and acute dropsy of the brain.

Symptoms.—These vary according to the number and location of the tubercles, and to the existence or non-existence of softening of the brain around them.

In one case, in a boy aged 3½ years, and in the left hemisphere of whose cerebellum WEST found a tubercle, there had been an almost constant and involuntary rotary motion of the head when lying down; but this is a rare symptom.

As they are generally seated near the surface of the brain, we would expect often to find delirium, stupor, or headache. In fact HENNIS GREEN mentions pain in the head as the most constant symptom of the early stages of the disease, having met with it as a prominent symptom in 17 cases out of 20. This pain is often very severe, so that during its continuance the child shrieks with the agony of the suffering; but singularly enough it does not continue with this intensity for more than a few hours, and on the next day the child may be found to be no worse than usual. Vomiting in many instances attends these exacerbations of pain.

In other instances a general dulness steals over all the faculties, and the child grows quite indifferent to what is going on around it; he may never complain of headache, but be fretful and cry if moved, yet be perfectly quiet if allowed to remain undisturbed, dozing for hours together.

According to GENDRIN when the tubercles are located in one cerebral peduncle, convulsions commence in one leg and from thence extend to the whole of the same side on which the peduncle is affected.

When they occupy the mesocephalon, the muscles of the face and especially of the mouth are most convulsed, and generally spasms only occur at a later period.

In a very few cases no symptoms are present; much more frequently, however, the signs of disturbance of the brain, though not entirely absent, are too vague to excite much attention and too slight to occasion much suffering, so that if they do not wholly escape notice, they are confounded with other indications of ill-health attendant upon the general tubercularization with which this disease of the brain is frequently associated. In these latent, or semi-latent cases death finally takes place rather suddenly, under the indications of the most serious brain-disease. This acute stage sometimes lasts for a few hours only, and a child who had shown no sign of head-affection, though probably the symptoms of tubercular disease of the lungs or other organs had long been present, suddenly sinks into a state of stupor, which soon deepens into a profound and fatal coma. In another set of cases convulsions take place suddenly, followed by paralysis of one limb, or of the whole of one side, and either is immediately succeeded by coma, or this does not come on till after the fits have recurred several times. In a third variety of cases death is preceded by symptoms of acute dropsy of the brain. This sudden outbreak of symptoms may take place without evident cause, or follow a not very severe blow or fall upon the head.—WEST.

When headache, nausea and vomiting are present, the case may still be obscure; for some delicate children have irregular attacks of violent headache, off and on for years, accompanied with vomiting, from slight causes or no apparent cause at all, and finally recover as their health becomes more robust. Some children may even have headache aggravated at intervals and associated with occasional convulsive movements of one limb, and even with attacks of an epileptic character, and yet show by the confirmed health they subsequently attain to, that some cause of a less abiding nature than a tubercular deposit must have given rise to the disturbance of the brain.—West.

Affections of the motor system are, however, often among the earliest indications of this disease; convulsive movements are the most frequent of these; paralysis of a limb, or impaired power over it, usually succeeds the convulsions, and but seldom take place independently of them. Sometimes we observe nothing more than an occasional convulsive twitching of one limb, more frequently of the arm than of the leg, unattended with any loss of consciousness, or impairment of the intellect; but the seizure is more frequently attended with stupor, though the convulsive action may be confined to one side, or even to one limb. When convulsions, whether general or partial, have once occurred they are seldom absent for many days together.

The transition from the premonitory to the acute stage sometimes takes place gradually, the convulsions becoming more and more frequent, and the other brain symptoms more serious, and the intervals of freedom from suffering shorter; or the change takes place suddenly, and without such previous increase in the severity of the child's suffering as to make one anticipate its approaching death; and yet we cannot always discover such differences between the morbid appearances in the two cases as should explain the dissimilar course of the disease.—West.

When tubercles are seated solely in the corpus-striatum, there will probably be convulsive movements when a portion only is involved, and paralysis if the disease includes the whole of the organ.

If located in the optic thalami, there will be more or less loss of sensation.

Tubercular disease of the medulla-oblongata and pons-varolii, is attended with difficulty and irregularity of breathing.

Disease of the crus-cerebri is followed by convulsions or paralysis of the opposite side; also when the white substance of the brain is involved. The symptoms of tuberculosis of other parts of the brain will be similar to those which have been observed when hydatids are present.

Treatment.—The infants of tuberculous mothers should be weaned early, or given to a healthy wet-nurse, or what perhaps would be better still, they should be fed upon diluted cream; as milk, both human and animal, contains a large proportion of albumen and caseine, it should be entirely avoided. Milk, as is well-known, is a watery liquid, having in solution a certain amount of caseine, sugar of milk or lactine, extractive matter, together with several inorganic salts, (such as the Phosphates of Lime, Magnesia, and of the Per-oxide of Iron, the Chlorides of Potassium and Sodium, and Pure-soda,) and holding in suspension myriads of extremely minute globules of fatty matter, plainly visible through the microscope. Fresh milk is almost invariably slightly alkaline, but on exposure to air, especially in warm weather, it rapidly becomes acid, owing to the conversion of the sugar of milk or lactine, into lactic acid, under the influence of the caseine which acts as a ferment. If the milk has been long retained in the breast, this change occasionally takes place before being drawn; and in some morbid conditions also, the milk is found to have an acid reaction even when freshly drawn. Such milk would be especially injurious to children with a tendency to tuberculous ailments; if milk be used at all, the mother should be supplied with litimus paper to test each specimen before it is given to the babe.

Acidity of the stomach and bowels should be carefully obviated and prevented; still ordinary acidity of the digestive organs will not necessarily produce tuberculous disease. As the Chlorides and Phosphates of Soda and Potassa are deficient in tuberculous blood, it might be advisable to use these salts to correct or prevent acidity of the stomach and bowels.

As Iron is decidedly deficient in the blood of tuberculous subjects I have long been in the habit of using a combination of equal parts of Phosphate of Iron and Phosphate of Lime or Soda, thoroughly triturated together, and mixed with double its weight of Sugar, in order to prevent acidity of the stomach, and supply the requisite quantity of Iron to the system. Phosphate of Lime ought also be an excellent dietetic and preventive, if not curative remedy against tuberculous acidity. According to Ancell crude tubercle contains but a very small proportion of Phosphate and Carbonate of Lime—say one per cent.—

whereas, chalky tubercles frequently weigh 10, 20 or 30 grains. Hence in order to form chalky concretions, the deposition and resorption of animal matter, such as Albumen and Caseine must have taken place to a very great extent, or for a considerable period. It appears to ANCELL that where the tendency to cretaceous aggregation has existed in the highest degree, the blood must have wholly or partially lost its tuberculous quality; and that after having secreted intractable tubercle, owing to this favorable change it pours out a blastema, which depositing its earthy salts, is in the main susceptible of resorption, and is actually absorbed, the earthy particles gradually accumulating in the tuberculous cavity. That some such process as this occurs, he thinks, follows from a consideration of the whole series of chemical facts. Supplying an excess of Phosphate of Lime to the system may perhaps favor and hasten these beneficial changes.

The acids in the normal gastric juice are: the Muriatic, Lactic and Acetic; the Muriatic generally predominates, although either may be in excess and require peculiar treatment. The chyme which is made from the fibrine of meat and coagulated albumen, contains much Muriatic acid; that which is made from quite fresh meat and milk contains an excess of Lactic acid; while that which is made from amylaceous and farinaceous substances and vegetables contains much Acetic acid. In some states of the system quite new and unusual acids are found, or get into the stomach, such as: Phosphoric, Uric, Oleic or Butyric, and even Fluoric acid. It is not yet known positively which one of these acids predominates in the tuberculous dyscrasia, but they all require their peculiar and specific antidotes. The best antidotes of Muriatic acid are: Zincum, Ferrum, Argentum and Ammonia; Soda, Plumbum and Baryta are the best antidotes for Phosphoric acid; the tendency to the formation of Uric acid in the stomach is best antidoted by Cuprum and Colchicum; while an excess of Lactic acid is best met with Zincum.—(See Treatise on Diseases of Married Females, p. 52.)

Hepar-sulphur. may correct acidity of the stomach, and neutralize the predominance of albumen in the blood, besides having a symptomatic relation to tubercular disease.

When deposits of tubercle have actually taken place, they cannot be removed by any known solvent. Still trials may be made with at least a shadow of a hope of success. Thus, if we admit with Hecht and Scharlau that tubercle contains 30 per cent. of Fibrine, the solvents of Fibrine may be used. According to Denis if moist Fibrine be digested in a solution of Nitrate of Potash containing a little Soda, it gradually becomes converted into a substance in almost every respect identical with Albumen; being soluble in water, and coagulable by heat. Again, the alkalies and their carbonates and acetates entirely prevent the coagulation of Fibrine; and tolerably strong solutions of Nitrate of Potash, Nitrate of Lime, and Muriate of Ammonia, retard it for a long time; the Muriate of Ammonia, indeed, gradually dissolves Fibrine, after it has been allowed to coagulate.

If we assume that tubercle consists in an excessive formation and deposition of Albumen, the solvents of Albumen may be tried. Hepar-sulphur. has already been alluded to. Coagulated Albumen is also readily soluble in Potash and other alkaline solutions; the Phosphoric, Acetic and Tartaric acids, also appear to exercise a decided solvent action upon it, and when present even prevent its coagulating on the application of heat. On the other hand, the Nitric and Muriatic acids, the Bichloride of Mercury, and Ferrocyanide of Potassium coagulate and precipitate Albumen and hence may be more homœopathic to Albuminous tubercles.

Finally, if we assume that tubercle consists merely of Caseine, we may be obliged to resort to Acetic, or some other acid, for although Caseine coagulates and is precipitated by Acetic acid, it redissolves if the acid be added in decided excess. In fact, although Caseine is precipitated and coagulated by Acetic and nearly all the acids, it redissolves in a considerable excess of most of them.

The experienced physician can easily decide when to give the preference to one or the other of these remedies; or to use two or several of them in alternation or combination; also when it will be advisable to use the inhalation of the vapors of these medicines in combination with their internal use; and finally when to rely upon infinitessimal quantities in order to overcome a qualitative or dynamic predisposition or tendency to tubercular disease, and when to give more massive quantities in order to remove absolutely material and quantitative deposits.

CANCER OF THE BRAIN.

THE symptoms of cancer of the brain and its membranes are similar if not identical with those of tubercles or other tumors of these parts. An accurate diagnosis is seldom more than conjectured, except when the cerebral symptoms happen to coincide with the phenomena observed in other parts of the body, which may serve as a clue to the disease going on in the brain. Thus, tubercles in the brain are more common in children and young adults; hard cancer, is more common in persons over 40, while medullary cancer may occur in young subjects. In tubercular disease the skin is apt to present a pasty or doughy appearance; in cancer it often presents a peculiar straw-yellow color. As WATSON truly observes various local diseases and tumors of the brain, do not disclose their precise nature by any peculiar symptoms or succession of symptoms; but if we detect signs of tuberculous or cancerous disease in other parts of the body, we may safely infer that the symptoms which denote disease of the brain are caused by tuberculous or cancerous disease there situated; but from the symptoms alone, we can only learn that there is some morbid condition of the brain. If there be signs of disease of the lungs, bronchial glands, peritonæum or bowels, the probability is that the disease is tuberculous. If there be disease of the breasts, axillary glands, womb, &c., &c., the probability is that the disease is cancerous.

Hence the treatment, although it may be homœopathic, must not be merely symptomatic; it must be directed against the nature of the disease, and not merely against its symptoms or manifestations.

However similar the symptoms of tubercular and cancerous disease of the brain may be, viz.: headache, blindness, paralysis, convulsions, &c., &c. yet there is a decided antagonism not only in the nature of the two diseases, but also in the localities which they prefer: thus, cancer of the breast, stomach, liver, large bowels and womb, is very common; tubercular disease of these organs is very rare; tubercular disease of the lungs, spleen, small bowels, bronchial glands, peritonæum, &c., is sufficiently common, while cancerous affections of these organs is decidedly rare. Hence the remedies for cancerous disease may or must be injurious in tubercular disease, and vice versa.

In tuberculosis, the cellular, vascular, albuminous and glandular tissues are most apt to be affected; in cancerous disease, the gelatiniform, fibrous, albuminous or medullary and glandular parts. Caseine and Albumen are the predominant elements in the tuberculous dyscrasia; Gelatine, Fibrine, Phosphorised fat, Cholesterine, and perhaps Albumen are the most abundant constituents in cancer. Caseine is never found in cancer.

In scirrhus we may find from 0.2144 to 0.2778 of Gelatine; 0.1428 of Fibrine; 0.1388 of Phosphorized fat; and 0.0278 of Albumen; the rest water and salts.

Treatment.—The best remedies against the cancerous dyscrasia, are: Arsenicum, Alumina, Carbo-animalis, Soot, Calendula, Muriates of Gold and Soda, Donovan's Solution, &c.

ON THE

HOMŒOPATHIC TREATMENT

OF

INFLAMMATION AND DROPSY OF THE BRAIN,

&c., &c.

THE following remedies have been used most frequently, viz.: Aconite, Arnica, Belladonna, Bryonia, Chamomilla, Cuprum, Digitalis, Hellebore, Hyosciamus, Iodine, Opium, Rhus, Spts.-Nit.-dulc., Stramonium, Sulphur, Veratrum and Zinc.

ACONITE.

GENERAL REMARKS.—According to WARING the comparative activity of the different parts of the plant has been closely examined by Drs. FLEMING and TURNBULL. They agree that the *root* is the part which is most energetic, certain and eligible for medicinal use; the *seeds* rank second; the *leaves* third; the *flowers* fourth, and the *fruit* and *stem* last. The homœopathic tincture which is made from the whole plant is much weaker and more inefficient than the tincture of the root, because the root contains a much larger proportion of the active principle of the plant, (Aconitine,) than any other part, or all other parts combined. When the homœopathic tincture is diluted one-half, or even twenty times as it frequently is, it becomes a very uncertain and weak preparation to combat acute congestive or inflammatory affections, because Aconite is antipathic rather than homœopathic to these affections, and hence tangible or even massive doses are required. Although Aconite resembles Digitalis and Tobacco in its action upon the heart and arteries and is not strictly homœopathic to inflammatory or actively congestive diseases, still it is used as a matter of course, or of routine, by the majority of homœopathists against the majority of these affections; consequently it frequently fails to produce any good effect, especially when the dilutions, either high or low are used. Lately, Dr. HENRY, homœopathic physician in Montgomery, Alabama, has found out that the Veratrum-viride, exerts a still more powerful action upon the heart and arteries; predicts that it will soon stand as a great rival to the long tried Aconite; and asserts that he prefers it to Aconite, and has never failed in reducing the action of the heart with it. Singularly enough, Veratrum-viride is quite as antipathic to fever and inflammation as Aconite.

According to FLEMING and WARING, when a small piece of the root of Aconite is chewed, it causes an increased flow of saliva, a peculiar numbness of the lips and tongue, with a tingling sensation, and partial loss of use of the lips. Its topical application is unaccompanied by either pain, redness or swelling, even when its pathogenetic effects are developed to the fullest extent; proving that it is not homœopathic to inflammation, but that it exerts a depressing and benumbing, or paralyzing effect upon the vascular system and nerves of sensation.

Given internally, Dr. FLEMING, divides its operation into four degrees:

First Degree.—Half an hour after a dose of 5 drops of the Tincture of the Root, warmth is felt in the stomach, with slight nausea, oppression of breathing, general warmth of the body, numbness, tingling and a sense of distension of the throat, lips and tongue. There is also a tingling at the tips of the fingers, with a peculiar sensation at the roots of the teeth; slight muscular weakness is generally experienced, with indisposition for exertion, either mental or bodily. In about half an hour more, the pulse will be found diminished in strength, and in another hour both the pulse and breathing will have become less frequent, viz.: the pulse will have fallen from 72 to 64, and the breathing from 18 to 15 or 16.

Second Degree.—If 10 drops be taken at first, or the original dose of 5 drops, be followed in two hours by another of equal amount, the above symptoms will supervene more rapidly and with greater severity. The tingling will extend up along the arms, and the sensitiveness of the skin is more or less impaired. In one and a half hours, the pulse will probably have fallen to about 56 beats per minute and become smaller and weaker, still maintaining, however, perfect regularity. The respirations will be about 13 per minute and laboring, attended with great muscular debility, giddiness and confusion of sight, with lethargy, coldness of the skin and extremities.

Larger doses will be followed by the same symptoms to a more severe extent. The pulse occasionally falls to 40, or even 36, but more generally rises to 70 or 80, becoming small, weak and irregular; respiration is oppressed, and the skin becomes moist and cold.—FLEMING.

Of the allied remedies of Aconite, *Tobacco* acts specifically upon the stomach, solar plexus of nerves, heart, arteries and nerves of motion and muscular system. *Digitalis* acts principally upon the heart, arteries, kidneys, and serous membranes. *Veratrum-viride* upon the stomach, liver, bowels, heart and arteries. *Colchicum* upon the liver, kidneys, heart, arteries and fibrous tissues. *Tartar-emetic* and *Ipecac.* upon the stomach, solar plexus, skin and muscular system. *Aconite* upon the skin, sero-fibrous tissues, heart and arteries. All these remedies depress the action of the heart and arteries in a similar and specific manner.

Although I believe that the majority of TESTE's remarks on the Materia Medica are flippant and insincere, still I agree with him when he says, that of all the medicines used by homœopathic physicians, Aconite is the one which they use erroneously most frequently. As it only possesses the power of perturbating or depressing the action of the heart and arteries, and is not homœopathic to inflammatory local lesions, whenever inflammatory fever and local inflammation have already acquired a certain degree of intensity, infinitessimal doses cannot be administered without involving a loss of very precious time. Either, some decidedly homœopathic remedy must be used in small quantities; or more massive doses of Aconite must be given. TESSIER found that when inflammation of the lungs was at its height, the high dilutions only produced some slight effect upon the pulse, none upon the disease.—PETERS.

a. In opposition to the above, KREUSSLER says: whenever traces merely of inflammation of the brain present themselves, or whenever this disease seems fully developed, Aconite is the first remedy which ought to be given. It is not the question whether inflammatory fever is present or not, for pure inflammation of the brain or its membranes requires the use of this remedy from the very commencement of the disease, until effusions and exudations have taken place. Two or three doses of the 6th or 12th dilution may be given, and its action awaited for twelve or twenty-four hours. If not the least improvement occurs during this time, viz.: neither perspiration, sediment in the urine, nor bleeding of the nose, and the restlessness continues, followed by stupor and delirium, then another remedy must be used.—KREUSSLER. I venture to assert that either other remedies, or larger doses will be required in the majority of cases.—PETERS.

b. HEICHELHEIM says he has treated eight children in the first stage of dropsy of the brain and relieved them all with Aconite followed by Bellad.

c. SCHROEN asserts that when congestion of the brain with impending inflammation sets in during dentition of young children, he has always found *Aconite* useful; but large and repeated doses had to be given. KREUSSLER, with characteristic flippancy and dogmatism assumes that Aconite will not remove simple congestion, but only that stasis and congestion which is the first stage of acute inflammation.

CASE 1.—A girl, aged 10, had heat and redness of the whole body, especially of the head and eyes, contracted pupils, entire unconsciousness, delirium, dryness of the tongue, vomiting of greenish substances, subsultus, quickened respiration, pulse 120 to 130, with grasping at the head.

Treatment and Result.—Acon. 18, one drop in 6 spoonsful of water, 1 spoonful every half-hour; in six hours consciousness was restored, the fever and vomiting had ceased; *Bryonia* was given on the next day, and she was quite well in two days more. —GASTFREUND.

CASE 2.—A lady, aged 32, who had often suffered with severe headache, was suddenly attacked with symptoms which denoted approaching inflammation of the brain. She ran in perfect despair about the room, complained of pain in the forehead, as if everything would be forced out of it; her head was glowing hot; she had nausea, white coated tongue, pain in the back, constipation for two days; pulse tranquil, and skin natural.—[I have frequently seen similar attacks in nervous and hysterical females, but never supposed that I had either threatened or actual inflammation to deal with.]—PETERS.

Treatment.—Aconite 6, 1 drop; in five minutes the pain abated; the patient soon became composed and slept till morning, when she was quite restored.—KREUSSLER.

CASE 3.—A boy, aged 5 years, sickened with the usual signs of inflammation of the brain, of which the following were the most prominent:

Symptoms.—Spasms of the limbs, alternating with trembling motion of them; vomiting of food or mucus as soon as he raised his head; starting up from sleep with delirium, or pain in both sides of the head; dryness and heat of skin; much thirst; full, hard and quick pulse.

Treatment.—Aconite 30, in 2 ounces of water, 1 teaspoonful every hour at first, then every two hours, with perfect recovery in three days.—WEBER.

CASE 4.—A maiden, aged 14, had suffered for twenty-four hours with the following symptoms of brain-affection: vertigo and vomiting whenever she rose up; constant pain in the forehead; delirium, sopor, screaming and starting up from sleep, with fixedness of look; her face was pale at times, at others red; skin hot and dry; thirst, and constipation.

Treatment.—14 doses of Aconite 30, removed the whole disorder in three days. The constipation was removed by Nux. 30.—WEBER.

CASE 5.—A girl, aged nine years, was attacked with inflammation of the brain, for which she received Bell. 4, 1 drop every three hours, for thirty-one hours without benefit.

Symptoms.—Wandering of the mind; constant chewing motion of the lower jaw; incoherent muttering; the pupils were contracted; expression of the eyes unsteady and indifferent;

face moderately flushed; skin moist; pulse full, hard, quick and frequent.

Treatment.—Aconite 3, 1 drop every hour; in five hours she fell asleep and slept for four hours; she awoke conscious, and was gradually restored on the third day.—NOACK.

CASE 6.—HAUBOLD cured a case of acute hydrocephalus, attended with vomiting; boring of the very large head into the pillow; by means of three doses of Aconite in thirty-six hours, followed by 1 dose of Bellad.

CASE 7.—After a somewhat hard fall upon the head, a boy, aged 2 years, was attacked suddenly with the following:

Symptoms.—He dozed a great deal, but often awoke suddenly, raised himself up and vomited up a clear, watery fluid; his tongue was clean and he drank again immediately afterwards, then fell asleep and awoke vomiting at least three times in every hour. He frequently started in his sleep; had rolling of his half-opened eyes; bored the back of his head into the pillow; grasped at his head automatically; frequent alternations of the color of his face from pale to red; picking of his nose; and gritting of the teeth.

Treatment.—Two doses of Aconite 3, 1 drop per dose, every hour; followed by Bellad. 3, 1 drop every two hours. On the following day he was quite well.—FRANK.

CASE 8.—A child, aged 3 years, was attacked with inflammation of the membranes of the brain, which terminated in effusion into the ventricles. It was given up as hopeless by two physicians.

Treatment.—Aconite was then given every half-hour, until the quickness of the pulse was lessened; then *Bellad.* was given in the same way. The child improved in some days, and had completely recovered at the end of a fortnight.—DUNSFORD.

CASE 9.—YELDHAM thinks that many of the slighter affections of the brain, giving rise to headache, and other symptoms clearly referable to disorder of that organ, are doubtless of an inflammatory character. Hence he would doubtless meet with, and cure more cases of inflammation of the brain than most other physicians.—PETERS.

A hearty young man, aged 20, caught cold on his journey home, about a week ago; yesterday was seized with shivering and violent pain in the head; took pills which acted freely, but without relief; he lies with his neck stretched out and head thrown back on the pillow, from which position he cannot bear to move; complains of intense pain in the forehead over the eyes; cannot tolerate the least light or noise; his brow is knit; eyes red and angry; his skin, especially that of the forehead is hot and dry; pulse 95, full and hard; mouth and tongue dry, with incessant thirst; no other pain, but is liable to rush of blood to the head.

Treatment.—Aconite 3, directly followed by Bellad. 3, every two hours; was rather better the next day; head not so hot and painful; thirst not so urgent; pulse as frequent, but not so hard and throbbing; skin cooler.—Aconite 3, and Bellad. 3, in alternation every three hours; recovered entirely in two days more.

REVIEW.—Of nine cases, 7 were in children, and two in adults.

In case 7, a fall upon the head was the exciting cause.

Vomiting was present in 4 cases.

In most of the cases there was a state of excitement, with delirium, spasms, subsultus, &c., &c.; the pulse varied from 72 to 95, or even 120 or 130, and was full, hard, quick or suppressed. Yet in cases of poisoning with Aconite, the brain is remarkably undisturbed and clear, and the pulse is apt to be weak, small and slow.—PETERS.

The stage in which it proved most useful was that of irritation, only occasionally approaching that of exudation.

DOSES:—Aconite 3, was given twice, in repeated doses; Aconite 6, once; Aconite 18, once in solution, and repeated every half-hour; Aconite 30, twice in solution.

In 3 cases Aconite effected a cure alone.
" 5 " " was followed by Bellad.
" 1 " " " " " Bryon.

The *duration* of the attacks was twenty-four hours in 1 case; thirty-six hours in 1 case; three days in 5 cases; and fourteen days in 1 case.

Aconite probably acts as a powerful antiphlogistic sudorific, as it induces perspiration in the majority of acute cases in which it proves beneficial.

ARNICA.

According to SOBERNHEIM it facilitates the circulation of the lymph, and increases the absorbent powers of the collective lymphatic and venous systems. It was used and highly recommended in arachnitis with effusion by the celebrated GÖLIS of Vienna; he had the head of the patient freely and frequently bathed with an infusion of Arnica, when signs of effusion or exudation, or of a sub-paralytic state of the brain came on;—he also regarded it as the principal remedy against concussions of the brain, or spinal marrow; in sanguineous, or sero-lymphatic exudations from falls, blows, contusions, concussions, &c. It is very useful in low states of the system when there is dulness of the senses, dejection of spirits, drowsiness, sopor, or even stupor, or muttering delirium with dryness and blackness of the tongue, &c., &c. If it fails, Hydriodate of Potash may be used internally and externally, aided or not by a few doses of Iodide of Mercury, or of Apocynum-cannabinum.—PETERS.

CASE 10.—A delicate boy, aged 2½ years, was attacked with the following symptoms about five weeks after he had had an attack of measles.

He complained of pain in his head; squinted; was afraid of falling, and at times even fell backwards; he had attacks of vomiting, cramps of the hands, and fits of screaming; was only comfortable while lying upon his back; had attacks of unconsciousness, from which he could only be aroused by loud talking; his head was hot; pupils dilated; breathing anxious; urine scanty and red; pulse quick and small.

Treatment and Result.—Aconite 9, followed in three hours by Bellad. 12; but the disease increased steadily for nine hours, when he became exceedingly restless, with severe convulsions of the limbs, violent fits of screaming; he was only easy when lying on his right side, with his head bent far back; the pupils were very much dilated; eyes entirely insensible to light; he was perfectly unconscious, and grasped at his head.

Arnica 3, in 1 drop doses; by the next night he could open his eyes; his consciousness returned the next morning; he wished for food, and to be carried about, but was unable to hold his head up; the pupils were somewhat contracted; his urine turbid, with a yellow sediment; and he was very irritable. On the second day he attempted to stand, but fell over; Arnica 6 was given. On the third day, a return of fever was removed by Aconite. On the fifth day he seemed restored and had some appetite. Merc. 2 finally restored him perfectly in fourteen days.—MALY.

CASE 11.—In a case of acute hydrocephalus, in which Acon. and Bell. afforded no relief, Arnica 6, repeated every four hours, effected a rapid improvement.—HAUBOLD.

CASE 12.—Inflammation of the brain with violent symptoms in a maiden, aged 21, arising from a fall upon the head, was soon removed by several doses of Arnica 4; remaining blindness was cured by Bellad. and Opium.—THORER.

REVIEW.—It has been decidedly useful in the second stage of hydrocephalus, especially when induced by falls or blows upon the head.

ARSENICUM.

This remedy ought to prove one of the most efficient homœopathic remedies against serous inflammations in general and inflammatory dropsies. One of its most marked and frequent effects is to produce dropsical effusions about the head and face, attended with fever and great scantiness of the urine. It is most homœopathic to the acute variety of hydrocephalus, yet WAHLE only recommends it in the chronic form, after the previous use of Hellebore and Sulphur, and when the patient is peculiarly irritable and passionate.

CASE 13.—A boy, aged 6 years, had been drooping for some time, finally he had all the symptoms of brain-disease, accompanied by gastric derangement; he lay doubled up in bed, with his knees drawn up to his stomach; bowels very sensitive to touch; was drowsy and heavy, and lay in a stupor with half-closed eyes and open mouth, whenever he was not disturbed;

when aroused, and also at other times he often started and screamed out with a loud and piercing cry; his features were sunken; mouth and nostrils sore, dry and black; his tongue dry and parched, with a thick, brownish-yellow coating; red edges and papillæ. The skin of his whole body, but more particularly of the head and bowels was hot and dry; he was thirsty and had no appetite; his bowels loose and evacuations unhealthy; pulse 125, hard and incompressible; he was annoyed by a short hacking cough.

Treatment.—Arsenicum 6, every four hours; at the end of two days he seemed much the same, only his tongue appeared to be cleaning at the edges, and his thirst was not so great. The Arsenicum was continued for three days more, with only slight shades of amendment; he was then ordered Hellebore 6, every four hours, with decided improvement at the end of the second day; his tongue became moist and cleaned off rapidly; skin cool, thirst moderate, pulse less frequent and more soft, eyes clear, bright and intelligent, little or no screaming or drowsiness. He was perfectly restored in a few days more, under the continued use of Hellebore.—YELDHAM.

BELLADONNA.

GENERAL REMARKS.—*a.* This remedy acts specifically upon the blood, brain, nervous, muscular and lymphatic systems, also upon the throat, skin and kidneys.

Its action upon the *blood* is similar to that produced by Alcohol, or extreme heat of the sun; there is a commotion and actual expansion of the blood, as is shown by the quickness and fulness of the blood-vessels, heat and redness of the face and skin. It would seem to cause an intense arterial and inflammatory condition, but in fact it causes a tumultuous conversion of the arterial blood into venous, for after a while the apparent increased arterial action ceases, and excessive and predominant venosity supplies its place. The apparent arterial storm lasts for about twelve hours, when great venosity becomes apparent; the redness of the face gives place to lividity; the veins everywhere seem to be crowded and overfilled; the muscles become relaxed; confusion and stupefaction of the brain ensue; but finally profuse sweats and urination restore the balance of the system.

It may be that this powerful commotion and intoxication of the arterial system is removed by the exertions or natural functions of the venous and lymphatic systems, which absorb or remove the noxious element from the arterial system, and thus become contaminated themselves.

Its action upon the *brain* is that of a powerful irritant or stimulant, unless the dose be in great excess, when the powers of the brain are completely overcome or stupefied; Belladonna stupefaction may also arise from exhaustion from previous over-excitement.—(See Treatise on Mental Derangement.)

Its action upon the *muscular* system is rather depressing than exciting; Belladonna convulsions are rare, and when present slight; while paralysis of the sphincters, such as dilatation of the pupils, of the neck of the bladder, womb, and the rectum are common; besides it is one of the best palliatives against those wandering pains in rheumatism, which arise from spasmodic contraction of the muscles, caused by the fleeting irritation of the poison of rheumatism; also against rheumatic colicky pains from spasmodic contraction of the muscular coat of the stomach and bowels.

Its action upon the *throat* and *skin* is similar to that produced by the poison of scarlet fever.

Its action upon the kidneys is very decided; the secretion of urine is increased excessively.—PETERS.

b. LOBETHAL says he gives 2 or 3 drops of the tincture of Bellad. in several spoonsful of water, against violent congestion towards the head in young children, with threatening of inflammation or dropsy of the brain, with far more confidence than he does the 24th or 30th dilution. In slighter and more chronic cases, in some of the latter of which he has several times succeeded in effecting cures even when there was entire dulness of the senses, he prefers the 24th or 30th dilutions to the lower potencies.

c. KREUSSLER advises the 18th or 24th dilution, repeated twice a day, when there are aching and outward pressing pains with dull stitches in the head, preceded by dizziness and feeling of intoxication; when the patients stare fixedly before them, and their faces and eyes are much flushed; when infants bore with their heads into the pillow; also when there is retention of fæces and urine, which afterwards pass off involuntarily; the thirst being excessive, the pulse frequent and quick. When improvement sets in the doses are to be repeated less frequently than twice a day.

d. Knorre thinks that Bellad. is most indicated in the *first*, or inflammatory stage of hydrocephalus, when this is strongly marked and bears an arterial, or venous-inflammatory character rather than a torpid or sub-inflammatory. In the *second*, or incurable stage it is of no further avail, except that it sometimes relieves the vomiting, and that perhaps only imperfectly.

IN CHILDREN.

CASE 14.—A girl, aged 6 years, after several days' sickness, had the following:

Symptoms.—Acute fever, general heat of body, redness of the face, quick, hard pulse, quick breathing, sleepy-drowsiness, frequent vomiting, gritting of the teeth, and great anxiety and restlessness while awake.

Treatment.—Bellad. 3, 15 drops in 3 ounces of water, 1 teaspoonful every hour; with relief in twenty-four hours and speedy recovery.—Elwert.

CASE 15.—A boy, aged 6, had been sick for six or eight hours, with violent fever, quick pulse, hurried breathing, trembling, great redness of face, general dry heat of skin, drowsiness, frequent starting, fixed and glassy look, cramp of the jaws.

Treatment.—Bellad. 3 relieved him in twenty-four hours.—Elwert.

CASE 16.—A boy, aged 5, had suffered for several hours with active fever and nervous excitement. He received Aconite 3, followed by general perspiration and by increase of the disease; he was aroused with difficulty, stared fixedly, and did not understand when spoken to, had startings and tremblings of the limbs, jerks, twitchings of the muscles of the face; pulse not to be counted and respiration hurried.

Treatment.—Bellad. 3, 10 drops in 3 ounces of water, 1 teaspoonful every half-hour, with evident improvement in twenty-four hours.—ELWERT.

CASES 17 and 18.—Two similar cases were treated with Bellad., one with 15 drops of the tincture in two ounces of water, the other with the second dilution; the doses were repeated every quarter or half-hour.—ELWERT.

CASE 19.—A girl, aged 5 years, had been sick for twenty-four hours; she had passed a sleepless night, screamed, raged, spoke in a confused manner, her face was bright red, forehead hot, eyes glassy, protruding and injected, the carotids beat violently, pulse could not be felt on account of her restlessness; urination involuntary.

Treatment.—3 doses of Bellad. 30, cured her so quickly that she could leave her bed on the fifth day.—SCHWARZE.

CASE 20.—A male infant, aged 13 weeks, had three attacks at short intervals of time, as follows:

Symptoms.—Red, scarlet-colored spots appeared upon the abdomen, and after they disappeared he had constant drowsiness, squinting and rolling of the eyes, frothy mucus before the mouth, green stools and whitish urine; he was only aroused from his stupor by attacks of suffocative cough.

Treatment.—6 doses of Bellad. 30, 1 dose every twenty-four, thirty-six or forty-eight hours removed the brain-affection in six days; the suffocative cough, with vomiting, greenish and fluid stools were removed by Ipecac. 30, followed in twenty-four hours by Veratrum, in the course of five days more.—Dr. B. in D——.

CASE 21.—A delicate boy, aged 8, played for a long time in the sun on a hot July day; soon after he was attacked with violent headache, fever, drowsiness and stupor; every quarter or half-hour he would start up suddenly, with shrill screams, then mutter several words, and grasp at his head; his pupils were unequally dilated, especially the right; his face much reddened; skin burning hot; and fever ran very high.

Treatment.—Bellad. and Acon. 6, in solution, every two hours; after a few doses, profuse perspiration set in and lasted all night; he awoke in the morning as after a long sleep, and was quite restored in the course of the day.—RAMPAL.

CASE 22.—A 4 year old, spongy and ricketty child, was attacked with fever attended with evening and night-aggravations, violent headache, and inability to sit up.

Treatment.—1 dose of Bellad. 24, benefitted him so much in twenty-four hours that all danger seemed over. A similar attack in a healthy 3 year old child, was cured by the same treatment.—MORITZ MÜLLER.

CASE 23.—A healthy girl, aged 8, was exposed to the hot sun in July, and became sick on the following night; she was treated allopathically for several days, and was left with the following:

Symptoms.—Violent headache, face pale and suffering, unconsciousness, with delirium about food; she was constantly boring her fingers in her nose, had great heat of the body with thirst, and some perspiration upon the head.

Treatment.—Bell. 30, followed by sound sleep for several hours, from which she awoke better, but with a violent cough, which caused severe pains in the head. Bryon. 12, 2 doses in twenty-four hours completed the cure.—SEGIN.

CASE 24.—A delicate child, aged 3 years, who had had two attacks of inflammatory brain-affection, and recovered under allopathic treatment, was taken with a third and very violent paroxysm. Bellad. 3, 1 drop in divided doses soon relieved her. —SEGIN.

It is doubtful whether any child would survive three attacks of inflammation of the brain under any mode of treatment.—PETERS.

CASE 25.—A strong and well-nourished child, aged nine months, became restless, coughed much, started in its sleep, and was attacked with repeated convulsive movements of the face and limbs.

Treatment.—Bellad. 30, produced rapid relief; a similar attack, eight days after, was relieved in the same way; but in two days more there was a second relapse, attended with a red, psydracious eruption. Bellad. 30, followed by Sulph. 30, effected a radical cure.—SEGIN.

CASE 26.—A male child, aged 3 years, whose brother had died a year before of inflammation of the brain, was attacked with similar signs of commencing disease.

Treatment.—Bellad. 30, only relieved the vomiting; but after 4 doses of Aconite 24, followed on the next day by Bellad. 30, a rapid improvement ensued, and perfect recovery on the fourth day.—SEGIN.

CASE 27.—A robust boy, aged 10 months, had been sick for two days.

Symptoms.—Lachrymose, irritable and restless at night; sleeplessness, or half-slumber with frequent startings; pungent, dry heat; hanging backwards of the head; jaws dropped; and seemed to have thirst, but rejected the proffered drink; loose stools, with some straining.

Treatment.—Bellad. 30, at night; his sleep was more quiet, was more lively in the morning, but still irritable and inclined to cry. A violent increase of fever was relieved by 2 doses of Aconite 24, and on the fifth day of the disease the fever was very slight, but the irritability and depression were great. Bellad. 30, was followed by quiet sleep, pleasant awaking, moderate heat, profuse sweat and urination during the day, and greater clearness of mind. Recovery on the fourth day of treatment, and sixth day of the disease.—SEGIN.

CASE 28.—A child, aged 2½ years, whose sister had died one year before of inflammation of the brain under allopathic treatment, was treated allopathically for several days, constantly growing worse.

Symptoms.—Sensitive, irritable, lachrymose, half-slumber from which it often started up in a fright; frequent flushes of fever; a red, moist eruption behind the ears.

Treatment.—Bellad. 12, repeated in three hours; in five hours after the second dose, she was more quiet; 3 more doses of Bellad. were followed by quiet night sleep, and earache in the morning. Sulph. 12, was followed by boring with the fingers in the mouth, nose and ears, and profuse urination. Bellad.

12, followed in twenty-four hours by Merc. 1 and Sulphur, effected a recovery on the fifteenth day of treatment.—SEGIN.

CASE 29.—A boy, aged 7 months, was suddenly attacked with frequently repeated vomitings, high fever and involuntary movements of the facial muscles and arms; also with great restlessness, constant boring of the head in the pillow, and remarkably dilated pupils.

Treatment.—Bellad. 5, four doses, one every two hours, from evening until midnight; after two o'clock at night, all these threatening symptoms subsided, and he was quite well on the next day.—SEGIN.

CASE 30.—A boy, aged 7 years, very sensitive and delicate, with tendency to scrofula, was attacked suddenly, five weeks after having the measles, with violent fever, pulse full and 100, skin dry and hot, especially on the head and stomach, eyes brilliant and injected, also sensitive to light, pupils contracted, thirst and constipation.

Treatment.—Aconite 1st dilution, 6 drops in solution, 1 teaspoonful every half-hour; at the end of four hours the symptoms had much increased, pulse was very hard, full and 150, with violent throbbing of the carotid and temporal arteries; the skin of the whole body was glowing hot and dry; face red and bloated; eyes still more reddened, and sensitive to light, and only one-half closed during sleep; there was deliriun, with grasping of the hands at the bed clothes; and great dryness of the tongue.

Treatment.—Bellad., 1st dilution, 10 drops in water, 1 teaspoonful every half-hour in alternation with Aconite, also cold applications to the head; perspiration sat in some time after midnight, followed by greater quiet, and return of consciousness in the morning; the pulse was soft and had fallen to 120; after a restless night he had a movement of the bowels on the third morning and pulse fell to 100. Bellad. 3, three drops in solution, one teaspoonful every hour, was followed by recovery on the fourth day.—SCHWEICKERT.

CASE 31.—A girl aged 5, had been sick for three days.

Symptoms.—Face hot, red and bloated; boring with the head into the pillow; eyes half open during sleep, or else much distorted; much thirst, no appetite, stools seldom and in small hard lumps; jaw dropped; nose quite dry; grasping at the head, during the heavy sleep; sudden starting up in a fright, with anxious staring about, and quick relapse into stupor.

Treatment.—Bellad. 30, followed by sound sleep for two hours, and speedy recovery.—BETHMANN.

CASE 32.—A little girl, aged 2½ years, had been failing in health for some time; three nights ago became hot and feverish, and soon became very ill indeed; lying about the room, complaining of headache, and referring all her suffering to her head, she was drowsy and heavy; eyelids drooping; eyes sunk deep in their sockets; mouth parched; cheeks flushed; head and body dry and hot; pulse quick and throbbing; tongue white, with red points upon it; great thirst; quick breathing, some cough; bowels quite regular; she avoided light and was distressed at the least noise; starts suddenly from her sleep, and screams as if frightened.

Treatment.—Aconite 12, every four hours, without benefit, as she still remained drowsy, with constant starting and screaming, heat and thirst. Belladonna 6, every two hours, followed by great relief, fever and thirst diminished, slept well, did not scream or start, tongue cleaning, her look was placid and intelligent, and she was able to sit up a little. Continued Bellad. 6, three times a day, and was quite restored on the sixth day.—YELDHAM.

CASE 33.—Threatened hydrocephalus. A delicate boy, aged 5, has been complaining for some time of headache, loss of appetite and listlessness; is now quite chilly, creeping into the fire, although a very warm day; has a staring, unmeaning look; does not answer when spoken to; pupils sluggish; pulse slow and feeble. The parents state that they have already lost two children with dropsy of the brain, and fear that this little boy is going off in the same manner.

Treatment.—Bellad. 3, and Ipecac. 3, in alternation; on the next day there was some improvement. Bellad. 3, and Tinct.-sulph. in alternation; in five days more he was almost well, and the cure was completed by Pulsatilla 3.

Subsequently his little sister was affected in much the same way, and was restored by similar treatment.—Brit. Jour. Hom. Vol. 9, p. 585.—Dr. SHARP.

Cases which approach the second stage of Acute Hydrocephalus.

CASE 34.—A boy, aged 3½ years, after headache for several days, was attacked with violent vomiting, heavy stupor with snoring, from which he could hardly be roused; convulsive starts shook his whole body occasionally; his head was glowing hot, and thrown backwards; his cheeks alternated from glowing red, to pale; eyes rigid, insensible, glassy, somewhat reddened, half-open, and turned upwards; pupils dilated, at times insensible to light; breathing quick, deep, heavy and hot; pulse full and hard at times, at others small and contracted; skin hot, and dry; entire unconsciousness, confused speech, startings and vomiting.

Treatment.—Bellad. 400, in a wine-glass half-full of water, one teaspoonful every hour; in six hours he was much better and the Bellad. was omitted. In fifteen hours consciousness was restored, and fever lessened; well on third day.—STAPF.

CASE 35.—A girl, aged 3 years, was attacked from taking cold during the desquamation of scarlet fever, with:

Symptoms.—Great restlessness, drowsiness, unconsciousness, boring with the head in the pillow, parchment-like dryness of the skin, with large drops of perspiration upon the face, constant rolling of the eyes, great thirst, and frequent vomiting.

Treatment.—Tinct. Bellad., one drop per dose, every hour, for five hours; pimples broke out upon the scalp, the glands of the neck swelled, loose stools set in, and quiet sleep, followed by return of consciousness and great relief. Several doses of Bellad. 3, completed the cure.—F. MÜLLER.

CASE 36.—A boy, aged 3 years, was attacked with an inflammatory affection of the brain, during the period of desquamation of scarlet fever.

Symptoms.—Swelling of the parotid and cervical glands; he lay constantly in a soporose slumber with bloated and red face; short, rattling and groaning respiration; involuntary stools; loss of speech and consciousness; inflammation of the mouth; thin offensive stools; red and hot urine.

Treatment.—Bellad. 30, 20 doses, one every four or six hours; consciousness commenced to return in twelve hours, followed by more quiet sleep and voluntary evacuations. Profound sleep was removed by two doses of Tartar-emetic 12.—GROSS.

CASE 37.—A previously healthy girl, aged 2½ years, was attacked with vomiting, convulsions and fever; on the second day she had the following:

Symptoms.—She lay in a soporose slumber, from which she started up at times, grasped at her head, which was very hot; bored with her head into the pillow; rolled her head about; when roused she only opened her eyes one-half, stared stupidly before her; pupils dilated, with squinting; paleness of the face; nose pinched, dry and stopped up; lips covered with a brown crust; skin parched and hot, with traces of a purplish scarlet-rash; abdomen sunken; constipation for six days; involuntary urination. Her head fell back whenever it was raised up; she uttered a peculiar cry and was very uneasy whenever she was raised up from the horizontal position, or even moved. Did not answer questions or pay any attention to what was going on around her.

Treatment.—Bellad. 3, one drop four times a day; after the first three doses violent convulsions sat in, and then the disease gradually subsided, until the fifth day when she was quite restored.—KNORRE.

CASE 38.—A girl, aged 15 months, was attacked with fever and stupor, and was treated allopathically for six days, when she presented the following:

Symptoms.—She lay with closed and agglutinated eyes, when they were opened they looked dim; constantly groaning; heard nothing; wished for nothing, and could not speak a loud word; tossed the left arm and leg about, and held them up in the air; her face was pale and sunken; skin and nostrils dry;

breath short and quick; tongue moist; she could drink when raised up, but let her head fall back immediately; pulse very frequent and irritable, with a false hardness, beating more violently in the right, than in the left arm; abdomen drawn in, and painful to touch; stools and urine were passed involuntarily.

Treatment.—Bellad. 24, one drop; in five hours frequent greenish stools sat in, followed in twelve hours by relief, and ability to open the eyes, although the left eye was only half opened. On the eighth day, Chamomilla 12. was given with transient relief, followed on the tenth day by increased restlessness, whimpering during the attacks of diarrhœa, tossing off of the bed-clothes; the skin was dry and torpid; cough spasmodic; breathing quick and short; nose reddened. Bellad. 30, 1 drop, was followed by recovery on the fourteenth day. —MORITZ MÜLLER.

CASE 39.—A boy, aged 3½ years, was attacked during the period of desquamation of scarlet fever, with discharge from the ears, and inflammation of the brain sat in when this ceased. He was treated allopathically and left in the following condition:

Symptoms.—Restlessness; tossing about of the body; grasping at the head with the hands; paleness and shrunken state of the face, with pinched nose; dilatation of the pupils; boring of the head into the pillow; heat of the head; stupefaction; brown and blackish tongue; the child desired nothing, but drank water when it was offered; skin dry and burning hot; pulse small and frequent; some œdema of the scalp.

Treatment.—Tinct.-Bellad., half-drop, every two hours; the following night was very restless, but perspiration followed by some repose ensued; boils broke out upon the scalp and back; re-appearance of the discharge from the ear. Bellad. 3, one drop every four hours, followed by quiet sleep, perfect restoration of consciousness; desire for food; offensive stools; Bellad. 3, every night and morning only, was succeeded by perfect recovery in ten days.—F. MÜLLER.

CASE 40.—A little girl, aged 2½ years, previously healthy and intelligent, had been sick for five days, notwithstanding the use of Aconite, Pulsat., several doses of Calomel, again followed by Aconite. The exciting cause of the attack was measles with scanty and livid eruption.

Symptoms.—Stupefaction; slumber with half-opened eyes; gritting of the teeth; starting up from sleep; whimpering, alternating with violent motions of the limbs; tossing to and fro of the body; attempts to get out of bed; wild delirium; congestion to the head; violent pulsation of the carotids; boring of the head into the pillow; grasping at the head; alternating paleness and circumscribed redness of the face; squinting; very frequent and irregular pulse.

Treatment.—Bellad. 2, every three hours; the second dose was followed by more quiet sleep and improvement of most of the symptoms; on the eighth day of the disease, after a fresh exacerbation, sweat sat in at night, and quiet sleep was followed by gradual improvement. She recovered entirely under the continued use of two doses of Bellad., daily.—DIEZ.

CASE 41.—Bellad. 30, in 1 drop doses acted very favorably and promptly in a case of acute dropsy of the ventricles, attended with opisthotonos, and unconscious stupefaction in which the patient lay part of the time as if in an apoplexy, but from which it started up occasionally in great alarm and agony as if from severe pain.—KAMMERER.

CASE 42.—A boy, aged 2½ years, had been treated allopathically without avail, but was restored in fourteen days with Aconite and Bellad.; Hyosciamus and Veratrum were also somewhat useful; but repeated doses of Bellad. effected the most good.—SCHINDLER.

CASE 43.—A girl, aged 18 months, took cold during an attack of measles, and the eruption receded.

Symptoms.—Much thirst; squinting; boring of the head in the pillow; dripping perspiration on the head; spasms, during which the head was drawn back to the spine; she lay constantly in a stupor with half closed eyes, and widely dilated pupils.

Treatment.—Bellad. 30; on the next day there were no convulsions and all the other symptoms were improved; it was soon out of danger, and recovered entirely on the fourth day.—BETHMAN.

CASE 44.—A child had lain for two days in a deep stupor, with convulsions and slow pulse; the eyes were half closed, covered with mucus, and squinting.

Treatment.—Several doses of Bellad. 30, effected a cure in three days.—BICKING.

CASE 45.—A boy, aged 4 years, was attacked six weeks after having the measles with Encephal. insolationis, attended with violent tonic and clonic cramps; pulse hard, small and from 160 to 170.

Treatment.—Aconite 1, ten drops in water, and Bellad. 1, in the same doses, in alternation, every half, one, or one and a quarter hours, a teaspoonful at a time. Recovery on the fifth day.—SCHWEICKERT, Jr.

CASE 46.—A one year old boy, had all the signs of effusion into the ventricles.

Treatment.—Bellad. 1, in solution, one teaspoonful every two hours, followed by Sulphur 3, and again by Bellad. A cure was effected in four weeks, and no relapse had occurred at the end of seven months.—HEICHELHEIM.

CASE 47.—A girl, aged 5, had been sick for three days; she neither spoke nor ate; her head was hot and drawn backwards; pupils much dilated and insensible; pulse quick and moderately full.

Treatment.—Bellad. 12, 3 drops in a glass of water, one teaspoonful every two hours; the patient recovered quickly.—SCHROEN.

IN ADULTS.

CASE 48.—A powerful man, aged 30, sickened suddenly after taking cold; on the second day he had:

Symptoms.—Sleeplessness; dizziness on attempting to sit up; violent delirium; raging, screaming, attempting to get out of bed, tossing off the bed clothes, and tossing to and fro; eyes painful, reddened, intolerant of light, wild and rolling; pupils contracted; sparks and flames before the eyes; hearing acute and sensitive, with roaring and tinkling sounds before the ears; face hot and red, although at times moist and sticky. In his clear moments he complained of confusion in the head; of frightful, fixed, burning, aching and piercing pains therein; he had fits of sneezing and of bleeding from the nose; his lips were red, hot and dry; tongue red and covered with a little tough mucus; throat contracted, with urging to swallow; disgust for food; yellow and slimy vomits; hiccough; constipation; red and hot urine; breathing anxious, sobbing and interrupted; voice hoarse and speaking difficult; pulse quick, hard and spasmodic; skin dry, hot, red and tense.

Treatment.—Bellad. 30, 1 drop; followed by great improvement in twelve hours; on the seventh day of the disease the patient was able to leave his bed for a short time. One dose of Bryon. completed the cure.—SCHUBERT.

CASE 49.—A servant girl, aged 28, after suffering with headache for eight days, was attacked with the following:

Symptoms.—Head hot; violent pain in the forehead as if the blood were violently forced into it; protrusion of the eyes; frequent vomiting of greenish fluid, excited by every movement of the head, and only abating when she was lying quietly on her back; pulse full and slow; constipation.

Treatment.—Nux-vom. 3, was given without benefit; on the next day the symptoms increased and unconsciousness with quiet delirium sat in. Bellad. 1, every two hours, was followed by gradual and steady recovery at the end of seven days.—ROTHANSL.

CASE 50.—A man aged 30, was attacked after taking cold with fever, signs of inflammation of the brain, &c.; after bleeding blistering and leeching, he was left with the following:

Symptoms.—Violent fury, he sprang up, broke the windows, and had to be bound.

Treatment.—Bellad. 18, every quarter of an hour; followed by improvement in a few hours; he was entirely restored at the end of eight days.—IVANOVICH.

CASE 51.—A man, aged 40, was taken with signs of arachnitis after an attack of erysipelas of the face.

Symptoms.—His eyes stood wide open, and were dull; the pupils dilated; nose dry; tongue with a whitish yellow coating;

thirst moderate; constipation for thirty-six hours; urine light yellow and clear; breathing irregular, at times quick, at others slow, now deep and anxious, and then scarcely perceptible; pulse contracted and small, but quick and hard; at times he could speak rationally, but always hastily; at others he would stare horribly at one place where he seemed to see some frightful object, then would spring up from the bed, strike around him and attempt to escape, followed by attacks of trembling and ability to speak quietly and rationally again.

Treatment.—Bellad. 3, was followed by an aggravation for one hour, and then immediately by improvement; on the second day after the use of Bellad., Cocculus 6, was given on account of the presence of pressing headache, noises in the ears, irritable, sensitive and vexatious disposition. In two days more he was entirely restored.—RAU.

CASE 52.—Mrs. S., aged 67; particularly liable to head attacks, for which she has been repeatedly cupped, leeched and blistered.

Symptoms.—Her head has not been right for the last week, and for three days past it has grown much worse; is now confined to bed, complaining of a throbbing and hard aching pain right through the head, from back to front; light and noise distract her; she can get no sleep, and feels as if she would lose her senses; sees everything double; her forehead and top of head are burning hot to the hand; pulse hard, full and 100; she is very thirsty; tongue foul, but moist; she had a shivering fit the day before and then vomited.

Treatment.—She had taken aperient and other medicines and used cold applications to the head without benefit. Aconite 3, one dose, to be repeated in four hours and then followed by Bellad. 3, every four hours; on the next day she was much better, had no headache, her forehead was cool, she could bear light without inconvenience, pulse soft and only 65, no nausea. She continued the use of Bellad. and on the third day took Pulsat. 6, and Sulphur 12, for some pain in the stomach and slight confusion of the head.—YELDHAM.

REVIEW.—Of RÜCKERT'S 37 cases, 33 were children, viz.: 15 boys and 11 girls from the age of 13 weeks to 7 years; and

4 were adults, viz.: 3 males and 1 female from the age of 28 to 40 years.

As *causes* of the disease we find: taking cold in 2 cases; suppressed measles in 1 instance; sun-stroke in 3 cases; during measles in 1 case; after measles in 2 cases; during the desquamation of scarlet fever in 3 cases.

The above cases prove incontestibly that Bellad. has proved useful not only in the first but also in the *second* stage of hydrocephalus; it has frequently removed redness and heat of the face, throbbing of the carotids, squinting, and also involuntary urination.

The inflammation in two of the adult cases had reached a great height.

Dose.—In 29 cases:

The *Tincture* was given in 3; viz.: 15 drops in solution in 1 case; ½ and 1 drop doses each in 1 case.

The 1st *dilution* in 4 cases, 3 times in solution.
" 2d " " 2 " once " "
" 3d " " 5 " twice " " and twice in drop doses.

The 6th, 12th and 18th each in 1 case.
" 24th dilution in 2 cases.
" 30th " " 9 " 5 times in single doses and 4 " " solution.
" 400th " " 1 "

Hence the doses varied from the strong tincture through all the dilutions to the highest potencies, and generally with satisfactory results; as aggravations only occurred in two instances from the use of the 3d dilution. Lobethal even prefers the pure tincture in solution to the higher dilutions.

In these 37 cases, Bellad. effected the cure alone in 21; in 6 instances, Aconite was given with advantage in alternation every half, or two hours; Tart.-emet. was given in 1 case after Bellad. to remove drowsiness; in 1 case Sulphur was given between two doses of Bellad; and Cocculus in 1 case to remove a remaining peculiarly irritable state of mind.

In the first stage of dropsy of the brain Belladonna generally removed all danger in twenty-four hours; in 5 cases, however, from two to six days were required. In the second stage, three, four, five or even fourteen days were required, and in one case even four weeks. In adults from five to eight days were necessary.

BRYONIA-ALBA.

The root which is the only part used in medicine bears a sufficient resemblance to a thick turnip to have given rise to very alarming mistakes; hence it has received the common name Devil's turnip. Some French peasants use it fresh as a purgative. Allopathic physicians look upon it as a drastic purgative and as a substitute for Colocynth, Elaterium, &c. Towards the end of the last century, Dr. DE MONTGAMY fancied that Bryonia contained all the therapeutic properties of Ipecac. and proposed its substitution. In all probability it is very similar in its action to Colchicum, Helleborus-niger, and Veratrum-album. At least it acts decidedly upon the stomach, liver and bowels, also upon the serous and fibrous tissues, and probably upon the kidneys.

It has principally been used against rheumatism; mild typhus fever, which commences with pains in the limbs and bones; against inflammatory swelling of the joints, œdema of the legs and pleurisy; the ancients often employed it internally against dropsy, and more particularly in hydrothorax, of which it must have effected many cures. DE MONTGAMY says he has frequently cured bilious fevers, vomiting, colic, diarrhœa and dysentery with it; hence TESTE terms it an emetic which cures vomiting and a drastic which stops diarrhœa and colic. HAHNEMANN probably got the hint for its use against pleurisy, from the ancient use of it against hydrothorax. KASPAR says it is homœopathic to infiltrations into the cellular tissue and serous effusions into the serous cavities; but not to plastic and fibrinous exudations. In dropsy of the head, chest, &c., if small doses do not suffice, it may be allowable to use it in large doses after the manner of the ancients in these diseases, in fact, so as to produce a decided action upon the liver, bowels and kidneys.—PETERS.

According to the Oestreichische Zeitschrift, the pathological appearances produced by Bryonia, together with the symptomatic phenomena, point to congestion and inflammation of the brain.

According to KREUSSLER, Bryonia is indicated when there is great restlessness, tossing about in bed, especially at night, troublesome and frightful dreams, extremely irritable state of mind, heat of the head, greater redness of the cheeks than of the rest of the face, violent and piercing pains in the head, nausea and constipation. He prefers the 12th or 18th dilutions, repeated twice a day.

According to WAHLE it often happens that Aconite and Belladonna, even when given in the first stage, will not prevent effusion and exudation. Then Bryonia will often effect wonders when the face is very red or almost mahogany colored, the eyes rolling about, at times closed and at others wide open, the lips dry, tongue dry and brownish yellow, abdomen distended, bowels constipated, urine suppressed or sharp and burning, skin of the whole body dry and hot, breathing quick, anxious and groaning, thirst excessive and urgent.

He prefers a few globules of the 30th dilution. If Bryonia be given too late, which may easily happen, as the first occurrence of effusion is often overlooked, so that a cure is not effected in twelve or twenty-four hours, then some other remedy must be resorted to.

CASE 53.—A powerful man after lying drunken in the snow for six hours, had the following:

Symptoms.—Heat and redness of the head and face; great thirst, chilliness, constant inclination to sleep, starting up in affright, screaming out, delirium, complains of frightful images before his sight, frightful dreams, cold sweat on the forehead, pains in the head and limbs.

Treatment.—Tinct.-Bryonia in one drop doses; followed by an aggravation in two hours; after this he drank water freely, broke out into a profuse and offensive perspiration, so that he had to change his shirt five times in fifteen hours, and was completely restored in several days.—SCHULER.

CASE 54.—A youth, aged 18, had suffered with a discharge from the ear, which became suppressed by cold.

Symptoms.—Violent piercing and insupportable pains darting from one ear to the other through the head; high fever, intolerance of light with very moveable pupils, sleeplessness or starting up from slumber, violent cough with pain in the forehead; constipation.

Treatment.—Bryonia 2, one-sixth of a drop every two hours; at the end of twenty-four hours the discharge from the ear had returned, he had profuse perspiration especially upon the head, the pain and fever were but slight, the skin only moderately warm, thirst not urgent, but he was restless, tossed about, thought he was going to die, slumbered a good deal, and had an involuntary discharge of mucus from the bowels. *Hyosciamus* 2d dilution, followed by the 1st, removed all danger in three days, and the patient was well in six.—SEGIN.

CASE 55.—A man, aged 37, of nervous-venous constitution and afflicted with piles, had had inflammation of the brain three years before, and was attacked with acute arachnitis fourteen days after the suppression of the hæmorrhoidal flow.

Symptoms.—Restless sleep, typhoid delirium with spasmodic twitchings of the fingers, constant thirst, redness of the face, heat of the head, jerking of the hands, contraction of the abdomen, with sensitiveness to pressure, profuse perspiration, pulse large soft and quick, 100 per minute; if spoken to sharply he started up, answered yes or no in broken tones, then fell into a slumber again, but complained of violent pains in the head, his eyes closed spasmodically, pupils were contracted, tongue moist and broad.

Treatment.—Bellad. 4, one drop every two hours; in two days there was some improvement, he could speak more connectedly, his urine commenced to deposit a sediment, but his pulse remained frequent and quick and he soon relapsed; violent drawing and beating pains shot from one temple to the other, and his pulse became quicker, smaller and harder. *Bryonia* 2, was then given, one drop every two hours the first day, every three hours on the second, and night and morning on the third day, with progressive improvement; the patient only complained of a sense of fluctuation in the head, with slight dizziness when he sat up, and some pain in the right temple. A fit of vexation caused a fresh relapse which was quickly cured by Bellad. 4, one drop every two hours.—NOACK.

REVIEW.—The above 3 cases all occurred in adult males; 2 cases were in the first stage, and in the other the presence of effusion was feared. In every case Bryonia was the decisive remedy; in one instance it effected a cure alone; in one case Hyosciamus had to be used; and in the other, Bellad. had been used with only transient benefit.

Taking cold was the exciting cause in two cases; while suppression of an ear and hæmorrhoidal discharge complicated the others.

WAHLE'S exact indications for the use of Bryonia are very important; he lays stress upon the presence of a red, almost mahogany-color of the face, while KREUSSLER prefers redness of the cheeks, rather than of the whole face as an indication; the violent pains from the ears and temples through the head were well marked in one case.

DOSE.—The curative doses were the 1st and 2d dilutions; although KREUSSLER prefers the 12th or 18th dilution, and WAHLE the 30th, from notional and theoretical grounds.

CUPRUM.

Cuprum is homœopathic when there is a febrile-inflammatory affection, attended with quite severe pain in the forehead, with paleness and sunkenness of the face, warmth and dryness of the skin and some quickness of the pulse.

Also when there is a remitting or mild typhoid-like form of fever, with great weakness and lassitude of the limbs, vertigo, heaviness in the head and headache, pains in the stomach and bowels and constipation. Also, when the patient is so dizzy that he cannot sit up, with occasional headache, restless sleep disturbed by dreams, slight delirium, or constant slumber, which may increase to perfect coma; or there may be entire sleeplessness, with paleness of the face, with expression of extreme prostration or entire stupidity, the eyes being sunken and dull, and the pupils dilated. Or there may be a sensation of utter exhaustion and lassitude, which may be increased to the point of fainting, from slight exertion. The tongue may be red at the edges, or red, dry and rough with enlargement of the papillæ; the thirst great, appetite extinct, with disgust for food, skin warm and moist; pulse quick; urine turbid and jumentous. If these symptoms pass off, vertigo and confusion of the head will remain, with long-continued and obstinate weakness and lassitude.

When there is frequent and violent vomiting, or persistent nausea. The pulse may be full, hard and frequent, or weak and slow.

In almost all copper-cases there will be headache, at times violent and generally seated in the forehead and vertex; this headache may abate in a few days to return again. In the milder cases there will only be aching and heaviness in the head, with decided and obstinate dizziness, and a certain amount of stupefaction. In the majority of cases the patient will lie still and apathetic, with dull and unexpressive eyes, stupid and relaxed expression of countenance and great inclination to slumber, but the sleep will be disturbed by dreams, restless and not refreshing. In some there will be a well-marked soporose condition; in others, entire sleeplessness for three or four days, attended with a feeling of internal restlessness and anxiety. Actual delirium occurred only 7 times out of 38, and generally was of the quiet kind, interrupted by mutterings and occasional groans. In one case furious delirium was present. In all cases loud speaking to them would break up their delirium, but they were obliged to collect themselves for a long time before they could answer questions.

There may be darkness or flimmering and sparks before the eyes; the pupils are generally and widely dilated, but not insensible to light; but when the congestion to the head is very great the pupils may be contracted.

In the *ears* there may be roaring and tinkling in many cases, and long-continued deafness.—LANGENBECK.

Cuprum is supposed to be peculiarly homœopathic when there is vomiting of greenish substances, followed by copious, green, offensive and liquid stools. Hence in the brain-affections which follow cholera infantum.

It proved homœopathic in one case in which there was colic and anxiety, great rigidity of the body, coldness of the hands, swelling and redness of the face with great drops of perspiration upon it, eyes fixed and dull, tongue swollen and stiff, pulse full and hard, breathing short and heavy, followed by oppression of the chest, throbbing and roaring in the head, surprising dulness of the intellect, so that everything which the patient said was erroneous.

It proved homœopathic to severe pain in the stomach, followed by violent convulsions, especially affecting the abdomen, arms and legs, attended with frightful and violent cries, or howling or croaking, also with disturbance of the intellect, appearance of fright and attempts to escape; the eyes were brilliant and seemed as if they would start out of the head. Also to severe vomiting, violent cramps in both of the great toes which were drawn tetanically towards the soles of the feet, with excessive pain.

According to Christison and Orfila it is homœopathic to insensibility, almost always to convulsions, to rigidity of the body and even tetanus; also to violent convulsions and insensibility. According to Blake, however, the salts of copper when injected into the blood-vessels act with peculiar force in exhausting muscular irritability and paralyzing the heart; the force of the heart's contractions are speedily reduced, allowing of distension of the heart from loss of contractility. It is also homœopathic to vomiting, difficulty of breathing and stiffness of the limbs. It is peculiarly homœopathic to violent headache, vomiting, cutting pains in the bowels, followed by cramps in the legs, and pains in the thighs, especially if associated with bilious derangement and jaundice; also to severe headache, with great prostration of strength.

It is indicated when there is insensibility, with the jaws locked, muscles rigid and frequently convulsed, breathing interrupted and pulse small and slow; or by convulsions and loss of consciousness, followed by extraordinary paralytic weakness of the arms and legs, especially if there be pains the stomach, an eruption over the breast, general shooting pains, thirst, frequent small pulse, vomiting, hiccough and purging.

Copper, or more especially Brass, is homœopathic to irritation about the genitals, a vesicular eruption about the hairs on the pubes, with loss of appetite, tendency to vomiting, obstinate constipation, soreness and dryness of the throat and irritation of the nose, and great want of sleep.

Among the pathological lesions it is homœopathic to Jaundice, congestion of the surface of the brain, perforation of the bowels by ulceration; especially of the rectum.—PETERS.

Concerning the adaptation of this remedy in inflammatory diseases of the brain, we find only a general remark, and one case where it had been given and then in frequent alternation with Stramon. and Bellad., so that in regard to Cuprum and its influence little is to be learned; it requires further examination by practitioners.—RÜCKERT.

GENERAL REMARKS.—SCHMID has alluded to a particular kind of affection of the brain, developing itself in children during febrile catarrh, difficult dentition, and eruptive diseases, which finds its remedy in Cuprum-acet. The following are characteristic:

Symptoms.—The little patients have a surly, very irritable temper, or are indifferent and feeble, with restless sleep, tossing about in the same, are sleepy, without being able to sleep; unable to hold their heads up while awake; dryness of the mouth, disgust for food, nausea, vomiting, constipation, scanty urine; chilliness accompanied by heat; heat, generally slight, but at times burning; pulse very changeable, moderately full and irritated, with evening exacerbations; convulsions, gritting of the teeth.

Bell. does not afford relief; the exacerbations may be moderated by Aconite; but Cuprum acet. is the most reliable remedy. —Hyg. 12, 2, 116.

CASE 55.—R., a large-headed, robust boy, 4 years of age, formerly atrophical, was attacked on the evening of the 30th of June, with general convulsions.

Treatment.—Acon. 1, and Bell. 1, aided by sponging the head with cold water. At nine o'clock in the evening he had the following:

Symptoms.—The burning heat existing before sponging with cold water was changed to a moderate temperature of the skin; pulse quick, hard, almost uncountable. General convulsions of the limbs from time to time; on the left side the spasms were more clonic, on the right more tonic; spasmodic convulsive movements of the muscles of the face; eyes mostly open and staring, but at times closed by the convulsion of the muscles of the face, attended with squinting. The pupils were fully dilated and insensible to light. Lower jaw tightly pressed against the upper one, with gnashing of the teeth. Respiration very heavy, accompanied by rattling in the chest, and intermitting at times for eight to ten seconds, as in the dying. Palsy of the lungs was momentarily expected.

Prescription and Result.—Cuprum-acet. 1, 1 gr. per dose, dry upon the tongue, followed in ten minutes after by Tinct. Stram. 1, and cold applications to the head.

After the second dose of each medicine an intermission of the convulsions was followed by coldness and relaxation of the limbs and apparent cessation of the respiration, so that paralysis of the nerv. vag. seemed imminent. Phosph. Tinct. was then given; some contraction of the pupils was soon observed, and the Phosphor. was continued after the lapse of a quarter of an hour, in alternation with Cuprum and Stram. At twelve o'clock at night there was an important intermission of convulsions, but frightful reaction of the blood-vessels, the face and body became glowing hot and dark red, the carotids throbbed violently, the eyes were decidedly injected and the pupils contracted. The child was conscious and screamed when sprinkled with cold water.

Cupr. S., 2 gr. per dose, in alternation with 10 drops Bell. (in solution.) On the following morning the little patient was sitting up and playing in the bed, his pulse was still 120, but the hardness was diminished, and his eyes yet somewhat staring.—Both remedies were continued till the 3d of July, when the boy was dismissed cured.—SCHWEICKERT.

DIGITALIS-PURP.

This remedy has long enjoyed a high reputation against many dropsical affections, and also in dropsy of the brain. According to WARING it has been found serviceable by WITHERING,

Brown, Whyte, Cheyne and Gölis. The latter however, without appearing to place much faith in its efficacy, advises gr. ¼ of the pounded leaves, with gr. ½ of Calomel, every second hour. He gave it, both in the inflammatory stage, and in that of effusion; in the latter, chiefly as a palliative, to moderate the violence of the convulsions. Kleber advises its external application, in combination with Squills to the scalp. Merriman treated cases successfully with Digitalis and Calomel as advised by Gölis. Of 92 cases of dropsy of all kinds collected by Bayle, 65 are said to have been cured by Digitalis, 15 improved and 11 not cured. Withering, of 126 cases, in the last stages of dropsy, cured 48 with Digitalis alone; Ferria of 20 cases, cured 8 perfectly, improved 8 materially, and only failed entirely in 4 cases; Jones of 24 cases cured 15 perfectly, improved 4, and saw no good effects in 5 cases only; in 7 other cases out of 12 of ascites, it acted as a diuretic; also in 6 cases out of 15 of hydrothorax. Hence we may agree with Pereira, who says, of all the remedies for dropsy, none have gained more and few so much celebrity as Digitalis.

We propose next to inquire whether it has been found most useful in inflammatory or dyscratic dropsies. It is a decidedly antipathic remedy to fever and inflammation, as in full doses its most ordinary effects are: nausea or actual vomiting, slow and often irregular pulse, coldness of the limbs, fainting, or a tendency to it, giddiness and confusion of vision. Yet Waring says, experience has shown that although it exercises a powerfully depressing action upon the heart, it possesses little or no power in controlling inflammatory action. Pereira says that in violent and acute inflammation accompanied with great excitement of the general circulation, especially in plethoric subjects, Digitalis is in some cases hurtful; in others it is a trivial and unimportant remedy, and fox-glove if serviceable at all, can only be used successfully after other and more powerful antiphlogistic measures. Again, he says: inflammation of a chronic kind may be going on in one part of the body, to an extent sufficient to produce complete disorganization, and ultimately to cause the death of the patient without the action of the larger arteries or vascular system generally being remarkably increased; in such cases Digitalis is for the most part of little use. Finally, Pereira decrees that as a remedy for inflammation, fox-glove is principally useful in less violent cases, particularly when accompanied with increased frequency of the pulse, and occurring in subjects not able to support copious blood-letting. Still he admits that it has some influence over inflammation of the arachnoid, and is certainly a most valuable agent in arachnitis of children; while its specific influence over the brain would make it a doubtful remedy in phrenitis.

There is one stage of dropsy of the brain in which it is peculiarly homœopathic. In the *second* stage, the pulse becomes slow, labored, intermitting and irregular, but is easily quickened by motion or mental disturbance to double its previous amount of pulsations; in this stage the pulse falls from 120 or 140, to 80, or even as low as 54, and this is the time in which Digitalis is peculiarly homœopathic; if rightly given it may prevent the second quickening of the pulse, or at least prevent it from rising again to 140 or 160, which it is very apt to do. Dr. Baildon first noticed the effect of posture in ascertaining the real effects of Digitalis on the pulse; when by gradually increased doses, he took it to the extent of gr. vj. in the day, the pulse fell from 110 to 40; when it was actually 40, the erect posture would raise it to 100; when sitting it was 72; and on again lying down it fell to 40. Digitalis acts specifically upon the par-vagum, and the slowness of the breathing and pulse in the second stage of dropsy of the brain, is produced by pressure upon this nerve at the base of the brain.

Pereira and Holland have both observed several times in patients affected with a slow, intermittent and otherwise irregular pulse, that Digitalis would produce regularity of pulsation. If it will remove the symptom it may also remove the cause upon which the symptom depends; besides, Digitalis produces absorption and acts profusely upon the kidneys, and hence may remove the slow pulse of hydrocephalus, by producing absorption of the dropsical effusion. It is not advisable to use Digitalis in the first stage, if for no other reason than that given by Hope, who says in no disease do the symptoms more require to be kept, as far as practicable in a simple, uncomplicated, and intelligible state, and no remedy is so calculated to confuse them as Digitalis. The reduction of the pulse which it occasions cannot be discriminated with any degree of certainty, from that occasioned by the supervention of pressure in the second stage; again, Digitalis is apt to produce vertigo, faintness and nausea, and how, asks Dr. HOPE, are these symptoms artificially excited, to be distinguished from the same results of inflammation and dropsy of the brain? Easily, by not using Digitalis at all, during the first or inflammatory stage; but by giving it boldly and perseveringly in the *second* or dropsical stage. PEREIRA says the quantity of Digitalis that may be given to a patient without destroying life, is much greater than is ordinarily imagined. In one instance he saw 20 drops of the tincture given to an infant laboring under hydrocephalus, three times daily for a fortnight, at the end of which time the little patient was completely recovered without one untoward symptom. I do not propose that Digitalis should always be given in such large doses; but if smaller ones will not suffice, larger ones should be made to do the work, and effect the cures they have accomplished before. It is exceedingly doubtful whether Digitalis can be given usefully during the first or inflammatory stage; WITHERING has correctly observed that it seldom succeeds in dropsical persons of great natural strength, of tense fibre, of warm skin, of florid complexion, or in those with a tight and cordy pulse; on the contrary, he says, experience teaches that if the pulse be feeble or intermitting, the countenance pale, the lips livid, and the skin cold, we may expect the diuretic effects to follow in a kindly manner. In short, when nature or disease brings the pulse and general system into that condition which is most peculiarly apt to be produced by Digitalis, then the other and curative effects of the drug may be expected to follow promptly and from moderate doses.

It is surprising how frequently a symptomatic similarity between the action of a drug and of a disease, affords a hint for the selection of a curative remedy. Thus the principal diseases of the valves of the heart are contraction and patency of the Aortic valves and of the Mitral. The slighter degrees of contraction of the *Aortic* valves have little or no effect upon the pulse, which will remain *firm* and *full* as long as the contraction of the valves is not so great as to prevent the left ventricle from emptying itself; again, Aortic-regurgitation produces a preeminently jerking pulse, for the beat of the artery is short and quick, as if the blood were smartly jerked or shot under the finger. Hence the homœopathist would conclude from the pulse alone, that Digitalis will rarely prove useful in diseases of the *Aortic* valves, and old school experience has already shown that it is rarely useful when the pulse is hard, tight or corded.—But when the *Mitral* valve is contracted, and also when it admits of free regurgitation, the pulse is in various degrees small, weak, irregular, intermitting and unequal, i. e. the pulse resembles that produced by Digitalis. From the pulse alone the homœopathist would conclude that Digitalis ought to prove useful if not curative, in diseases of the Mitral valve. What does experience teach on this point? CORRIGAN was the first to allude to the *injurious* effects of Digitalis in diseases of the *Aortic* valves, while he found the most *favorable* results to follow its use in affections of the *Mitral* valves. In patency, admitting of regurgitation through the *Aortic* valves, the less frequently the heart beats, the greater will be the opportunity for regurgitation, and hence the prolonged employment of Digitalis, so as to lessen the frequency and force of the heart's action, cannot fail to be injurious. On the other hand in contraction of the *Mitral* valve, the lengthened interval between the contractions of the heart, produced by Digitalis, permits the left ventricle to become more fully distended, while it also lessens the frequency of the interruptions to the passage of the blood, and hence the pulse becomes fuller, stronger, and more regular. Again, in patency of the Mitral valve, Digitalis prevents the regurgitation from being so frequently repeated.

Slowness and intermittence of the pulse in the second stage of hydrocephalus, are probably as safe guides for the use of Digitalis as they are in disease of the Mitral valve; at least as Digitalis does not generally exert its absorbent and diuretic action until it has lowered the pulse and reduced the system, it will of course be more apt to produce absorption of the hydrocephalic fluid, when the pulse has already become slow, weak and irregular or intermitting from the effects of disease.—PETERS.

In conclusion, Digitalis has long retained a reputation against scrofulous affections, and hence it may be suitable in scrofulous meningitis. VOGT says: next to its diuretic action it exerts a decidedly powerful action upon the lymphatic glands and the whole lymphatic system. From its great curative powers against scrofula we can conclude that it fluidizes the lymph, facilitates its circulation, and removes obstructions of it. Next to the vascular, urinary and lymphatic systems it acts especially upon the serous membranes. In the second degree of the action of Digitalis, pains are often felt in the lymphatic glands, and also a very abundant flow of saliva; hence it also acts upon the salivary glands, and perhaps upon the pancreas.—VOGT.

Digitalis may prove to be one of the most homœopathic remedies against *sick*-headache, especially in that variety which is attended with disturbance of the urinary secretion. Even in small doses it causes headache especially in the temples and back of the head; decided disturbance of vision, such as clouds, sparks, flimmering or colors before the eyes, with sensitiveness to light; also paleness and coolness of the skin, weakness of the pulse, general prostration, nausea and vomiting; with a peculiar disturbance of the urinary organs. Many persons, subject to sick-headaches, will have their urine clear and abundant when they are well; when the headaches occur frequently and severely their urine is apt to be thick and dark, like coffee or brandy, with more or less brick-dust, or other sediment. When the headache comes on, the urine will again become clear, and be like spring-water and abundant; when the headache is going off, the urine becomes thick and dark. In another class of headaches the urine acts entirely differently, being scanty and irritating during the headache, and becoming clear and abundant when the headache passes off. In one or both of these forms of headache, Digitalis will prove useful. It would seem that many headaches arise from derangement of the kidneys and retention of urea, or some other effete substance in the blood.—PETERS.

CASE 56.—A little girl, 2 years of age, blond, of delicate constitution, and merry disposition, fell into the second stage of hydrocephalus, with the following:

Symptoms.—Head hot, falling backwards on lifting up the child; sleep-like condition, with half-opened eyes and widely dilated pupils; look staring, with squinting; dulness and rolling of the eyes; convulsions of the muscles of the face; great thirst, constipation; urine scanty, leaving on the chamber a glossy, glimmer-like deposit; skin, sometimes hot and dry, sometimes cold and covered with sweat; pulse irregular, weak and soft; convulsions of the limbs during sleep; piercing cries.

Treatment.—Bell. 9. in water, four hourly; the first and second day without result, afterwards Digit. 3., also four hourly. The following day improved consciousness, increased flow of urine; soft, slimy stools, followed by green, looser, more slimy passages, preceded each time by crying, drawing up of the legs, screaming and convulsions of the limbs. After three days' use of the Digitalis, Cham. 3. was given, followed by sleep for five or six hours, from which she awoke conscious, with appetite, natural expression, pulse more regular and stronger. Still some Sb. Cham. 3. On the twentieth day of the treatment the recovered child went into the fresh air.—Y. 95.

HELLEBORUS-NIGER.

General Remarks.—According to Vogt and Pereira in small doses it acts as a mild stimulant to the stomach, bowels and abdominal nerves, also quite especially upon the pelvic nerves and those of the rectum and genital organs; in short, it is a powerful alterative remedy for the abdominal nervous system. In somewhat larger doses it increases the secretions from the stomach, and causes the excretion of a larger quantity of fluid bile; it arouses the circulation in the portal system, and in the liver and spleen. It acts less powerfully upon the abdominal lymphatic system, and very little if at all upon the kidneys. Next to its action upon the abdominal nervous system, its effects upon the skin are most decided.

It is much more apt to excite vomiting in large doses than purging, and Emmert found it more apt to excite vomiting when injected into the veins, than any other drug. In excessive doses it causes most violent vomiting and purging.

It is one of the oldest medicines used in the practice of medicine. Thus, about the year 1500 before the Christian era, a certain Melampus, son of Armithaon, a most celebrated augur and physician, is said to have cured the daughters of Proctus, king of the Argivans, who in consequence of remaining unmarried were seized with an amorous furor and a wandering mania. They were cured by means of Hellebore given in the milk of goats. From this circumstance the great fame of this plant is derived. In the course of time the use of Hellebore became so frequent, that every year a large concourse of patients flocked to Anticyra, where this plant grew in great abundance and perfection, in order to be cured with it of mania, melancholy and other mental affections. At first it was thought to be especially useful in cases with derangement of the pelvic organs, and even in later times it was greatly esteemed by MEAD as an emmenagogue, and is still much valued by some practitioners. He gave two teaspoonsful of the tincture in a glass of warm water, twice a day.

But soon it was conjectured that Black Hellebore possessed the power of carrying off black bile easily and promptly, and hence its use was extended to liver and spleen diseases, and such cases of epilepsy, mania and melancholy as were supposed to proceed from the presence of black bile.

Finally it was regarded as simply an evacuant remedy, and given against dropsy, jaundice, suppressed menses and hæmorrhoids, worms, obstinate eruptions, chronic gout and rheumatism, and fever and ague. And against diseases arising from the suppression of eruptions, or accustomed hæmorrhagies.

HAHNEMANN says: if it is used for a long time it will cause severe headaches and a fever; hence he infers its usefulness against chronic headaches, mental affections, quartan fevers and dropsy, as proven by old school experience, i. e., because a remedy which acts upon the head and causes headache, it may cure mental affections homœopathically; a remedy which simply causes fever, may cure quartan fever homœopathically; and last of all dropsy, because the worst kinds of dropsy are always accompanied by remitting fever—certainly never have such wholesale assumptions been made from such slight premises; yet such overstrained attempts to fasten a homœopathic explanation upon allopathic cures are not at all uncommon with HAHNEMANN.—See Lesser Writings, p. 292.

a. BREDENOLL says; since I have been a homœopathic

physician, (fifteen years,) I have frequently treated patients, suffering with hydroceph. acut., and have cured at least twelve. The principal remedy is and remains Helleb. I never have seen any result from Bryon. and Sulph. if I abandoned Helleb. —N. Arch. 3, 3, 46.

b. WAHLE says; if the first stage of effusion has already begun, and Bryon. was not given at the proper time, so as to effect a cure in the course of twelve to twenty-four hours, and there appeared during an intermission of the fever, the well-known symptoms of effusion, such as heavy breathing, unconsciousness, trembling, and putting of the hands to the head, squinting, indifference to light, chewing motions of the mouth, sopor, then one dose of Helleb.-nig. 30. will often remove all danger in the course of a few hours.—Arch. 15, 2, 23.

CASE 57.—A boy, 2½ years of age, was treated for inflammation of the brain, for fourteen days with Mercur., Moschus, leeches, &c. On the 31st of July he was in the following condition:

Symptoms.—He had lain for six days in a soporific state; the eyes could only be half-opened; eye-lids were stuck together and dry; the eye-balls reddish, glassy and turned upwards; the pupils dilated; no sign of consciousness; face pale and disfigured; head hanging down behind; pulse, weak, quick and irregular.

Prescription.—Hell. 3. a few drops in a wine-glass of water, a teaspoonful to be taken every half-hour.

On the 2d of August there were signs of consciousness; the eyes were less fixed; he commenced to take food; on the 3d of August, state improving in general, but there were frequent convulsions of the right arm, convulsive pain in the limbs, and sudden starting up from sleep. Hyosc. 3. and Helleb. in alternation till the 8th, with continual improvement. Then he was conscious and without fever, still the convulsive movements had abated but little, saliva accumulated in the mouth, his speech was indistinct, voice groaning, he coughed at night, with severe vomiting. Bell. was given morning and evening, one drop per dose for four days, when the recovery was complete.—ELWERT.

CASE 58.—A little girl, 2¼ years of age, sickened with all the signs of disease of the brain, and the following symptoms were present on the sixteenth day of her illness:

Symptoms.—She has been lying for a week upon her back, apparently in slumber, her eyes only half-shut, pupils contracted, cornea and albuginea dim as if covered with dust; in the corners of the lids dry mucus, squinting, eyes turned inwards, sunken and surrounded by blue circles; face pale and thin, nose pinched; nostrils covered with sordes; lips chapped and dry; body emaciated, covered with loose, harsh skin. The pit of the stomach drawn in, legs extended, the legs were drawn up to the thighs at every attempt to change the posture.—Groaning; painful, lamentable crying; face distorted by pain; the head fell back involuntarily; eyes wide opened, with enlarged pupils; oscillationof the iris; access to light, speaking and calling did not arouse the patient. He drank largely, biting violently at the spoon, without arousing from his unconscious state; distortion of the face, chewing with the mouth; grasped with the hands at his head, had cramps in the dorsal muscles, gritting of the teeth, constipation, involuntary urination, partial sweat on the scalp; pulse quick, weak and intermitting.

Prescription.—Tinct. Helleb.-nig. Gtt. ij., to be taken every two hours, day and night, for six days, finally every three to six hours.

On the third day the brilliancy of the eyes had returned, he cried out seldom, gave attention to objects, and from the sixth day of the treatment, the improvement advanced so rapidly that no other remedy was required.—Allg. Hom. Ztg. 19, 39.—KNORRE.

CASE 59.—A boy, aged 6 years, had been drooping for some time, and finally got all the symptoms of brain-disease, attended with gastric derangement; he lay doubled up in bed, with his knees drawn up to his stomach, and could not bear his abdomen to be touched; he was very drowsy and heavy, and when not disturbed, remained constantly in a stupor with half-closed eyes and open mouth; when roused, and also at other times, he started up and screamed out with loud piercing cries; his features were sharp and sunken; his mouth and nostrils sore, dry and black; his tongue dry and parched, also thickly coated brown and yellow, the edges and papillæ being of a deep red color; the skin of the whole body, but more particularly of the head and bowels, was dry and hot; he was thirsty and had no appetite; bowels loose and evacuations unhealthy; pulse 125, and hard; he was also harassed by a short, hacking cough.

Treatment.—Arsenicum 6., every four hours; at the end of two days he was much the same, except that the tongue appeared somewhat clearer, and he was not so thirsty; continue Arsen. 6., every four hours; in three days more there were only some shades of amendment. Then Hellebore 6. was given every four hours, and in two days there was a decided improvement, and in a few days more he was perfectly restored.—YELDHAM.

CASE 60.—A boy, aged 3 years, was taken sick three or four days ago, with disordered bowels, and soon fell into a drowsy and heavy state, in which he hangs back on his mother's arm, shewing the greatest repugnance to being moved or disturbed; his brow was knit and frowning; his eye-lids drooping, pupils contracted, eyes dull and unexpressive; his head as well as body generally hot and dry; breathing short and quick, pulse 160 and throbbing; was very thirsty, could not bear the least noise and avoided the light; his tongue was white and thickly coated; bowels loose; he was exceedingly weak, and had commenced to emaciate.

Treatment.—Aconite 12. and Bellad. 12. in alternation every four hours; the next night he was quite delirious, but much improved in the morning, his skin was cool, pulse only 100, thirst less, eyes still heavy and frowning; omit Acon. and continue Bellad.; on the next day there was an increase of stupor, but his skin was still cool and pulse laboring; gave Hellebore 6. every four hours with marked improvement in twenty-four hours and rapid recovery.—YELDHAM.

CASE 61.—A girl, aged 7, had been failing for some time; bowels relaxed and passages unhealthy.

Treatment.—Mercurius 6., three times a day; in two days was considerably worse, stupid, heavy and lethargic; started and screamed; her head was hot, and she was feverish and thirsty; her tongue coated brown and dry. Bellad. 6., every four hours; at the end of three days more she was still worse, was perfectly lethargic and unconscious of everything; she screamed and started terribly, and rolled her head; her lips, tongue and teeth were black and dry, and covered with a thick, hard and offensive matter; pulse very rapid, and skin and head very hot. Then took Hellebore 12. and Rhus. 12., every four hours in alternation, with decided improvement at the end of two days, when her lips and tongue were moist and cleaning, mind more quiet and intelligent, no more screaming. The medicines were continued for five days more, when she was quite restored.

HYOSCIAMUS.

The most marked effects observed by Greding were:

1. *Perspiration.* Seven patients out of forty had a profuse dripping perspiration on the first night; and two-thirds of all the others had more or less sweat; they perspired not only in summer, but also in the fall and winter; the perspirations were *sour* at times.

2. *Sleep.* A quiet, refreshing and deep sleep, generally attended with breaking out of the perspiration; many patients slept the first night, but more, viz.: twenty out of forty, slept better afterwards.

3. Happiness of mind, activity of body, and greater clearness of intellect; fourteen out of forty patients experienced the former, and nine the latter.

4. Dulness and heaviness of the head occurred in four cases.

5. Headache in fifteen cases.

6. Dizziness in eight cases.

7. Torpor of mind in three cases.

8. Eruptions occurred in five cases, viz.: brown spots, or liver-spots, small pustules, boils, and also swelling of the left parotid gland.

9. Profuse urination occurred in three cases, on the first day; and finally in at least one-third of all the cases.

10. Diarrhœa more or less profuse and continuous occurred in twenty-three cases; with expulsion of worms in three cases;

with vomiting of bile and mucus in ten cases; with colic and rumbling in six cases; with nausea in five cases. Constipation only took place in two cases, and then only in a slight degree.

11. Menstruation was brought on, or increased in twelve cases; in one case it was brought on after a suppression of five months.

12. Salivation occurred in one case.

13. Profuse catarrh in one case.

14. Rheumatic pains in seven cases.

15. Dry, convulsive cough in two cases.

16. Hiccough in three cases, in one with involuntary urination.

In one case, in an adult woman, an overdose of the Root produced, slight and then increased stupefaction; flimmering before the eyes, brilliancy of the eyes, double vision; considerable dilatation of the pupils; dimness of sight; dizziness; great dryness of the mouth; trembling of the limbs and staggering; small, scarcely perceptible, frequently intermitting and moderately slow pulse.

In a girl, aged 4 years, a large quantity of unripe seeds, produced unsteadiness of gait, small, white blisters on the lips, and flushed face; at the end of three hours the face was very red, the eyes injected, the pupils extremely dilated and insensible to light, the tongue coated, pulse small and moderately frequent; heart beating violently and irregularly; there was entire loss of consciousness; frequent groaning; grasping about, with outstretched fingers, as if something had to be seized suddenly; frightful gritting of the teeth; frequent jerking of the hands and feet; constant incomprehensible babbling; skin almost natural; abdomen soft.

In a boy, aged 3 years, the seeds caused him to fall down senseless upon the floor; he thrashed around him; frothed at the mouth; his face was much reddened; and he had alternate convulsive movements of the face and limbs.

In a girl, aged 6, the seeds caused paleness of the face without heat of the head; great dilatation of the pupils; smallness and quickness of the pulse; throbbing of the heart; coldness of the hands and feet; slight convulsions of the limbs; squinting; gritting of the teeth; and unconsciousness.

In a girl, aged 6, the seeds caused: heat of the head and whole body; redness and bloating of the face; fulness, without quickness of the pulse; violent and irregular action of the heart; protrusion with great redness of the eyes and much dilatation of the pupils; the most happy delirium, so that she sang and spoke and babbled constantly, but very hastily and indistinctly; but she became very violent, and struck around her whenever she was spoken to loudly or taken hold of.

In an adult, three ounces of the seeds, made the face bluish; the eyes red, wild and sparkling; the veins of the neck and limbs, but especially of the face, much distended; the whole body was convulsed; frequently returning subsultus; and such a furious delirium that no one could hold him. During the intermissions the patient was occupied in trying to catch flies which seemed to be flying about, or in picking shreds out of his quilt. Afterwards he seemed much exhausted and breathed like one in an apoplexy, from which he was aroused by still more violent convulsions; the pulse was small, quick, contracted and distinctly intermitting; tongue dry and clean; hypogastric region much distended and very painful; urine very scanty; there was such excessive itching that he expended his little strength in scratching himself until the blood came; invincible horror for all liquids; afterwards perspiration sat in very profusely and lasted for two whole days, over the whole body, but especially on the legs, and a pimply eruption broke out upon the thighs, both before and behind, from the hips down to the knees; the pimples were large, red and confluent, like those of small-pox, but did not contain any fluid. His sight remained very dim for some time.—FRANK.

A coachman, from the herb, experienced confusion of the head, and such stiffness of the arms and legs that he could scarcely stand, and finally fell down; his eyes seemed inflamed for a long time afterwards.—FRANK.

SCHNELLER from four grain doses of Extract, experienced: mist before the eyes and weakness of sight; dryness of mouth;

yellow coated tongue; great distension of abdomen, with inclination to breathe deep; sour eructations; scanty stools; rather slow pulse; also left frontal headache, with ambliopia, frequent inclination to yawn and sleepiness, with evening nausea. Some of the doses were not followed by head-symptoms, but merely by frequent inclination to sneeze, with the feeling as if a catarrh of the head would set in; also frequent sour eructations, some little constipation, and good sleep.

In other experiments he had: tickling and burning in the throat, with increased secretion of mucus, dryness of the mouth, white tongue, hoarseness, loss of appetite, and some colic; also peculiar drawing and rending pains in the joints, especially in the wrists and knees.

Five grain doses caused: thick coating of the tongue, insipid taste, offensive breath, eruption of small boils upon the face, dimness of vision and redness of the eyes. Eleven grain doses caused: vertigo, gauze before the eyes, headache on the right side of the forehead, prickling feeling in the arms, followed by sticky perspiration, with heat, redness and turgor of the face. At other times he experienced: dryness of the nostrils, pain at the root of the nose, and excretion of a very little mucus mixed with blood, &c.—FRANK.

In an adult soldier, the young shoots caused some burning in the throat, stupefaction, and a dropsical swelling of the arms and hands.

Two other soldiers experienced: very violent dizziness, and they finally fell down as if deeply intoxicated; their eyes were wild, pupils much dilated, expression fixed and stupid, respiration difficult, pulse small and intermitting; loss of voice, lock-jaw, risus sardonicus, loss of sensation, typhomania, coldness of the limbs, paralysis of the legs, carphologia and convulsions of the arms. The patient who vomited least, had mania with delirium, but without fury, although it was difficult to hold him, when he sought to escape.

A girl, aged 4½ years, ate one root, and seemed as if intoxicated; she was awake, but without consciousness, did not answer questions, but looked around the room as if seeking something, made frequent, but not convulsive motions with the hands and feet; if she attempted to take hold of anything she grasped to one side of it; her eyes were wide open, pupils dilated, pulse natural, and face reddened.—FRANK.

Four children, from 4 to 8 years of age, ate of the leaves: They began to stagger, then fell down in convulsions; their faces were bloated, skin dry, pupils excessively dilated, eyes turned upwards and inwards. In one child the abdomen was so much distended that it seemed as if it would burst, but without pain; the tongue was stretched far out of its mouth, turned up, and occasionally thrown spasmodically against the nose. In the two youngest, such violent convulsive movements sat in at times that a strong man could scarcely prevent them from injuring themselves; when free from convulsions they spoke much, very hastily, and unconnectedly. The two oldest were affected quite differently; they lay quite quietly in a perfectly stupid and unconscious state. None of them seemed to be in pain; all seemed comfortable, and one was occasionally merry and silly.—FRANK.

Two girls, aged 5 years, ate several capsules, and were attacked with trembling of the limbs, anxiety, restlessness and confusion of words and actions; in six or eight hours they were talking incessantly and confusedly, they laughed and sang at times, did not know their relatives, had frequent spasms of the facial muscles, especially if one attempted to hold them or take anything out of their hands, when they became violent and attempted to bite, pinch and scratch; they seemed very strong in their hands and feet, and at times attempted to dance; they gritted their teeth, and had a spasmodic stretching out of their tongues, with a peculiar trembling motion of it; their eyes were brilliant and rolled about unsteadily, and were reddened; the pupils exceedingly dilated and insensible to light; pulse almost extinct, small, and very quick.—FRANK.

CASE 62.—A man, aged 24 years, healthy and strong, got sick after a severe chill. On the second day the malady was the following:

Symptoms.—He lay senseless with closed eyes, did not open them when spoken to; his mouth could be opened with difficulty; tongue, covered with a white, foamy slime; he dreamed about business affairs, animating his servant to work; he sang unintelligible songs; murmured, laughed and then became quiet again, started often, worked with his hands, as if he intended to prick on the ceiling; pupils enlarged, eyes dull, face red, skin dry and parched, breathing quick and anxious; pulse regular, but full, abdomen somewhat contracted, but he did not complain of pain if touched and pressed.

Prescription.—Hyosc. 6., one drop per dose, in half an hour after, slept for four hours, passed urine involuntarily; seven hours after, awaked with consciousness. On the following day, some signs of inflammation of the lungs were soon removed by Arnica.—Mossbauer.

CASE 63.—It was useful in an affection of the brain, attended with convulsions of the whole left side of the face and body; the right arm and the right leg constantly affected, although not spasmodically, while the limbs of the left side, without being paralysed, lay quite still. Ipecac. was of no use, but Hyosc. effected a speedy cure, and caused a quiet sleep.—Gross, Jr.

Review.—The presence of redness of the face, delirium, picking at the bed-clothes, fright, convulsions, are indications for the use of this remedy.

IODINE AND HYDRIODATE OF POTASH.

Iodine acts principally upon the absorbent system, and the particles absorbed are quickly ejected through the kidneys, as the urine is generally much increased in quantity; some persons experience this latter effect so instantaneously that Iodine has been detected in the urine almost immediately after each dose has been taken. This excessive absorption and drain from the system may lead to great emaciation, or it may excite an increased demand for food so that one of the first and most important effects of this remedy may be a great increase of appetite, which will enable us with ease to invigorate the constitution by wholesome and sufficient nourishment. Again, although it is well-known to all practical men that Iodine acts as a diuretic, it is not equally known that the Iodine-urine contains large quantities of urea. Now, urea is the product of the decomposition of the albuminous tissues, and as it has been clearly shown by chemical analysis that tubercle is composed chiefly of albumen and caseine, we can understand how Iodine acts by carrying a large quantity of albumen out of the system, thus retarding the growth and promoting the absorption of tuberculous matter.—GLOVER. We have already seen that Hepar.-sulphur diminishes the quantity of albumen in the blood; it might be advisable to put a tuberculous subject upon alternate courses of Hepar.-sulph. and Iodine; the one to diminish the quantity, and the other to expel the excess of albumen from the system.

WARING says: In *tubercular meningitis* or *acute hydrocephalus* Iodine has been used with benefit. Drs. CHRISTIE and WONINGER relate two cases which had reached the paralytic stage, but which recovered under the external and internal use of Iodine. Dr. BENNETT has derived decided benefit from Iodine and its preparations in this disease; and Dr. WILLSHIRE bears similar testimony; he advises the use of Iodine externally and internally in the early stages of the disease, before there is much evidence of congestion and inflammation; he applies the Iodine-ointment to the shaven scalp, and gives internally, gr. $\frac{1}{10}$ of Iodine and gr. iij. of Potass.-iod. in solution, every three hours; this, aided by turpentine enemas will be found in most cases a palliative, and in some a curative mode of treatment. Dr. RILLIET advises the use of Iodine frictions to the shaven scalp in the second and third stages of hydrocephalus.

ROWLAND HOSKINS relates a very aggravated and apparently hopeless case which yielded to the Iodide of Potassium in half-grain doses, every four hours; but Scammony was given at the same time as a purgative. Another case illustrative of the efficacy of this salt, is related by Dr. GUEROUD. Dr. COPELAND also states that he has prescribed it in small doses with evident advantage.

CASE 64.—A child, aged 2½ years, was attacked with fever and vomiting, followed on the third day by convulsions, and all the signs of dropsy of the brain; on the fourth day the eyes were open, squinting and dim; the pupils much dilated; there was unconsciousness with incessant screeching, without weeping; entire blindness; the eyes were moist, the edge of the lower lid relaxed and inverted, (entropium); the little patient lay on its back, with its head pressed back into the pillow; when it was raised up its head fell back hopelessly; there was entire paralysis of the right limbs, with partial palsy of the left; frequent, involuntary and automatic motions were made with the left arm and leg; drinks passed over the clean and dry tongue into the windpipe and excited spasmodic coughing; the urine was scanty; the cheeks which had been pale yesterday were red to-day; the pulse which had been slow and irregular yesterday was very quick to-day; the whole body was in a dripping perspiration, notwithstanding that ice was applied to the head. The last febrile reaction had taken place previous to dissolution.

Treatment.—Kali-hydr. 1 drachm in 2 oz. of water, 30 drops per dose, every hour; notwithstanding the difficulty of swallowing, the whole of the above medicine was given in less than twenty-four hours and the prescription repeated, without alteration of the symptoms except an increase of the dryness of the mouth and thirst; but on the tenth day of the disease, and the second day of this treatment, the first traces of improvement were observed in commencing contraction of the pupils; on the seventh day consciousness was restored, there was regular movement of the pupils, natural position of the eyes, the countenance was expressive, the little patient began to move the left hand and arm, and two days afterwards motion was also restored to the right side; great appetite set in, and many small *boils* broke out on the face and neck. Finally this critical eruption of boils became a perfect torture to the child, for at least one hundred large and small ones appeared first and last upon the head, back, neck, face and chest; shortly after the pimples appeared, they quickly changed without much redness or inflammation into larger or smaller abscesses, some of which attained the size of a hickory-nut and then burst.

At the end of four weeks the child was perfectly well of disease and eruption, after using about ten drachms of Iodide of Potash in the course of eleven days.—Frank's Magazine, Dr. ROESER.

CASE 65.—A case of hydrocephalus progressed notwithstanding the most active antiphlogistic and derivative treatment into the second stage, but after the use of half an oz. Iodide of Potash in the course of three days, consciousness had returned, the pulse was no longer irregular and intermitting, but still frequent; a perfect cure was effected in six days by smaller quantities—about two drachms more. Tartar-emetic ointment had also been applied to the nape of the neck.—Dr. VEIT.

CASE 66.—A girl, aged 6 years, after eight days of sickness, lay in a deep stupor, from which she occasionally started up with screaming; the pupils were dilated, one considerably more than the other; the eyes were insensible to light, with squinting; she could be rendered conscious for a short time by shaking and loud talking; she gritted her teeth in her sleep; the pulse was quick and irregular; she could still move her limbs, hold up her head, and swallow.

Treatment.—Kali-hydriod. was used without aid from any other medicine; at the end of two days and after taking drachms ij., all dangerous symptoms had disappeared, the position of the eyes was natural, the pupils normal, and stools regular. But great redness of the cheeks and strong pulsation of the carotids set in, calling for the omission of Kali-hydriod. and the use of Calomel, leeches and cold applications to the head; on the next day this congestive and febrile paroxysm had subsided, and the face was again pale, but the stupor sat in again, and the pupils became dilated and sluggish. Kali-hydriod. was resumed, and in five days more perfect recovery had taken place.—Dr. VEIT.

CASE 67.—A boy, aged 3½ years, of strong constitution and active temperament, but who had frequently suffered with crusta-serpiginosa and catarrho-scrofulous opthalmia, was attacked with incipient inflammation of the brain, and treated with Calomel, &c., from the 17th to the 26th of June, when all the signs of effusion sat in; he was entirely unconscious; tossed about the right leg in a restless manner, while the left lay paralysed and motionless; occasionally sudden starts of the whole body, and screaming fits; the eyeballs were drawn spasmodically upwards, and only partially covered by the lids; the pupils were entirely immovable and very widely dilated; the conjunctiva was reddened and the cornea and edges of the lids covered with purulent mucus; the nostrils were dry; face pale and sunken; mouth distorted and partly opened, with frequent sucking motion of the lips; tongue moist; gums touched, and together with the teeth and lips were covered with brown sordes; there was frequent gritting of the teeth; slow and unfrequent pulse; dry skin; great thirst; constipation and almost entire suppression of urine.

Treatment.—Kali-hydriod., half a drachm in three ounces of water, and one ounce of simple syrup, a moderate tablespoonful every two hours. On the next day, with the exception of some congestion of the head, for which seven leeches were applied to the mastoid processes, there was evident improvement, which progressed steadily under a renewal of the prescription on the 28th and 30th of June, and 2d of July. The critical appearances were a profuse secretion of urine, which was at first turbid, but soon became clear; several semi-fluid stools; moderate warm perspiration, some white miliary eruption upon the chest and neck, especially in the outbreak of *boils* upon the forehead, scalp and nape of neck; these were of various sizes, some as large as a hazel-nut; they suppurated and ulcerated, and their irruption was aided by the application of Tartar-emetic ointment for several days. Dryness of the mouth, and a frequent, dry cough, were also noticed as effects of the remedy. The child was entirely restored in eighteen days, under the use of half an ounce of Hydriodate of Potash.—AMELUNG.

CASE 68.—A little boy, aged 2⅓ years, suffering with dropsy of the brain and consumption, was so far restored by the use of six drachms of Kali-hydriod. in four days, that there seemed but little doubt that he would recover from the brain disease. The pupils became regular, consciousness was restored, although the little patient could not speak, he could hold up his head somewhat, and move his emaciated limbs, he passed much urine, had several stools per day, and pimples and boils commenced to break out upon his head, aided by the application of Tartar-emetic ointment. Finally the hydrocephalic symptoms disappeared entirely, but the child ultimately died of consumption.—Dr. ROESER.

CASE 69.—A boy, aged 2½ years, previously quite healthy,

was attacked with decided inflammation of the brain attended with fever, headache, contracted pupils, intolerance of light, vomiting and constipation.

Treatment and Result.—Eight leeches were applied to the temples, and two grains of Calomel given every two hours; the Mercury had not operated upon the bowels at the end of several days, the vomiting had ceased, the headache persisted, also the stupor, from which, however, the little patient occasionally started up with frightful screams. Ice was applied to the head, six more leeches to the temples and a blister to the back of the neck. After the use of several drachms of Calomel, the constipation persisted and the most decided signs of dropsy of the brain sat in. There was constant stupor, squinting, very much dilated and insensible pupils, frequent automatic screaming, dirty and dry tongue and slowness of the pulse.

Treatment.—Kali-hydriod., two drachms in one and a half ounces of water, twenty to thirty drops per dose, every hour; the whole quantity to be used every twenty-four hours. At the end of two days several loose stools had occurred, the pulse was fuller, harder and quicker, the pupils somewhat contracted and sensitive to light, gums touched by Mercury. At the end of nine days consciousness was entirely restored, pupils natural, sopor gone, and there was only a little squinting with one eye.

Violent mercurial gangrene of the mouth was followed by great restlessness and delirium; and the Hydriodate of Potash was stopped, but had to be resumed again in seven days on account of a return of the brain symptoms; two drachms were used per day with rapid improvement for seventeen days, when the patient had perfect possession of his mental faculties, was stout and blooming, but some of his teeth had fallen out, and part of his jaw-bone was loose.—Dr. ROESER.

N. B.—Since ROESER has resorted to such heroic doses of Hydriodate of Potash, sometimes using three ounces and six drachms in one case, he has only met with three fatal cases out of many; in one of these cases a post mortem examination revealed tubercles and ulceration of the lungs; in the two other cases the remedy was given too late and quite irregularly.

CASE 70.—A boy, aged 5 years, was attacked with violent inflammation of the brain, eight days after a fall upon the head.

Symptoms.—Perfect stupefaction and blindness, heat of the head, immoveableness of the pupils, entire suppression of all the secretions, quickened pulse, and violent, finally incessant convulsions, passing over into opisthotonos.

Treatment.—After the fruitless use of leeches, ice to the head, Calomel and Sublimate in unction, Kali-hydriod. was given, one to two drachms in two ounces of water, a teaspoonful per dose. At first the symptoms were rather aggravated, but improvement soon sat in after the occurrence of profuse urination and copious discharge from the nose.—ZIMMERMANN.

CASE 71.—A boy, aged 2 years, previously afflicted with eruptions upon the head and face, was attacked with violent inflammation of the brain, apparently in consequence of repeated falls upon the head. Very active antiphlogistic and counter-irritant treatment had produced no good effect at the end of five days, on the contrary all the signs of effusion had taken place.

Symptoms.—The eyes were fixed and watery; pupils immoveable and widely dilated; absolute blindness; tetanic rigidity of the muscles of the nape; retraction of the head; paralysis of the left side; deep stupor; slow pulse, down to 50; frequent screaming and vomiting.

Treatment.—Kali-hydriod., one drachm in half an oz. of water, forty and finally fifty drops per dose, every two hours; without improvement for the first three days; but on the fourth day of the Potash treatment and ninth of the disease, profuse secretion of urine sat in, with evident improvement in all the alarming symptoms; after the use of two drachms of the Hydriodate he was almost out of danger on the twelfth day of the attack.—Frank's Magazine.—Dr. WOENIGER.

CASE 72.—The head of the patient at birth was unusually large and the fontanelles widely separated, the membranous portions being quite protuberant, with fluctuation; the child had had frequent convulsions and occasional paralysis. When Dr. BARBOUR saw the case, the head was of monstrous size; the fontanelles very large, the anterior being at least three inches in diameter, and occupied by a large fluctuating tumor, elevated about an inch above the level of the skull; the sagittal suture was widely open, and all the bones of the head quite moveable and compressible; his neck was remarkably emaciated and slender, so much so, that the weighty head could only be sustained by the shoulder on which it constantly leaned. Chronic diarrhœa also existed, attended with general emaciation, tumid abdomen and irritative fever; in fact he presented the most prominent symptoms of marasmus in connection with chronic dropsy of the brain.

Treatment.—In order to improve the secretions and check the diarrhœa Hydrarg.-cicuta and Pulv.-dover, grs. xv., made into twelve powders, one every six hours; this had such decided effect that an occasional laxative had to be given. To promote the absorption of the fluid and improve the general constitution, Hydriod.-potass., half a drachm in 2 ounces water, one teaspoonful three times a day was given. A blister was applied to the head, and frequent effusions of cold water were used. This course was continued for six weeks, and the result was highly gratifying; the irritative fever gradually yielded; the head diminished in size, day by day; the fontanelles became gradually reduced to their natural size; the convulsions did not recur; and the little boy gained flesh, strength and color, and finally appeared perfectly well. Dr. BARBOUR's great reliance, at least theoretically, was upon the Hydriodate of Potash.

CASE 73.—A girl, 12 years of age, was attacked with arthrit. acut. vaga. About midnight on the 16th of January, she became delirious and restless, sometimes sitting up in bed, at others lying down again. The inflammation of the wrists had ceased, and appeared to settle in the meninges; the patient was nearly given up.

Treatment—Iod.-solut., (ten gran. in half ounce of Alcohol,) two drops, p. d., to be taken half-hourly, for one day; on the second day, hourly; on the two following days every two hours. On the 17th the consciousness was already regained, the right hand had re-inflamed, the meninges were free. She then took Ant.-cr. and Bryon., and on the 26th was also recovered from the arthritis.—SCHMID, 130.

NATURAL CURES.

CASE 74.—A boy, aged 2½ years, robust, with a large head, and prominent forehead, was taken sick on the eighth of December. Six days afterwards acute hydrocephalus, was fully developed; the fontanelles were still widely open; leeches, Calomel, &c. were given without benefit, and on the eighteenth day the boy lay helpless and stupefied; his head and face were alternately hot and red; he gritted his teeth; the pupils were dilated and insensible to light; he swallowed fluids hastily: this state lasted two days more, when a larger quantity of clear watery fluid flowed from the ear, and the patient improved on the same evening; profuse flow of urine also sat in and lasted for several days; in a few days more the little patient was decidedly convalescent, and recovered perfectly in six weeks. Two profusely suppurating spots also formed on the back of the head. The author had previously witnessed a similar case.—RIECKE.

CASE 75.—A little girl, aged 4 years, had been sick for five days with inflammation of the brain, for which she had received no medical treatment, and now seemed at the point of death. Her face was red; eyes rigid and immoveable; breathing frequent and irregular; pulse hard and intermitting; for two days everything that she had swallowed had been ejected again through the nostrils. Ice to the head, leeches and injections were used without benefit; at the end of eight days more, her face was pale and sunken; nose and ears cold; pupils dilated; eyes turned up; mouth open; breathing scarcely perceptible; pulse small, frequent and intermitting; constipation for eight days, and no urine had been passed for three days; the right arm and leg were moved automatically; the whole left side seemed paralyzed. On the next day the whole scalp was slightly reddened and covered with an immense number of small miliary vesicles, which increased in size for two days more, then ran together, burst and discharged a large quantity of yellowish watery fluid, followed by improvement of the brain symptoms. At the end of a few days more the whole head and face were covered with a thick scab, through the fissures of which a bloody serous fluid exuded; evacuations from the bowels and bladder had commenced. In eight days more the little patient was out of danger; but she did not recover her speech or the use of the left side until after the lapse of many weeks.—MALIN.

CASE 76.—A little boy, aged 1½ years, became sick two weeks after an attack of scarlet fever; gradually all the signs of dropsy of the brain developed themselves; his face became pale; pupils dilated and fixed; the conjunctiva reddened; cornea dull and coated with mucus; entire stupor for three days; convulsions of the right side; boring of the head into the pillow; vomiting and constipation had been followed by involuntary diarrhœa; pulse was small and frequent, with occasional intermissions. Elder tea caused such a profuse perspiration that a large bed was saturated both above and below, and the child speedily recovered.—RITSCHER.

CASE 77.—A boy, aged 1½ years, had so large and heavy a hydrocephalic head that he could not hold it up without support; the head was soft and doughy to the feel; the fontanelles were wide open; the rest of the body delicate and relaxed. At the end of five years the reporter was surprised to find him alive and well; the head was only a little larger than natural; the bones were firm and closed; the body well nourished; the mental faculties moderately developed; the parents assured him that no medicine had been given and that everything had been left to nature.—Frank's Magazine.—DORFMÜLLER.

CASE 78.—An infant, aged 6 months, had suffered severely during the month from cold, which resulted in an enlargement of the head, which was one-third larger than natural; the sutures were all widely open, the fissure commencing at the root of the nose and extending up the forehead, being one inch across; the anterior fontanelle was capacious enough to admit three fingers; the coronal and sagittal sutures were also widely extended; the scalp covering these broad fissures was puffed and elastic to the touch, indicating the presence of fluid beneath. Dilatation of the pupils, squinting, jerking of the limbs, screaming, tossing of the arms upwards, plainly denoted the dropsical nature of the little patient's brain affection; the bowels were also costive, and vomiting frequently occurred.

Treatment.—Kali-hydriod., twenty-five grains, gradually increased to forty grains to the ounce of lard, to be rubbed over the whole head, twice in twenty-four hours; also a solution of 20 grains to the ounce of water, ten drops to be given morning and evening. This treatment was continued for nearly one month without benefit; then blisters were ordered to the head, first on one entire half, and then on the other, so that one side was always under the influence of the irritant; two grains of blue pill were given twice daily; but in spite of this, general anasarca sat in, and Hydriodate of Potash ointment was applied over the whole chest and abdomen. And now appeared the crisis of the case, for a vesicular eruption broke out over the whole body, the vesicles bursting and discharging pure lymph. From this critical discharge, the convalescence of the patient commenced, but the remedies were still continued for four months, when the child was perfectly healthy and sprightly, although there was still some obliquity of vision.

Dr. KENNEDY asks: Is the treatment of the more ordinary or sub-acute form of hydrocephalus too heroic? He believes it to be so, in the allopathic school, and that a better prospect of cure will be held out by a treatment a good deal modified from that in common use. Of *bleeding* he is fully satisfied that very little of it will answer every purpose; he has even noticed that cases left to themselves, without treatment for days, did not appear to run a more rapid course than those where active measures had been adopted from the outset. To *Mercury* similar remarks, Dr. KENNEDY thinks, apply. It would seem, as far as he has seen, to be used as a sine qua non; and yet the results do not appear to justify such faith in it; he has notes of more than twenty cases of hydrocephalus, in which the specific effects of Mercury were produced, and yet in not one of these cases was the result favorable, to say nothing of others, where salivation could not be induced. Is it right to give Mercury to weak and strumous children, he would ask, and do our utmost to induce its specific effects? The answer to this must be in the negative. KENNEDY gives four cases, which include all those of recovery which he has seen in a period of several years, after the disease had passed into the second stage, that is when the pulse had fallen. Now it is specially worthy of notice that three out of four had never been salivated, and in the fourth salivation was produced more by accident than design.

Treatment.—All four cases were leeched; the grey powder in very minute doses, as an alterative was administered in antimonial powder; blistering was very freely used, at first in the ordinary mode, and subsequently in two cases, under the form of the Tartar-emetic plaster applied to the head; and in this way a constant discharge was kept up. But, in addition to these measures, particular attention was paid to keep up the strength; some got beef-tea and others wine, and this while the disease was still present. A child of six years of age, got two ounces of wine, which was increased to three in the day, and this while the pupils were still dilated, while the screaming was constant and the convulsions persisted; and it was apparently under its use that this child rallied.

Several of the natural cures took place after the outbreak of pustules upon the head, or eruptions over the body. Dr. HAHN has saved fourteen cases by means of frictions of the scalp with Tartar-emetic ointment, repeated every two hours, until pustulation is established; he claims to have saved fourteen cases in apparently a hopeless state of coma.

CASE 79.—A fine boy, aged 9 months, was suddenly attacked with convulsions; he recovered from these and cut his first teeth shortly afterwards; but soon began to fall away, to become listless and lose his appetite; his bowels became constipated; pulse irregular; he also began to vomit and to become torpid; fever was soon added to his symptoms, and it was evident that he was the subject of meningitis.

Treatment.—Leeches were applied, and Calomel given, but in spite of this treatment he lapsed into complete coma. As soon as the coma became distinct, Tartar-emetic ointment was rubbed into the scalp every four hours, over a space the size of a crown piece; free suppuration ensued and signs of improvement were speedily witnessed; the child gradually became more conscious, his appetite returned, and in two weeks all traces of his disease had vanished.

OPIUM.

General Remarks.—According to Waring Opium is generally contra-indicated in acute inflammation of the brain, which tends to produce death by coma; there are, however, occasional exceptions to this rule; as, for instance, in inflammation of the brain, in which Dr. Griffin states that Opium, given in combination with Tartar-emetic, exerts an extraordinary power in allaying nervous irritation, quieting increased action in the capillaries, and inducing sound and refreshing sleep. It should, however, be employed with extreme caution, and only by one whose experience in this class of diseases gives him a title to depart from what is generally regarded as safe practice.

In delirium occasioned by inflammatory action of the brain, or its membranes, particularly when it assumes a maniacal or violent character, and after depletions have been carried as far as may be thought prudent, and the bowels have been freely evacuated, Dr. Copeland states that he has frequently seen a full dose of Opium or Hyosciamus, given either alone, or with Antimony and Camphor, produce the happiest effect. Any unpleasant symptoms which may result, either from too large doses of these narcotics, or from their inappropriate use, will readily be removed by the cold or tepid affusion upon the head. —Waring.

In hydrocephalus, Opium has sometimes been employed in the second and third stages, to lessen the acute pain in the head, convulsions and irritability of the stomach and bowels; and may be given with this view, at an early period when dropsy of the brain depends upon exhaustion and debility uncomplicated with inflammation. It has often succeeded, observes Dr. Bennett, in effecting this without in any way interfering with the action of other remedies, or inducing constipation when moderately employed. At the early period of the second stage, it may be given with Calomel, James' powder, or Tartar-emetic, in doses varying from gr. $\frac{1}{8}$ to gr. $\frac{1}{4}$, every four hours. According to Crampton and Cheyne, contraction of the pupils following the exhibition of this remedy indicates that it has been pushed sufficiently far. Dr. Risdon Bennett has since stated, that, avoiding its use when the pupil is contracted, he has employed Opium with the best effect, and has sometimes saved an apparently hopeless case. Drop doses may be repeated every four hours, if no unpleasant symptoms present themselves.—WARING.

WEST says: In the treatment of many diseases you see physicians destroy pain by narcotics, and the question naturally suggests itself to you whether you may not sometimes venture in the management of hydrocephalus to mitigate by their means your patients sufferings? The inquiry is one not very easy to reply to satisfactorily. I think, however, that there are two conditions under which you will be justified in trying the experiment of giving them. Sometimes the disease sets in with great excitement, and a condition closely resembling mania in the adult, symptoms which may have been ushered in by convulsions. In such a case although the heat of the head and flush of the face may have disappeared after free depletion and purgation, and though the pulse is feeble as well as frequent, yet the excitement may be scarcely if at all diminished. Here an opiate will sometimes give relief which nothing else would procure; your patient will fall asleep and wake tranquilized in the course of two or three hours. In other cases which do not set in thus violently, restlessness, talkativeness, or a kind of half-delirious consciousness of pain in the head, become very distressing as the disease advances, being always aggravated at night, so that your patient's condition seems one of constant suffering. Under these circumstances, I [WEST] have sometimes given a full dose of Morphia, and have continued it every night for several nights together with manifest relief.——PETERS.

CASE 80.—GROSS observed during the winter months in a number of children, under 7 years of age, a rheumatic-inflammatory affection of the meninges, which he treated according to circumstances with Bellad., &c. In some, the following condition prevailed: They were continually in slumber, with snoring and half-opened eyes, were awakened with difficulty, on awaking, insensible, complaining of nothing, wanted nothing, but vomited frequently.

Treatment.—Opium 6., cured generally within a few hours. —Arch. 9, 2, 140.

CASE 81.—A boy, aged 4 years, after a fall upon the head, got an attack of hydroceph. ac.—Acon. was taken first, then Bell. 30., and after fourteen hours he appeared to be out of danger. The recovery progressed until the fifth day of the disease; but there still existed a state of apathy, accompanied by a short, dry cough, constipation, all of which were relieved after Bryon 30. had been taken. On the seventh day of the malady he had the following:

Symptoms.—An increased condition of stupefaction, the Iris more insensible than in the last few days, the eyes not quite closed in sleeping. Three large worms passed without excrement through the fundament.

Treatment.—Opium 6. followed by sixteen hours sleep and after awaking by a profuse sweat, when the brain was entirely relieved.—BETHMANN.

CASE 82.—A girl, aged 17 years, of delicate phlegmatic constitution, whose sister had died with hydroceph. acut., complained of dizziness, headache, and vomiting, which increased daily; for four weeks she had been surly, and had lost her good looks; her cheeks were hollow, face pale yellow; eyes weak and without expression; the brain appeared as if oppressed by a heavy burden.

Treatment.—Bell. 18. in solution; she soon became unable to speak; was continually drowsy; she stared vaguely when spoken to, without giving any answer; all the former symptoms remained. Opium 4. in solution, two spoonsful morning and evening, was followed by a tolerable state of quietness, and the excessive desire for sleep disappeared; the patient improved rapidly.—MOOR.

REVIEW.—In the foregoing cases we find an amazed and stupid state, continual slumbering with half-opened eyes, snoring, and insensibility of the iris. GROSS observed principally a rheumatic-inflammatory irritation of the meninges; in one case a fall upon the head preceded the attack, and Acon., Bell. and Bryon. were given, with little effect; in another Bell. was prescribed without benefit. The *doses*, Opium 6. in two cases; the 4th dilution, in solution, in one case. This remedy is so decidedly homœopathic to congestions of the brain, that it deserves more frequent trials.

RHUS-TOXICODENDRON.

General Remarks.—Rhus is peculiarly homœopathic to inflammatory œdema, and to all inflammations attended with a copious effusion of serum; hence to all inflammatory dropsies, and to dropsy and œdema of the brain. In this respect it is the analogue of Arsenicum and Cantharides. If it were possible to obtain and retain the recent juice in all its original activity, it would probably form a more efficient external application than Cantharides, Croton-oil or Tartar-emetic.

It will perhaps prove most useful in the paralytic stage of hydrocephalus, and in those cases which arise from the suppression or retention of eruptive diseases. At least Dufresnoy, army physician and professor of botany in Valenciennes, employed it with success against *tetters* and *paralysis*. Of the twelve cases he published in 1788, seven refer to cutaneous affections, and five to paralysis consequent upon convulsions. Pontagnon of Montpelier cured a paralytic patient in a fortnight; and Gonan cured a young lady in a few weeks of hemiphlegia. Verdegen, Kok and Van Baerlem obtained similar results. Finally Alderson of England has published seventeen cases which go to prove the efficacy of Rhus against paralysis, and in general against all affections characterized by debility of the muscles. Hull and Duncan also advise it. It proved successful in four cases in which it was employed by Duncan; in each, a peculiar feeling of pricking or twitching, preceded permanent benefit. This sensation was so unpleasant that Dr. Duncan was obliged to discontinue it in one case. In general it operated as a gentle aperient, notwithstanding the torpid state of the bowels of such patients. In bad cases it may be commenced in doses of gr. j. of the dried leaves, and continued until grs. iv. or v. are taken daily, or until a pricking sensation is experienced in the affected part. Frictions with oil in which the fresh leaves have been digested may be employed at the same time.—Peters.

In the inflammatory dropsy of the brain, Rhus is, particularly in the second stage, or that of the effusion, one of the most important remedies. It is indicated when there is a soporific condition, inclination to paralysis, with a continuance of the sensorial activity; when there is a sense of fluctuating of the head, turning dizziness, and a painful, anxious disturbance, principally on the hind-head, where the patient feels the fluctuating; when there are convulsive motions of the limbs, with great complaint of severe headache; when the patient lies for a time in a state of dizziness, until the more severe attacks are renewed in shorter intervals; this hopeless state may often be cured within a few hours with this remedy.—HARTMANN.

CASE 83.—A little girl, 8 years of age, suffering for ten days with inflammation of the brain, showed the following:

Symptoms.—Loss of consciousness for two days; the right upper and lower limbs paralyzed; pulse quick, trembling, scarcely perceptible; urine passed involuntarily; slow breathing with frequent sighing; general appearance cadaverous; eyelids œdematous and swollen; body cold.

Treatment.—Arsen., Digit. and Merc.-s. produced but transient improvement.—Rhus. 6. one drop in one ounce of water, every four hours a teaspoonful, led within twelve days to a complete recovery. The second day after commencing the Rhus., a moist cough appeared, which is to be considered as a favorable sign.—STURM.

STURM remarks, that in eight cases of Hydroceph. ac. which he had treated, (the above one is the third,) were under the unfavorable circumstances of the already existing second stage, a recovery was obtained. In the first case Digit. and Hyosc.—in the second Merc., Arnica and Sulph. were the efficient remedies; the other five cases came under treatment at the beginning of the disease.

REVIEW.—But little, yet enough is to be remarked, in regard to the use of Rhus., in the second stage of inflammation of the brain. HARTMANN says it removes an inclination to paralysis, and STURM that it cured paralysis of the upper and lower limbs. The cadaverous appearance, œdematous and swollen eyelids, are symptoms we often meet with in cases cured with Rhus.

STRAMONIUM.

General Remarks.—The action of this remedy is very similar to that of Belladonna, (see page 514); it seems to act principally upon the blood and many of the ramifications of the great sympathetic nerve, especially in the brain, eyes, throat and genital organs. Its action upon the throat and skin is similar to that produced by the poison of scarlet fever; it is apt, like Belladonna, to produce paralysis of all the involuntary muscles, or those supplied by the sympathetic nerve, while its action upon the motor or spinal system of nerves, is nearly the opposite of this, or that of an irritant: thus it produces dilatation of the pupils, spasmodic contraction of the muscles of the face, relaxation of the cardiac and pyloric orifices of the stomach and of the muscular coat of the stomach and bowels, while it causes violent spasmodic contraction of the muscles of the throat; it will allay spasms of the bronchi, and excite cramps of the muscles of the limbs, &c., &c. It does not act upon the glands like Belladonna.

A tablespoonful of the seeds produced in a man aged 60, and his wife: vertigo, stupefaction, coma and spasms; their respiration was stertorous, they were completely unconscious, with hanging down of the lower jaw; they had cramps in the hands and feet, and rolling of the eyes with dilated pupils and intolerance of light; they made automatic motions and graspings with the hands, sometimes towards the nose, ears or head; the skin was cool, pulse somewhat quickened, with occasional intermissions; the swallowing of fluids was very difficult. After vomiting and purging there was some return of consciousness, with abatement of the cramps, but the face and hands remained cold; they had some burning pain in the distended abdomen, and their voices were hoarse and lisping; swallowing was painful and difficult.—Frank.

A girl, aged 4, ate of the seeds; she complained of pain in the ears and was put to bed; but instead of sleeping she became more and more excited and began to sing and speak confused stuff; her eyes were bright, pupils dilated and almost entirely insensible to light; pulse tranquil and skin cool; she began to talk almost incessantly in a most confused and incomprehensible manner, and often wept; she grasped frequently with her hands into the empty air, as if she would seize something, and occasionally seemed to be seeking something in the bed with her fingers; she could not stand for her knees bent under her immediately when she attempted it, and when she tried to rise she fell staggering about as if intoxicated; the abdomen was soft and painless and she was not thirsty. She recovered after free vomiting.—Frank.

A boy, aged 4 years, from eating the seeds, was found sitting up in bed, entirely unconscious, with flushed face, restless and brilliant eyes, widely dilated and rigid pupils, a peculiar and drunken look; he chattered incessantly without rhyme or reason and entirely without connection; he frequently sprang upwards hastily and anxiously, grasped about with his hands, and snatched at the air; he had no fever and his pulse was sluggish and slow; still he had a hot perspiration and drank eagerly, but these arose from his violent muscular exertions and from dryness of his throat. He recovered after free vomiting and purging.—Frank.

A robust boy, aged 3 years, ate of the seeds; soon after he complained of scratching in his throat and wished to be put to bed; he laid down upon his stomach, bored with his head into the pillow, and his hands and feet commenced to tremble; in half an hour afterwards he became unconscious and fell into the most violent spasms; his head was very hot, face dark red, his limbs redder than natural, his pupils greatly dilated, and he had profuse salivation; gritting of the teeth, violent trembling, convulsive attacks and paroxysms of great anxiety sat in, during which the child constantly exposed his genitals; the abdomen was distended, but not painful. Free vomiting and purging, with cold applications to the head, produced much relief; the intense redness of the face and the convulsions abated first, but the other symptoms persisted, especially the excitement, for the child continued to sing, scream and moved its eyes and hands for several hours, until it finally fell into a refreshing sleep, but the singing and screaming were still present on the next day, after which he slept for eight hours, and awoke quite restored. —Frank.

The leaves produced in four persons: sudden mental derangement, they made laughable movements, had vertigo, dilated pupils and distended abdomens.—FRANK.

Three cupsful of an infusion of the plant and seeds produced: nausea and great anxiety; the patient a robust and plethoric woman was found lying unconscious with closed eyes and mouth, violent throbbing of the pulse and spasms of the limbs; she was bled two pounds, when she opened her eyes, and stared wildly about her; her pupils were widely dilated and insensible to light and touch; the mouth could be opened, but the tongue was immoveable and she could utter no sound; the upper part of the body was drawn backwards spasmodically. Injections and counter irritation were followed by sleep and perspiration, with relief from the spasms.—FRANK.

A child, aged 1½ years, ate of the seeds, and was attacked with spasms and distension of the abdomen, followed by unconsciousness. It was restored by vomiting and purging.—FRANK.

A girl, aged 3 years, ate a considerable number of the seeds: she was attacked with violent convulsions of the arms, paralysis of the legs, the tongue hung out of her mouth, her eyes were quite fixed, pupils widely dilated, with muttering and loss of consciousness. Vomiting and purging were followed by relief; but on the next day the child complained that it was very dark and wished candles to be lighted; the pupils still remained much dilated; she had several bloody stools and finally recovered on the third day.—FRANK.

A man, suffering with rheumatism of the head, took six drops of the Tincture every two hours, and was apparently cured in a few days; but he increased the doses three or four-fold, and was suddenly attacked with heaviness of the head, stupefaction, inclination to vomit, great debility and dejection, staggering walk and inability to walk even a few steps, dilatation of the pupils, dryness of the lips and tongue, violent delirium, hard and full pulse, and discharge of thin almost spring-water-like urine. He recovered in a few days and his head-rheumatism never returned.—FRANK.

From their tendency to produce eruptions upon the skin, the internal use of Belladonna and Stramonium may prove as useful as Croton oil or Tartar-emetic ointment applied externally. Thus, in one case in which the patient was quite stupid, with quick pulse, hot skin, constant motion of the head, and of the hands to the head, intolerance of light, &c., and all these symptoms became gradually aggravated for nine days when a well-marked eruption of measles appeared with improvement in all the head symptoms; the child appeared less stupid, somewhat conscious and could more readily distinguish those about her. In another case of strongly marked cerebral symptoms, simulating meningitis in a child five years old, where they appeared to depend upon a slight erythematous affection of the face imperfectly developing itself; there was great restlessness, high fever, extreme dilatation of the pupils, unconsciousness, insensibility to light, and incessant rolling of the head from one side to the other; these symptoms lasted five or six days and subsided on the appearance of a full eruption from Croton oil on the back of the neck.

Belladonna and Stramonium may have a homœopathic relation to a peculiar diagnostic sign in tubercular meningitis, first announced by Trousseau, and which consists in the appearance of a remarkable *red line* remaining upon the skin of the forehead, or of the abdomen, after drawing the finger across it. A female patient of Dr. Parkman's who had scrofulous disease of the clavicle, was, when about to undergo an operation seized with a fatal illness, which Dr. P. diagnosed as tuberculous meningitis, from the peculiar red line spoken of above.

The above remedies are also homœopathic to great dryness of the mouth and nose, and Dr. Romberg states that the condition of the nasal mucous membrane constitutes a good diagnostic sign in head-affections; if the secretion be arrested and the nose be dry, then meningitis is impending. Other signs of meningitis in infants, are: the continual attempt to bury the occiput in the pillow, and a frequent change of color in the cheeks, and especially in one cheek only. Vomiting is often observed, but with these peculiarities, that it occurred when the stomach was empty, without nausea, without straining, and was brought on by moving or shaking the head. The expression of the eyes is noticeable; children usually follow with their eyes the eyes of their attendants; in meningitis they cease to do this. —ROMBERG.

CASE 84.—A girl, suffering with small-pox and meningitis, was attacked with convulsive and paralytic symptoms.

Treatment.—Tinct.-stram., five drops, in spir.-vini. half an ounce, removed the dangerous condition instantly.—Arch. 20, 2, 145, GOULLON.

In cases, where during and after an attack of small-pox, the most violent and most dangerous affections of the brain set in, accompanied by delirium, STAPF found Stram. in the 12th potency a quick and lasting remedy.—Ibid.

CASE 85.—GROSS observed during the winter season, among children under seven years, a rheumatic-inflammatory affection of the meninges, with the following:

Symptoms.—Sleep was not very heavy and soporose, but frequent convulsions of the limbs sat in, attended with groaning; disturbance of the mind; on awaking there was a peculiar kind of fatuity; the look was staring, and the child had a desperate air, gazing fixedly at one point, this state sometimes disappeared slowly, sometimes it passed off with a severe fit of crying, during which the child clung to near objects; the whole attended with high fever, redness of the face and perspiration. Stramonium 9. removed this state quickly and completely.—Other persons between fifteen and twenty-five years suffered with extreme absence of mind, they slept little, were taciturn, did not feel inclined to answer questions, were almost insensible and immovable, without being unconscious. Spirit.-nitr.-æther. was more useful than Stramon.—Arch. 9, 2, 140.

REVIEW.—Both experience and the remarks of STAPF, tend to prove that Stram. in suitable cases, is peculiarly adapted to inflammation of the meninges. STAPF says Stram. is particularly useful when spasms of the bladder are present.

SULPHUR.

General Remarks.—*a.* In the period, says Wahle, where the signs of exudation, under the well-known phenomena have appeared, if Hell.-nig. does not remove the danger in the course of six or eight hours, we have still a good remedy in Sulph. 30. and 60. It ought not to be given internally, but a few globules only should be smelled at. (Bah !)—Arch. 15, 2, 23.

b. Rummel says, that a physician is frequently not sent for in diseases of children until convulsions have set in, and these then mask the real malady which existed previously. The principal remedy is, according to his experience, Sulph. 30. He has used it with good effects even when inflammatory and exudative affections of the brain were present. If this remedy produces no good effect, the patient is generally in a hopeless state; but occasionally he found the previous and alternate use of Acon. and Bell. somewhat useful. He did not use Sulphur in any other potency than the 30th, and found it more useful in the erethistic than in the torpid stage.—Allg. Hom. Ztg., 32, 345.

CASE 86.—Résumé of the symptoms of inflammation of the brain in thirteen children, from four to ten years of age, boys and girls, of whom only one died, on account of too late assistance.

Premonitory Symptoms.—A short time before the beginning of the attack there was observed an insignificant scurf upon the face, or a little roughness of the chin, ears or face, or scurfy pustules on the lips. The scurf fell off suddenly, the pustules dried up quickly and healed. One or two days before the beginning of the malady the patient had no appetite, with heaviness of the head, chilliness and debility.

Symptoms of the Attack.—Soporific sleep disturbed every ten to twenty minutes by a sudden awaking, with a heavy, audible crying, ah! ah! or: oh! dear me! or restlessness for several minutes, followed again by sopor; gnashing of the teeth, vomiting of the food, intolerance of light, constipation, weak and frequent pulse, thirst, dry and white coated tongue, sour smell of the mouth, redness of the cheeks, or one cheek red, the other pale, perspiration of the head, with a dry, more or less cool skin of the body; the perspiration of the head emitted a musk-like smell.

Treatment.—Acon. and Bell. without effect. Sulphur $\frac{3}{1500}$, every six to twelve hours, effected the cure; to one child, Phosphor. $\frac{3}{10}$ was given with the best effect.

Course of the Disease.—After giving Acon. and Bellad.; crying out in the sleep rarely took place, sleep became more natural, still the child complained about pain of the fore- and hind-head, as well as about the vertex. From the use of Sulphur and Phosphor., the vomiting ceased, constipation abated, the symptoms of fever ceased, as well as the heavy sweating of the head, the skin got moist and a cure followed. Some children were cured after sixteen, others after twelve, and still others after eight doses.—Arch. 16, 1, 61, WEBER.

CASE 87.—A boy, 2½ years of age, was taken sick with the following:

Symptoms.—Head so heavy that it could scarcely be kept straight and fell to the side; holding it erect produced vomiting of liquids, or of slime; the child slept most of the time; was frightened, as if from anxiety; the cheeks changed frequently from pale to red, or if one was red, the other was pale. The limbs were cold; there was perspiration only on the head, which was very hot; thirst; pulse 100.

Treatment.—Acon. $\frac{}{30}$, ten drops, every two hours, followed by Bell. 30. after eight hours, without effect. Afterwards Sulphur $\frac{}{1500}$, every twelve hours. After four doses the child was perfectly cured, with the exception of great debility. Bell. $\frac{}{30}$, removed the weakness within four days.—Arch. 16, 2, 3, WEBER.

CASE 88.—Three cases of inflammation of the brain, in the persons of a boy, aged three years, and two girls of five years.

Symptoms.—Could only lay the head in certain situations; it had to be kept low, otherwise the child would cry and vomit; deep sleep, interrupted by raving; awaking with a heavy start, although ordinary calling and speaking would not awaken the patient; penetrating sour smell of the mouth.

Treatment.—Acon. and Bellad. were of no use, but after several doses of Sulph. 1500. a cure began instantly.—Arch. 16, 2, 5–10, WEBER.

REVIEW.—Of no remedy have we so many observations as of Sulph.; it proved useful even when the disease was approaching to the second stage, and when Acon., Bell. and Hellebore had been given without effect. It was given in high potencies, the 30th, 60th or 1500th. Among the characteristic symptoms we do not find the boring with the head, but rather a sinking down from heaviness; sweat on the head with a musk-like smell; changing of the color of the face; sour smell of the mouth.

The cure was in all cases rapid and progressive.

The doses as above mentioned were all high potencies.

VERATRUM.

CASE 89.—A child, 11 months of age, had on the fifth day of illness the following:

Symptoms.—It lies slumbering upon its back; eyes half closed; face pale and thin; it rolled its head violently from side to side, with sharp screams; or bored into the pillow; transient redness of the cheeks; throwing off the bed-clothes; the head when raised fell down backwards, with convulsive motions of the limbs; the eyes were languid and lifeless, with greatly contracted pupils; the child noticed nothing; its eyes resembled a dull, gliding glass, covered with a thin transparent mucus, which dried into hard masses in the corners; it remained in a torpid state even when spoken to loudly; when it was raised up it had several convulsive shocks and inclination to vomit. At the beginning of the attack there were frequent paroxysms of vomiting and diarrhœa; the head was hot, the body almost cool; pulse without strength and of diminished frequency; it refused to nurse.

Treatment and Result.—Verat.-alb. 2., twenty drops in two ounces aq. d., a teaspoonful every three hours. At the end of twenty-four hours after the patient had received three doses, there seemed little chance of life; but on the fourth day of the treatment, the patient having taken the Veratrum regularly, the following state of things was present: when called, the child cast its eyes to the place where the call came from; the pupils were of natural size, eyes bright and expressive; the child was awake almost every hour; has taken the mother's breast; tried to hold its head up; there were thin discharges from the bowels. The recovery was soon perfected.—Allg. Hom. Ztg. 19, 38, KNORRE.

ZINCUM.

GENERAL REMARKS.—In the irritative stage, says HARTMANN, if Bell. is without effect, Zinc. is incomparable in the second to third triturations; it should be given every two hours. He has never given this medicine in vain, and generally after the lapse of twelve to twenty-four hours, the crisis was perfectly formed.—Dess. Therap. 1, 540.

GENERAL REVIEW,

BY RUECKERT.

The principal remedy was Bell. thirty-seven times. Sulph. sixteen times. Aconite fifteen times. Bryon. and Opium three times. Arn., Hell., Hyosc. and Stram. twice. Cupr., Digit., Iod., Rhus. and Verat. once. Zinc. is recommended. Opium, Stram. and Spir.-nitr.-dulc. were frequently used in some epidemics.

Form of inflammation:

1. In encephalitis: Bell., Bry., Hyosc.
2. In inflammation of the meninges: Bell., Bry., Iod., Op., Spir.-nitr.-dulc., Stram.
3. In hydrocephalus-acut.
   a. In the first stage: Acon.
   b. " second stage: Arn., Bell., Digit., Hell., Rhus., Sulph., Verat.
   c. In the third stage: Helleb.

In order to secure a quick survey of the principal indications, we append the annexed synopsis.

During and after acute exanthems, such as scarlet fever or measles, when inflammation of the brain appeared, Arn., Bell., Cupr.—From dentition, Acon., Cupr.—During febrile catarrh, Cupr.—After sun-stroke, Bell.—During and after small pox,

Stram. Reports of cases have been contributed by thirty-eight physicians.

DOSES.—The strong tincture was only used in a few cases; from the first to the third potencies 35 times, viz.: 5 times in drop doses, 14 times in single doses, and 15 times in solution and repeated doses. From the fourth to the high potencies were used in 58 cases. 24 times but one remedy was given, 10 times single doses, 7 times in solution, 17 times in high potency in repeated doses. Of the cases in which one remedy alone proved successful: Acon. was given in 3 cases.
Bell. " " " 21 "
Bryon. " " " 1 case.—25 cases. To these we may add the 16 cases treated with Sulph., in which Acon. and Bell. were given without effect; 16, without regarding many other cases in which other remedies were given without effect, thus we have in whole 41 cases cured by one remedy.

These cases deserve sufficient attention to encourage us to attempt to cure without a sudden change of remedies. In general we may say that 12 children were cured by taking Sulph. Some required 16, others 12, others eight doses to effect a cure.

Among 18 cases:

In 10 the cure was effected in from 4 to 12 hours.
" 6 " " " 15 to 24 "
" 2 " " " 3 to 5 days.

A complete cure was effected in 30 cases;

23 times in from 1 to 5 days.
6 " " 6 to 12 "
once in 4 weeks.

Most of the cases, after the dangerous signs had ceased, were cured gradually without particular crisis. In 7 cases there was a quiet, many hours' lasting sleep; in 5 cases sweat; in 2 cases diarrhœa; in 2 cases boils; in 2 cases discharge from the ears; in one case a loose cough.

SPECIAL INDICATIONS.

	Aconite.	*Arnica.*	*Bellad.*	*Bryon.*	*Cuprum.*	*Digital.*	*Hellebor.*	*Hyosc.*	*Iodine.*	*Opium.*	*Rhus.*	*Stram.*	*Sulph.*	*Verat.*
Headache, violent and piercing,	..	..	..	Bry.	..	..	..	..	..	..	..	..	..	..
In the head, like swinging,	..	..	Bell	Bry.	..	..	..	..	..	..	Rhus.	..	..	..
Head warm and body cold,	..	..	..	..	..	..	..	..	..	..	..	..	..	Vera.
Heat of the head,	Ac.	..	Bell.	Bry.	..	Dig.	..	..	..	..	..	..	..	..
Sweat of the head, smelling like musk,	..	..	..	..	..	..	..	..	..	..	..	..	Sulp.	..
Boring with the back of the head,	Ac.	..	Bell.	..	..	..	..	..	..	..	..	Str.	..	Vera.
Fluctuating, falling back of the head,	..	..	Bell	..	Cup	Dig.	Hell.	..	..	..	Rhus.	..	..	Vera.
Head, violent turning in,	..	..	..	..	..	..	..	..	..	..	..	..	..	Vera.
Face, red,	..	..	Bell	Bry.	..	..	..	Hyos.	..	..	..	Str.	..	..
" bright, nearly brown,	..	..	..	Bry.	..	..	..	..	..	..	..	Str.	..	..
" slightly red,	..	..	..	..	..	..	..	..	..	..	..	..	..	..
Cheeks red,	..	..	..	Bry.	..	..	..	..	..	..	..	..	..	..
Face hot,	..	..	Bell	..	..	..	..	..	..	..	..	..	..	..
" pale,	..	..	Bell.	..	..	..	Hell.	..	..	..	..	..	..	..
" changing color,	Ac.	..	..	..	..	..	..	..	..	..	..	..	Sulp.	..
Eyes rolling, turning,	Ac.	..	Bell	..	..	Dig.	Hell.	..	..	..	..	..	..	..
" squinting,	..	Arn.	Bell	..	..	Dig.	Hell.	..	..	..	..	..	..	..
" staring,	..	..	Bell	..	..	Dig.	..	..	..	..	..	Str.	..	..
" half open,	..	..	Bell.	Bry.	..	Dig.	Hell.	Hyos.	..	..	..	..	..	Vera.
" sparkling,	..	..	Bell	..	..	..	..	..	..	..	..	..	..	..
" dim, weak,	..	..	Bell.	..	..	..	Hell.	Hyos.	..	..	..	..	..	Vera.
Eyelids, œdematous,	..	..	..	..	..	..	..	..	..	..	Rhus.	..	..	..
Pupils enlarged,	..	Arn.	Bell	..	..	Dig.	Hell	Hyos.	..	..	..	..	..	..
" contracted,	Ac.	..	Bell	..	..	..	..	..	..	Op.	..	..	Sulp.	Vera.
Tongue, dry,	Ac.	..	Bell	Bry	..	..	..	..	..	..	..	..	Sulp.	..
" white coated,	..	..	Bell	..	..	..	..	..	..	..	..	..	Sulp.	..
Sour smell of the mouth,	..	..	..	..	..	..	..	..	..	..	..	..	Sulp.	..
Great thirst,	Ac.	..	Bell	Bry.	..	Dig.	..	..	..	..	..	..	Sulp.	..
Gnashing of the teeth,	..	..	Bell	..	..	..	..	..	..	..	..	..	Sulp.	..
Vomiting,	Ac.	..	Bell	..	Cup	..	..	Hyos.	..	Op.	..	..	Sulp.	..
" on rising up,	Ac.	..	Bell	..	..	..	..	..	..	..	..	..	..	..
Abdomen, painful and swollen,	..	..	Bell	Bry.	..	..	..	Hyos	..	..	..	..	..	..
Stool, hard, wanting,	..	..	Bell.	Bry.	..	Dig.	..	..	..	..	..	..	Sulp.	..
" involuntary,	..	..	Bell.	..	..	..	Hell.	..	..	..	..	..	..	..
Urination involuntary,	..	..	Bell.	..	..	..	Hell.	..	..	..	..	..	..	..
Breathing, anxious, groaning,	..	Arn.	Bell	Bry.	..	..	..	Hyos.	..	..	..	..	..	..
Breathing quickened,	..	..	Bell	..	..	..	..	Hyos.	..	..	..	..	..	..
Pulse, quick, weak,	..	Arn.	Bell	..	..	..	Hell.	..	..	..	..	..	Sulp.	..
" full, hard,	Ac.	..	Bell.	..	..	..	..	..	..	..	..	..	..	..
" trembling, intermitting,	..	..	..	..	..	..	Hell.	..	..	..	Rhus.	..	..	..
" scarcely perceptible,	..	..	..	..	..	..	..	..	..	..	Rhus.	..	..	..
Beating of the carotids,	..	..	Bell.	..	..	..	..	..	..	..	..	..	..	..
Convulsive fits,	..	Arn.	Bell.	..	..	Dig.	Hell.	..	..	..	..	..	..	..
Trembling of the limbs,	..	..	Bell	..	..	..	Hell.	..	..	..	..	..	..	..
Grasping with the hands at the head,	Ac.	..	Bell	..	..	..	Hell.	..	..	..	..	..	..	..
Cramps,	..	..	Bell.	..	..	..	..	Hyos.	..	..	Rhus.	Str.	..	..
Inclination to paralysis,	..	..	..	..	..	..	..	..	..	..	Rhus.	Str.	..	..
Heat, general,	Ac.	..	Bell	..	..	..	..	..	..	..	..	..	..	..
Skin, dry, hot,	..	..	Bell	..	..	Dig.	..	Hyos.	..	..	..	..	..	..
Sleep, with snoring,	..	..	Bell.	..	..	..	..	..	..	Op.	..	..	..	..
" " starting,	Ac.	..	Bell	Bry.	..	..	..	..	..	..	Rhus.	..	Sulp.	..
" " gnashing of the teeth,	Ac.	..	Bell.	..	..	..	..	..	..	..	..	..	Sulp.	..
Inclined to sleep, but not able,	..	..	..	Bry.	Cup	..	..	..	..	..	..	..	..	..
Sopor,	..	..	Bell.	..	..	Dig.	Hell.	..	..	Op.	Rhus.	Str	Sulp.	..
Delirium,	Ac.	..	Bell.	Bry.	..	..	..	Hyos.	Iod.	..	..	Str.	..	..
Passionate,	..	..	..	Bry.	..	..	..	..	..	..	..	..	..	..
Stupid,	..	..	Bell	..	Cup.	..	Hell.	..	..	Op.	..	Str.	..	..
Inclination to run away,	Ac.	..	Bell.	..	..	..	Hell.	..	..	..	..	..	..	..

INDEX.

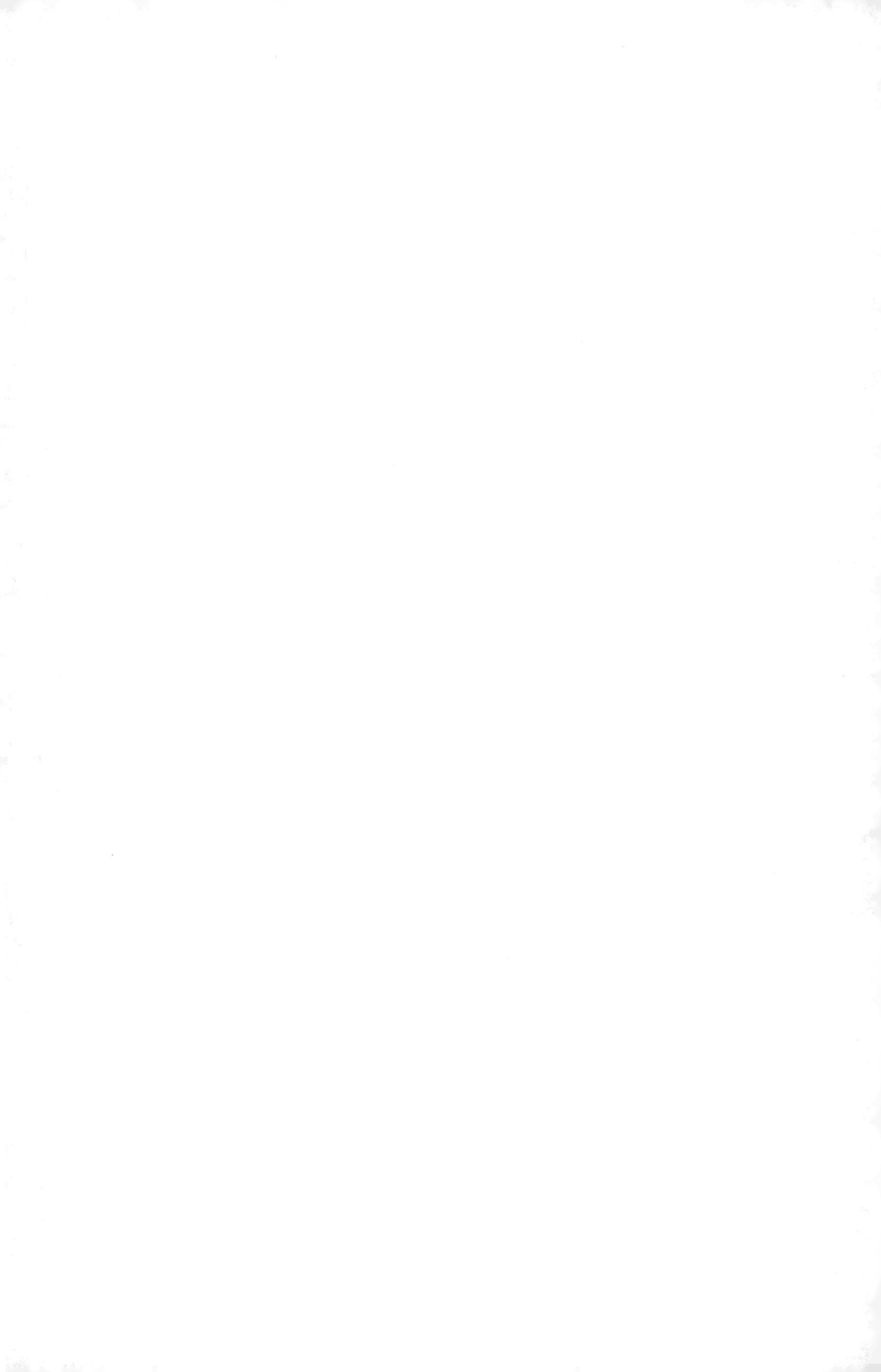

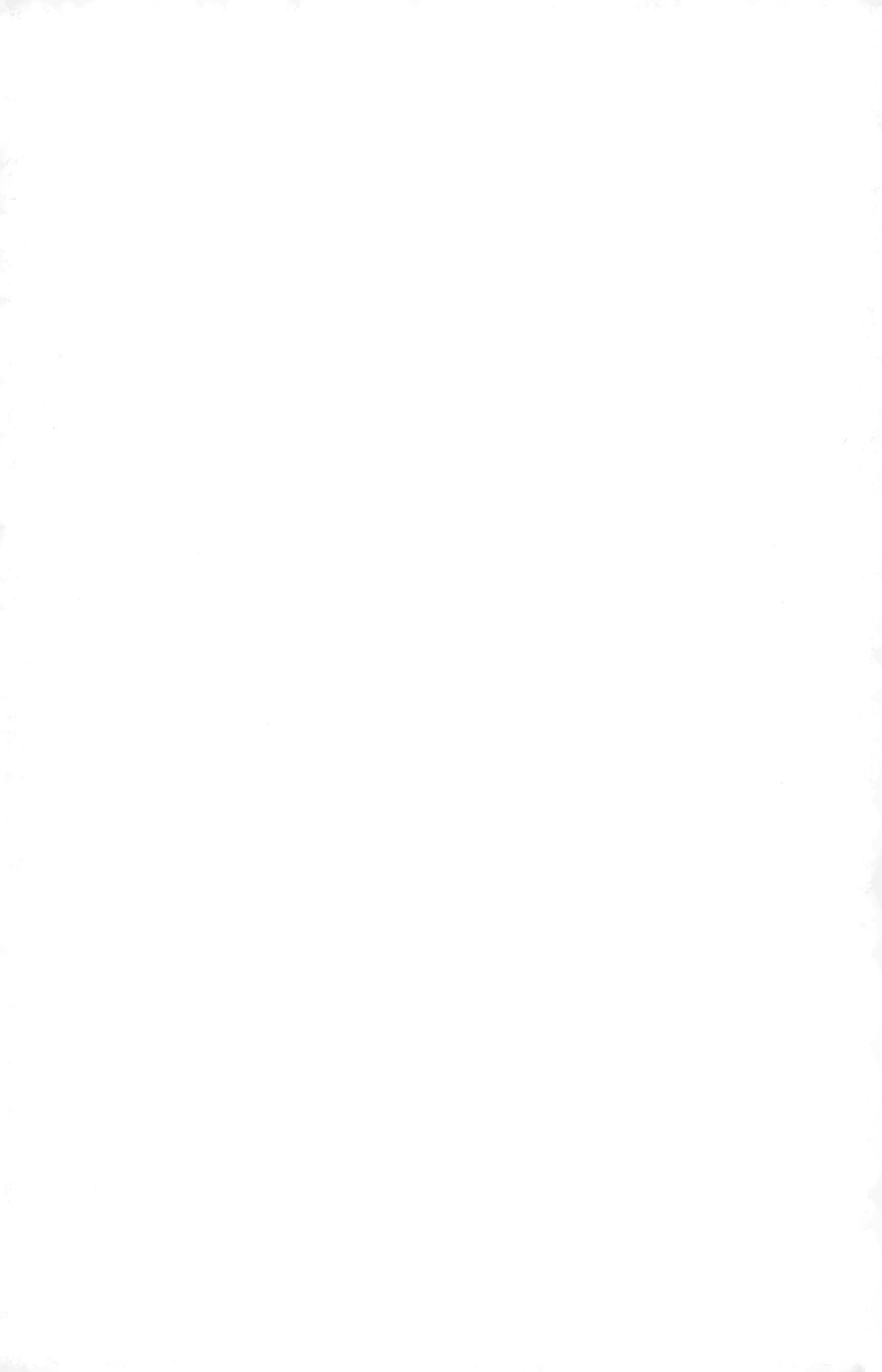

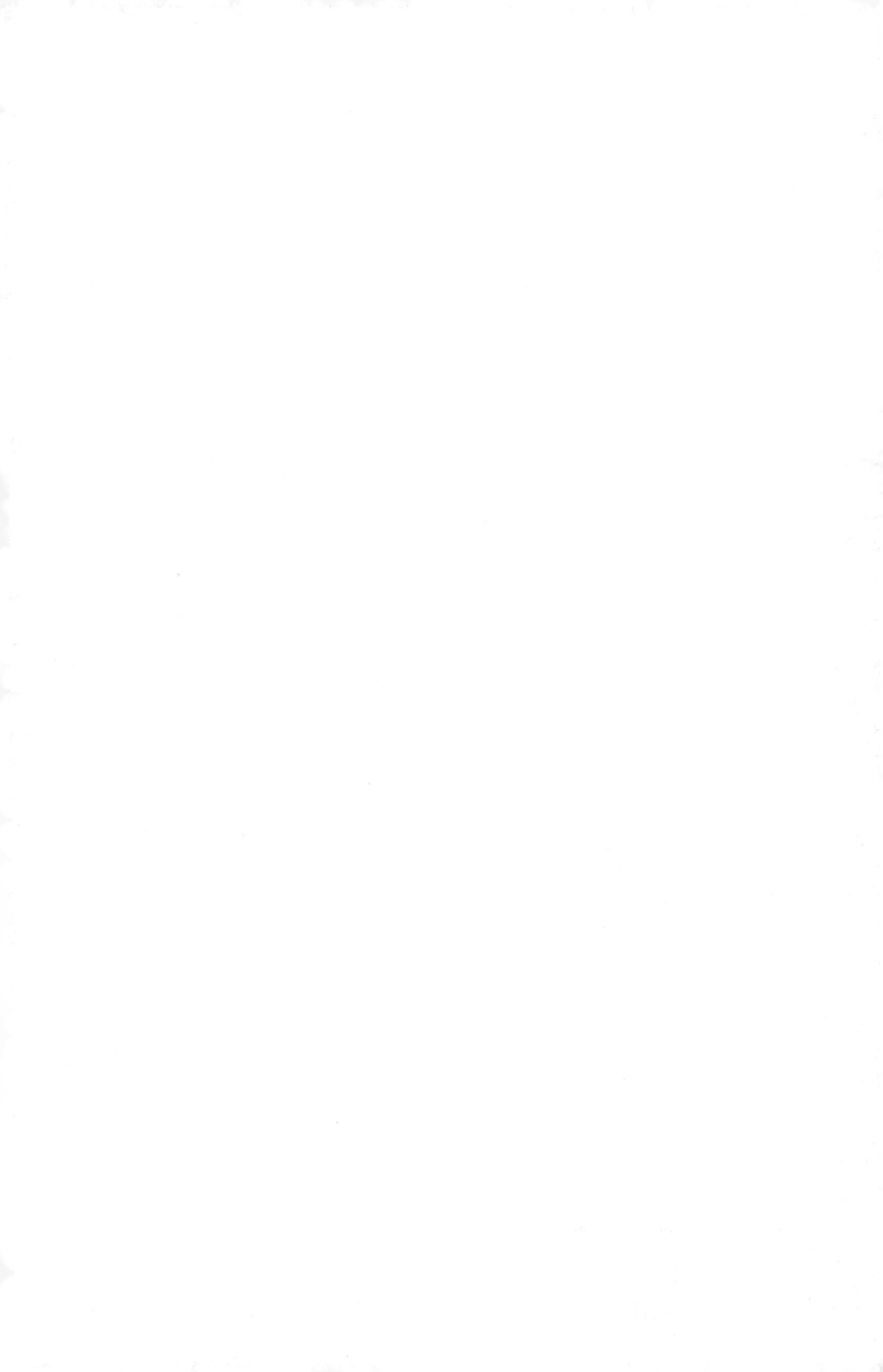

www.ingramcontent.com/pod-product-compliance
Lightning Source LLC
LaVergne TN
LVHW021101110826
845150LV00001B/138

* 9 7 8 1 4 2 5 5 6 6 0 8 1 *